2011
YEAR BOOK OF
UROLOGY®

The 2011 Year Book Series

Year Book of Anesthesiology and Pain Management™: Drs Chestnut, Abram, Black, Gravlee, Lien, Mathru, and Roizen

Year Book of Cardiology®: Drs Gersh, Cheitlin, Elliott, Gold, Graham, and Thourani

Year Book of Critical Care Medicine®: Drs Dellinger, Parrillo, Balk, Dorman, Dries, and Zanotti-Cavazzoni

Year Book of Dermatology and Dermatologic Surgery™: Dr Del Rosso

Year Book of Diagnostic Radiology®: Drs Osborn, Abbara, Elster, Manaster, Oestreich, Offiah, Rosado de Christenson, Stephens, and Walker

Year Book of Emergency Medicine®: Drs Hamilton, Bruno, Handly, Mullin, Quintana, and Ramoska

Year Book of Endocrinology®: Drs Schott, Apovian, Clarke, Eugster, Ludlam, Meikle, Schinner, Schteingart, and Toth

Year Book of Gastroenterology™: Drs Talley, DeVault, Harnois, Murray, Pearson, Philcox, Picco, and Smith

Year Book of Hand and Upper Limb Surgery®: Drs Yao and Steinmann

Year Book of Medicine®: Drs Barker, Garrick, Gersh, Khardori, LeRoith, Seo, Talley, and Thigpen

Year Book of Neonatal and Perinatal Medicine®: Drs Fanaroff, Benitz, Donn, Neu, Papile, Polin, and van Marter

Year Book of Neurology and Neurosurgery®: Drs Klimo and Rabinstein

Year Book of Obstetrics, Gynecology, and Women's Health®: Drs Dungan and Shulman

Year Book of Oncology®: Drs Arceci, Bauer, Chiorean, Gordon, Lawton, Murphy, Thigpen, and Tsao

Year Book of Ophthalmology®: Drs Rapuano, Cohen, Flanders, Fudemberg, Hammersmith, Milman, Myers, Nagra, Nelson, Penne, Pyfer, Sergott, Shields, Talekar, and Vander

Year Book of Orthopedics®: Drs Morrey, Beauchamp, Huddleston, Swiontkowski, and Trigg

Year Book of Otolaryngology-Head and Neck Surgery®: Drs Sindwani, Balough, Franco, Gapany, and Mitchell

Year Book of Pathology and Laboratory Medicine®: Drs Raab, Parwani, Bejarano, and Bissell

Year Book of Pediatrics®: Dr Stockman

Year Book of Plastic and Aesthetic Surgery™: Drs Miller, Gosain, Gurtner, Gutowski, Ruberg, Salisbury, and Smith

Year Book of Psychiatry and Applied Mental Health®: Drs Talbott, Ballenger, Buckley, Frances, Krupnick, and Mack

Year Book of Pulmonary Disease®: Drs Barker, Jones, Maurer, Raza, Tanoue, and Willsie

Year Book of Sports Medicine®: Drs Shephard, Cantu, Feldman, Jankowski, Khan, Lebrun, Nieman, Pierrynowski, and Rowland

Year Book of Surgery®: Drs Copeland, Behrns, Daly, Eberlein, Fahey, Huber, Klodell, Mozingo, and Pruett

Year Book of Urology®: Drs Andriole and Coplen

Year Book of Vascular Surgery®: Drs Moneta, Gillespie, Starnes, and Watkins

2011

The Year Book of UROLOGY®

Editors

Gerald L. Andriole, Jr, MD

Professor and Chief of Urology, Washington University School of Medicine; Chief of Urology, Barnes-Jewish Hospital, St Louis, Missouri

Douglas E. Coplen, MD

Associate Professor of Surgery (Urology), Washington University School of Medicine; Director of Pediatric Urology, St Louis Children's Hospital, St Louis, Missouri

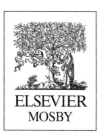

ELSEVIER
MOSBY

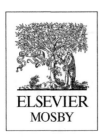

ELSEVIER
MOSBY

Vice President, Continuity: Kimberly Murphy
Editor: Yonah Korngold
Production Supervisor, Electronic Year Books: Donna M. Skelton
Electronic Article Manager: Mike Sheets
Illustrations and Permissions Coordinator: Dawn Vohsen

Composition by TNQ Books and Journals Pvt Ltd, India

Printed and bound by CPI Group (UK) Ltd, Croydon, CR0 4YY

Transferred to Digital Print 2011

Editorial Office:
Elsevier
Suite 1800
1600 John F. Kennedy Blvd
Philadelphia, PA 19103-2899

International Standard Serial Number: 0084-4071
International Standard Book Number: 978-0-323-08428-4

Contributors

Brian M. Benway, MD
Assistant Professor, Division of Urologic Surgery, Department of Surgery, Washington University School of Medicine, St Louis, Missouri

J. Quentin Clemens, MD
Associate Professor of Urology; Director, Division of Neurourology and Pelvic Reconstructive Surgery, University of Michigan, Ann Arbor, Michigan

Adam S. Kibel, MD
Associate Professor of Urologic Surgery, Washington University School of Medicine; Barnes-Jewish Hospital, St Louis, Missouri

Venkatesh Krishnamurthi, MD
Director, Kidney/Pancreas Transplant, Cleveland Clinic Foundation, Cleveland, Ohio

Eric S. Rovner, MD
Associate Professor of Urology, Medical University of South Carolina; Attending Surgeon, Medical University Hospital, Charleston, South Carolina

Alan Shindel, MD
Department of Surgery, Division of Urology, Washington University School of Medicine, St Louis, Missouri

Table of Contents

Journals Represented

Journals represented in this YEAR BOOK are listed below.

Acta Obstetricia et Gynecologica Scandinavica
Acta Paediatrica
AJR American Journal of Roentgenology
American Journal of Infection Control
American Journal of Obstetrics and Gynecology
American Journal of Preventive Medicine
American Journal of Rhinology & Allergy
American Journal of Transplantation
Annals of Internal Medicine
Archives of Surgery
British Journal of Urology International
British Medical Journal
Cancer
Cardiovascular and Interventional Radiology
Circulation
Clinical Infectious Diseases
European Urology
Fertility and Sterility
International Journal of Impotence Research
International Journal of Obstetrics & Gynaecology
International Journal of Radiation Oncology Biology Physics
Journal of Clinical Endocrinology & Metabolism
Journal of Clinical Oncology
Journal of General Internal Medicine
Journal of Neuroscience
Journal of Pediatric Surgery
Journal of Plastic, Reconstructive & Aesthetic Surgery
Journal of Sexual Medicine
Journal of the American Medical Association
Journal of the National Cancer Institute
Journal of Trauma
Journal of Urology
Lancet
Lancet Oncology
Nature
New England Journal of Medicine
Obstetrics & Gynecology
Pediatric Emergency Care
Pediatrics
Proceedings of the National Academy of Sciences of the United States of America
Scandinavian Journal of Urology and Nephrology
Urology

STANDARD ABBREVIATIONS

The following terms are abbreviated in this edition: acquired immunodeficiency syndrome (AIDS), cardiopulmonary resuscitation (CPR), central nervous system

(CNS), cerebrospinal fluid (CSF), computed tomography (CT), deoxyribonucleic acid (DNA), electrocardiography (ECG), health maintenance organization (HMO), human immunodeficiency virus (HIV), intensive care unit (ICU), intramuscular (IM), intravenous (IV), magnetic resonance (MR) imaging (MRI), ribonucleic acid (RNA), ultrasound (US), and ultraviolet (UV).

NOTE

The YEAR BOOK OF UROLOGY is a literature survey service providing abstracts of articles published in the professional literature. Every effort is made to assure the accuracy of the information presented in these pages. Neither the editors nor the publisher of the YEAR BOOK OF UROLOGY can be responsible for errors in the original materials. The editors' comments are their own opinions. Mention of specific products within this publication does not constitute endorsement.

To facilitate the use of the YEAR BOOK OF UROLOGY as a reference tool, all illustrations and tables included in this publication are now identified as they appear in the original article. This change is meant to help the reader recognize that any illustration or table appearing in the YEAR BOOK OF UROLOGY may be only one of many in the original article. For this reason, figure and table numbers will often appear to be out of sequence within the YEAR BOOK OF UROLOGY.

1 Clinical Outcomes

Effect of Amitriptyline on Symptoms in Treatment Naïve Patients With Interstitial Cystitis/Painful Bladder Syndrome

Foster HE Jr, the Interstitial Cystitis Collaborative Research Network (Yale Univ, New Haven, CT; et al)

J Urol 183:1853-1858, 2010

Purpose.—Amitriptyline is frequently used to treat patients with interstitial cystitis/painful bladder syndrome. The evidence to support this practice is derived mainly from a small, single site clinical trial and case reports.

Materials and Methods.—We conducted a multicenter, randomized, double-blind, placebo controlled clinical trial of amitriptyline in subjects with interstitial cystitis/painful bladder syndrome who were naïve to therapy. Study participants in both treatment arms received a standardized education and behavioral modification program. The drug dose was increased during a 6-week period from 10 up to 75 mg once daily. The primary outcome was a patient reported global response assessment of symptom improvement evaluated after 12 weeks of treatment.

Results.—A total of 271 subjects were randomized and 231 (85%) provided a global response assessment at 12 weeks of followup. Study participants were primarily women (83%) and white (74%), with a median age of 38 years. In an intent to treat analysis (271) the rate of response of subjects reporting moderate or marked improvement from baseline in the amitriptyline and placebo groups was 55% and 45%, respectively (p = 0.12). Of the subgroup of subjects (207) who achieved a drug dose of at least 50 mg, a significantly higher response rate was observed in the amitriptyline group (66%) compared to placebo (47%) (p = 0.01).

Conclusions.—When all randomized subjects were considered, amitriptyline plus an education and behavioral modification program did not significantly improve symptoms in treatment naïve patients with interstitial cystitis/painful bladder syndrome. However, amitriptyline may be beneficial in persons who can achieve a daily dose of 50 mg or greater, although this subgroup comparison was not specified in advance.

▶ This was a large, multisite, randomized, 12-week trial in which amitriptyline or placebo was administered to women with interstitial cystitis/painful bladder syndrome (IC/PBS) who had not previously received treatment for this condition. The amitriptyline dose started at 10 mg at bedtime and was then titrated up at weekly intervals to 25, 50, and then 75 mg at bedtime. In those who developed intolerable side effects, the dose was reduced back to the highest tolerable dose. The overall results of the study showed no difference between the 2 treatment groups. However, in the 76% of women who were able to tolerate the 50 or 75 mg doses, there was a significant improvement in their symptoms. Common side effects were fatigue/malaise, dry mouth, constipation, and dizziness, but these were modest. Based on these results and others, recent American Urological Association guidelines for the treatment of IC/PBS recommend amitriptyline as one of the first-line oral agents to consider (http://www. auanet.org/content/guidelines-and-quality-care/clinical-guidelines.cfm).

J. Q. Clemens, MD

2 Endourology and Stone Disease

Endourology

A short biodegradable helical spiral ureteric stent provides better antireflux and drainage properties than a double-J stent

Lumiaho J, Heino A, Aaltomaa S, et al (Kuopio Univ Hosp, Finland; et al)
Scand J Urol Nephrol 45:129-133, 2011

Objective.—The use of ureteric stents is a standard treatment for the relief of ureter blockages for benign or malignant reasons. The most common stent design in clinical use is a double-J stent with coiled ends to avoid stent displacement. However, there are a number of complications associated with stent use. A double-J stent design bypasses the ureterovesical junction, enables bladder pressure reflection to the renal pelvis and causes vesicoureteral reflux (VUR). This may result in scarring and renal failure.

Material and Methods.—An animal model was used to investigate whether VUR can be avoided in stented ureters using a short biodegradable partial helical spiral stent design that leaves the ureterovesical junction intact.

Materials and Methods.—Eight female pigs were used. Ureters on the left side were stented using a short helical spiral SR-PLGA stent (group A) and ureters on the right side using double-J stents (group B). Simulated voiding cystoureterography and standard intravenous urography examinations were performed on all eight animals at 4 weeks and on the remaining four animals at 8 weeks.

Results.—An SR-PLGA single coiled partial stent demonstrated superior drainage properties to a double-J stent at 4 weeks ($p = 0.020$). A marked but not statistically significant difference in favour of a SR-PLGA stent was also observed at 8 weeks ($p = 0.102$). A statistically significant difference was observed in VCUG findings in favour of group A at immediate postoperative control as well as in the 4 and 8 week follow-up studies ($p = 0.011$, $p = 0.010$, $p = 0.046$, respectively).

Conclusion.—A self-expandable, SR-PLGA partial ureteric stent presented with superior drainage and antireflux properties compared to a double-J stent. The reflux commonly related to double-J stent use can be minimized by using a partial ureteric stent design.

▶ In the described model, a double-J stent caused some obstructive changes in pigs without a preexisting anatomic abnormality. These changes were not as common in the pigs with a short biodegradable ureterovesical junction stent. Based on this, the authors conclude that the biodegradable stent has superior drainage properties. This observation may be more related to the model and not actually related to the properties of the stent. A rigorous comparative in vitro evaluation of fluid transport is needed. The authors also note that vesicoureteral reflux was more common in the double-J group. In humans, this has minimal clinical significance. If bladder function is normal, undue pressure is not transmitted up to the kidneys. The incidence of ascending urinary tract infection or renal failure in patients with an indwelling stent is very small. A biodegradable stent might be associated with lower morbidity than a standard double-J stent and would not require removal. In this model, a cystotomy was required for placement. If endoscopic placement is feasible and upper tract drainage/diversion is equivalent, then a biodegradable stent would be a significant improvement.

D. E. Coplen, MD

One Week of Nitrofurantoin Before Percutaneous Nephrolithotomy Significantly Reduces Upper Tract Infection and Urosepsis: A Prospective Controlled Study
Bag S, Kumar S, Taneja N, et al (Postgraduate Inst of Med Education and Res, Chandigarh, India)
Urology 77:45-49, 2011

Objectives.—To evaluate the role of nitrofurantoin (NFT) prophylaxis in a prospective randomized control study. Urosepsis is an important complication after percutaneous nephrolithotomy (PNL). Risk increases by around 4 times with larger stones and hydronephrosis (HDN).

Material and Methods.—Patients with stones ≥2.5 cm and/or HDN and sterile urine undergoing PNL were randomized into 2 groups. Standard perioperative antibiotic prophylaxis was the same in both groups. One group received sustained-released NFT 100 mg b.i.d. for 7 days preoperatively, and the other did not. Preoperative urine, intraoperative renal pelvic urine, and stone cultures were obtained. Postoperative occurrence of SIRS was considered urosepsis after excluding other causes. Serum samples were collected immediately after PNL and stored at −20°C. Serum endotoxin was estimated using Limulus Amoebocyte Lysate gelation technique (Sigma Aldrich, Saint Louis, Missouri). The operating surgeons and the microbiologist were blinded to the group distribution.

Results.—Of 101 patients, 48 received nitrofurantoin prophylaxis. Both groups were comparable for age, gender, stone burden, degree of HDN, duration of operation, and intraoperative blood loss. There was significantly low positive pelvic urine culture (0% vs 9.8%, RR 4.95, $P =.001$), positive stone culture (8.3% vs 30.2%, RR 3.64, $P =.001$), endotoxemia (17.5% vs 41.9%, OR 0.22, $P =.016$), and systemic inflammatory response system (19% vs 49%, OR 0.31, $P =.01$) in patients receiving NFT prophylaxis.

Conclusions.—Prophylaxis with NFT for a week before PNL is beneficial in the prevention of urosepsis and endotoxemia in patients with larger stones and HDN. NFT covers most of the urinary isolates and is preferred in areas of fluoroquinolone resistance.

▶ The authors present a randomized prospective trial evaluating the efficacy of preoperative empiric nitrofurantoin in preventing septic complications after percutaneous nephrolithotomy (PCNL). In a sample of 101 patients with large stone burden and/or hydronephrosis and negative voided urine cultures, roughly half were randomized to receive 7 days of twice-daily nitrofurantoin. Several assays, including renal pelvis urine and stone cultures, as well as endotoxin assay were assessed, along with clinical parameters. The authors found a decreased rate of renal pelvis and stone culture positivity, along with decreased positivity on endotoxin assays. However, despite this difference in culture and assay positivity, only 1 patient in the entire series (in the control group) developed true sepsis. As such, it is debatable whether or not any of the laboratory parameters the authors investigated truly influence clinical outcomes.

What is also not clear from this study is whether or not hydronephrosis alone (indicating obstruction that may lead to false-negative voided urine cultures) affected the risk of sepsis or indicators of sepsis. Such a distinction may be important, as it would help us to better identify those who are potentially at greater risk of occult infection.

While this is a very interesting and fairly low-risk proposed change in preoperative management, it remains to be seen if empiric administration of antibiotics before PCNL is capable of substantially affecting the risk of septic events. Moreover, it would be interesting to compare empiric antibiotic use with the preplacement of percutaneous access and culture directed preoperative antibiotics in those patients who appear to have clinically significant upper tract obstruction.

B. M. Benway, MD

Tubeless Procedure is Most Important Factor in Reducing Length of Hospitalization After Percutaneous Nephrolithotomy: Results of Univariable and Multivariable Models

Akman T, Binbay M, Yuruk E, et al (Haseki Training and Res Hosp, Istanbul, Turkey)
Urology 77:299-304, 2011

Objectives.—To evaluate the effects of kidney stones and patient-related parameters on the length of hospitalization (LOH), which is one important factor affecting the cost effectiveness of percutaneous nephrolithotomy (PCNL). Recently, increases in healthcare costs have highlighted the importance of evaluating the cost effectiveness of a treatment as much as its efficacy.

Material and Method.—During an 8-year period, the records of 1669 patients with renal calculi who underwent PCNL were reviewed retrospectively. Eleven patients with urosepsis were excluded from the present study. A total of 1658 patients were categorized into 2 groups (group 1 = ≤2 days; group 2 = >2 days) according to the median LOH (median = 2 days). Multivariate binary logistic regression analysis was used to detect the effects of independent variables, including the patient age, gender, body mass index, history of extracorporeal shock wave lithotripsy or open surgery, stone size and opacity, presence of hydronephrosis, and localization and number of accesses, on the LOH after PNL.

Results.—Overall success was achieved in 86.2% of cases after one session of PCNL. The mean length of hospitalization was 2.89 ± 1.66 days (range, 1-21). According to the outcome of the multivariate analysis, diabetes ($P = .0001$, OR = 1.67), impaired kidney function ($P = .03$, OR = 1.64), stone size ($P = .031$, OR = 1.31), number of accesses ($P = .001$, OR = 1.59), intercostal access ($P = .001$, OR = 1.79), and tubeless procedure ($P = .0001$, OR = 0.23) were variables influencing LOH.

Conclusions.—The presence of diabetes, a large stone burden, intercostals access, multiple accesses, and impaired kidney function prolong the LOH after PCNL. The use of the tubeless procedure was able to diminish the LOH.

▶ In the past few years, there have been several proposed techniques to reduce the footprint of percutaneous nephrolithotomy (PCNL). One of the more progressive techniques has been tubeless PCNL, in which patients emerge from the operating room without a percutaneous nephrostomy tube emanating from the tract. In this large retrospective evaluation of over 1600 patients who had undergone PCNL, the authors were able to identify a number of factors that may influence the length of hospitalization. Comorbidities, including diabetes and renal insufficiency, were found to increase length of stay, as were multiple accesses and large stone burdens. Tubeless procedures were associated with a nearly 5-fold decrease in hospital stay.

Naturally, length of stay is only 1 parameter by which success after PCNL may be measured, although it is one that is influenced by other critical parameters, including pain scores, transfusion rates, complication rates, and time to mobilization. Furthermore, tubeless procedures reduce the amount of additional procedures, such as stent internalization, that must be used, which also may account for the foreshortened stay.

Of course, not all patients are amenable to tubeless procedures. However, the high success rate of the authors' initial procedures suggest that for patients with moderate stone burden who have been cleared with confidence, tubeless procedures are appropriate.

B. M. Benway, MD

Complications of Stone Baskets: 14-Year Review of the Manufacturer and User Facility Device Experience Database

Chotikawanich E, Korman E, Monga M (Univ of Minnesota, Minneapolis)
J Urol 185:179-183, 2011

Purpose.—We categorized trends in failure of the stone baskets as reported in the United States Food and Drug Administration Manufacturer and User Facility Device Experience database.

Materials and Methods.—We queried the online database using the code for stone baskets (FFL) from January 1996 to December 2009. Variables extracted were the type of basket, malfunction and treatment, and patient outcome.

Results.—We identified 556 adverse events related to stone baskets. The device configuration was tipped in 48% of cases, tipless in 36%, forceps in 8% and the Stone Cone™ in 8%. Malfunction type included detachment of a portion of the basket in 49% of cases, breakage without detachment in 39% and inability to withdraw the basket in 12%. Compared to the early period studied (1996 to 2004) there was a 3-fold increase in adverse events from 2005 to 2007 and a 6-fold increase from 2008 to 2009. Of adverse events 79% and 11% were managed by endoscopy and open surgery, respectively. Of the patients 42 experienced serious complications requiring major surgery, including ureteral reconstruction in 7, reimplantation in 4 and nephrectomy in 7.

Conclusions.—With the increased use of stone baskets in the upper collecting system the number of adverse events has increased. Urologists should remain vigilant to prevent, recognize and manage these events.

▶ As ureteroscopic intervention for urolithiasis continues to become more commonplace, the authors have found that the utilization of baskets and graspers for stone extraction has also increased substantially over the past 15 years. Along with this increase is a sharp rise in the number of complications directly attributable to the use of these devices, some of which have had quite serious consequences. This is cause for alarm.

In reviewing the data, it appears that detachment, breakage, and inability to disengage are the 3 prevailing misadventures encountered when using these devices. All 3 are typically caused by overzealous attempts at extraction, trying to remove fragments that are too large, and placing excessive force on the stone as an extraction attempt is made. Pronged graspers confer a slight advantage in this regard, as they disengage the stone more readily, though they might be associated with a higher risk of mucosal damage.

The study is somewhat limited by the lack of a denominator. Nevertheless, the sharp increase in the absolute number of reported complications should caution surgeons who are considering stone extraction, especially in the upper tract.

Finally, we must revisit the discussion on whether to extract stones. While extraction may be tempting, it is important to remember that in a large prospective trial, extraction was not found to provide any improvement in stone-free rate over simple fragmentation.[1] It then begs the question: For upper tract stones, is extraction worth the risk?

B. M. Benway, MD

Reference

1. Pearle MS, Lingeman JE, Leveillee R, et al. Prospective, randomized trial comparing shock wave lithotripsy and ureteroscopy for lower pole caliceal calculi 1 cm or less. *J Urol.* 2005;173:2005-2009.

YouTube as a Source of Information on Kidney Stone Disease
Sood A, Sarangi S, Pandey A, et al (All India Inst of Med Sciences, New Delhi; Brigham and Women's Hosp, Boston, MA; et al)
Urology 77:558-563, 2011

Objective.—To look into effective use of popular Internet site YouTube as an information source on kidney stone disease. Urolithiasis is among the most common urological conditions, accounting for significant morbidity, however adequate education regarding simple lifestyle modifications and early recognition of symptoms can reduce recurrence and visits to emergency department.

Materials and Methods.—YouTube was searched using Keywords "nephrolithiasis"; "renal calculi"; "renal stones"; and "kidney stones" for videos uploaded containing relevant information about the disease. Only videos in English were included. Two physician viewers watched each video and classified them as useful; misleading; or personal experiences. The kappa-statistic was used to measure inter-observer variability. Total-viewership; duration; rating; days since upload; source; and information content were noted.

Results.—One-hundred ninety-nine videos had relevant information about nephrolithiasis; 58.3% of the videos had useful information and 18.1% were misleading. Useful videos had 47.2% of total viewership (i.e. total no. of views) share, whereas misleading videos had 2.8%, with statistically significant difference in viewership/day and rating among useful videos vs misleading videos. Universities'channel videos provided the best overall information coverage among the useful videos (prevention = 100%, symptoms = 80%, treatments = 60%, other information = 80%). No significant difference was seen in viewership/day or rating of useful videos based on the kind of information they contained.

Conclusions.—YouTube has a substantial amount of information on urolithiasis. Therefore, consumer-generated outlets such as YouTube have significant potential to sway individuals' attitudes both for and against the right choice. In view of this, authoritative videos by trusted sources should be posted for dissemination of reliable information.

▶ The amount of information available on the Internet continues to expand at an astounding rate, yet it would appear from this study that the medical profession has not yet caught up with the trend. The authors searched YouTube for videos relating to urolithiasis, finding that very few of the most useful videos came from medical professionals. Rather, individual users providing their own insights into stone disease tend to predominate the landscape. With nearly half of videos failing to provide useful and truthful information, perhaps this indicates a more critical need for reputable institutions to invest themselves more earnestly in social media.

B. M. Benway, MD

Shock Wave Lithotripsy

Shock Wave Lithotripsy is Not Predictive of Hypertension Among Community Stone Formers at Long-Term Followup
Krambeck AE, Rule AD, Li X, et al (Mayo Clinic School of Medicine, Rochester, MI)
J Urol 185:164-169, 2011

Purpose.—Concern exists over the subsequent development of hypertension after shock wave lithotripsy for the treatment of symptomatic urolithiasis. Referral bias and lack of long-term followup have been limitations of prior studies.

Materials and Methods.—We identified all Olmsted County, Minnesota residents with a diagnosis of urolithiasis from 1985 to 2008. The charts were electronically queried for hypertension and obesity by diagnostic codes, and use of shock wave lithotripsy by surgical codes. All patients first diagnosed with hypertension before or up to 90 days after the first documented kidney stone were considered to have prevalent hypertension and were excluded from analysis. Cox proportional hazards models were used to assess the association of shock wave lithotripsy with a subsequent diagnosis of hypertension.

Results.—We identified 6,077 patients with incident urolithiasis with more than 90 days of followup. We excluded 1,295 (21.3%) members of the population for prevalent hypertension leaving 4,782 patients with incident urolithiasis for analysis. During an average followup of 8.7 years new onset hypertension was diagnosed in 983 (20.6%) members of the cohort at a mean of 6.0 years from the index stone date. Only 400 (8.4%) patients in the cohort were treated with shock wave lithotripsy. There was no significant association between shock wave lithotripsy and the development of hypertension in univariate (p = 0.33) and multivariate modeling controlling for age, gender and obesity (HR 1.03; 95% CI 0.84, 1.27; p = 0.77).

Conclusions.—In a large population based cohort of kidney stone formers we failed to identify an association between shock wave lithotripsy and the subsequent long-term risk of hypertension.

▶ In a 2006 study,[1] Krambeck and colleagues presented an unsettling report linking shock wave lithotripsy (SWL) to the development of diabetes and hypertension. However, some critics took issue with this report, citing a patient population that skewed toward the complex and the potential for a response bias, as it was a questionnaire-based study. In this study, Krambeck and colleagues interrogated a comprehensive regional database to identify *International Classification of Diseases, Ninth Revision* codes to identify patients with urolithiasis and new diagnoses of hypertension. The authors found that treatment with SWL was not associated with an increased risk of hypertension compared with patients who did not undergo SWL. While further study is needed, this report helps restore the reputation of SWL as a safe means of treatment for patients with urolithiasis.

B. M. Benway, MD

Reference

1. Krambeck AE, Gettman MT, Rohlinger AL, Lohse CM, Patterson DE, Segura JW. Diabetes mellitus and hypertension associated with shock wave lithotripsy of renal and proximal ureteral stones at 19 years of followup. *J Urol.* 2006;175:1742-1747.

A Prospective Randomised Trial Comparing the Modified HM3 with the MODULITH® SLX-F2 Lithotripter

Zehnder P, Roth B, Birkhäuser F, et al (Univ of Bern, Switzerland)
Eur Urol 59:637-644, 2011

Background.—The relative efficacy of first- versus last-generation lithotripters is unknown.

Objectives.—To compare the clinical effectiveness and complications of the modified Dornier HM3 lithotripter (Dornier MedTech, Wessling, Germany) to the MODULITH® SLX-F2 lithotripter (Storz Medical AG, Tägerwilen, Switzerland) for extracorporeal shock wave lithotripsy (ESWL).

Design, Setting and Participants.—We conducted a prospective, randomised, single-institution trial that included elective and emergency patients.

Interventions.—Shock wave treatments were performed under anaesthesia.

Measurements.—Stone disintegration, residual fragments, collecting system dilatation, colic pain, and possible kidney haematoma were evaluated 1 d and 3 mo after ESWL. Complications, ESWL retreatments, and adjuvant procedures were documented.

Results and Limitations.—Patients treated with the HM3 lithotripter ($n = 405$) required fewer shock waves and shorter fluoroscopy times than patients treated with the MODULITH® SLX-F2 lithotripter ($n = 415$). For solitary kidney stones, the HM3 lithotripter produced a slightly higher stone-free rate ($p = 0.06$) on day 1; stone-free rates were not significantly different at 3 mo (HM3: 74% vs MODULITH® SLX-F2: 67%; $p = 0.36$). For solitary ureteral stones, the stone-free rate was higher at 3 mo with the HM3 lithotripter (HM3: 90% vs MODULITH® SLX-F2: 81%; $p = 0.05$). For solitary lower calyx stones, stone-free rates were equal at 3 mo

(63%). In patients with multiple stones, the HM3 lithotripter's stone-free rate was higher at 3 mo (HM3: 64% vs MODULITH® SLX-F2: 44%; $p = 0.003$). Overall, HM3 lithotripter led to fewer secondary treatments (HM3: 11% vs MODULITH® SLX-F2: 19%; $p = 0.001$) and fewer kidney haematomas (HM3: 1% vs. MODULITH® SLX-F2: 3%; $p = 0.02$).

Conclusions.—The modified HM3 lithotripter required fewer shock waves and shorter fluoroscopy times, showed higher stone-free rates for solitary ureteral stones and multiple stones, and led to fewer kidney haematomas and fewer secondary treatments than the MODULITH® SLX-F2 lithotripter. In patients with a solitary kidney and solitary lower calyx stones, results were comparable for both lithotripters.

▶ Generally, it is accepted that technology improves with time. However, this excellent study from Zehnder and colleagues challenges that notion. In a prospective randomized trial evaluating the efficacy of the first-generation Dornier HM3 lithotripter and the fourth-generation Storz Modulith SLX-F2 lithotripter, the authors found that the first-generation HM3 outperforms the fourth-generation lithotripter across several clinical scenarios. Improved stone-free rates were found for solitary ureteral calculi and patients with multiple calculi, while providing equivalent stone-free rate for solitary kidney stones and stones in the lower pole calyx. Finally, treatment on the HM3 was associated with a significantly lower rate of hematoma. The strength of this analysis lay in its prospective randomized design and large patient accrual, and the authors should be commended on an excellent study. It will be interesting to see if studies like this prompt a retro revival in the field of shockwave lithotripsy.

B. M. Benway, MD

3 Transplantation

Laparoscopic Live Donor Nephrectomy with Vaginal Extraction: Initial Report
Allaf ME, Singer A, Shen W, et al (Johns Hopkins Med Insts, Baltimore, MD)
Am J Transplant 10:1473-1477, 2010

The recent decrease in the total number of living kidney transplants coupled with the increase in the number of candidates on the waiting list underscores the importance of eliminating barriers to living kidney donation. We report what we believe to be the first pure right-sided laparoscopic live donor nephrectomy with extraction of the kidney through the vagina. The warm ischemia time was 3 min and the renal vessels and ureter of the procured kidney were of adequate length for routine transplantation. The donor did not receive any postoperative parenteral narcotic analgesia, was discharged home within 24 h and was back to normal activity in 14 days. The kidney functioned well with no complications or infections. Laparoscopic live donor nephrectomy with vaginal extraction may be a viable alternative to open and standard laparoscopic approaches. Potential advantages include reduced postoperative pain, shorter hospital stay and convalescence and a more desirable cosmetic result. These possible, but yet unproven, advantages may encourage more individuals to consider live donation.

▶ This article, along with another in this Year Book titled "Robotic-Assisted Laparoscopic Donor Nephrectomy with Transvaginal Extraction of the Kidney", demonstrate another advance in live donor nephrectomy surgery. Specifically, both groups show that vaginal extraction of a live-donor allograft can be safely performed with both a laparoscopic approach and a robotic-assisted laparoscopic approach. From both reports, minimal morbidity was encountered by the kidney donors, and both grafts functioned well. Of note, the second group expanded the applicability of vaginal extraction by performing the procedure in a patient with a uterus in place.

These authors are to be commended on advancing the field by demonstrating a new technique. What remains in doubt, however, is the widespread applicability of this new approach. For a new technique to become an equivalent standard of care, it must have a complication rate equal to that of the current technique. At present, laparoscopic donor nephrectomy has a very low complication rate, with most donors being discharged within 48 hours and approaching baseline status by 2 weeks. It is difficult to envision vaginal extraction substantially improving upon this already high standard. Additionally, the infectious risks to the recipient, following allograft extraction from the vagina, are not well delineated and will require focused and lengthy follow-up.

The significance of these articles is in their demonstration of technical feasibility and potential applicability to a, as of now undefined, specific patient population.

V. Krishnamurthi, MD

Embolization of Polycystic Kidneys as an Alternative to Nephrectomy Before Renal Transplantation: A Pilot Study

Cornelis F, Couzi L, Le Bras Y, et al (Bordeaux Univ Hosp, Place Amélie Raba Léon, France)
Am J Transplant 10:2363-2369, 2010

In autosomal polycystic kidney disease, nephrectomy is required before transplantation if kidney volume is excessive. We evaluated the effectiveness of transcatheter arterial embolization (TAE) to obtain sufficient volume reduction for graft implantation. From March 2007 to December 2009, 25 patients with kidneys descending below the iliac crest had unilateral renal TAE associated with a postembolization syndrome protocol. Volume reduction was evaluated by CT before, 3, and 6 months after embolization. The strategy was considered a success if the temporary contraindication for renal transplantation could be withdrawn within 6 months after TAE. TAE was well tolerated and the objective was reached in 21 patients. The temporary contraindication for transplantation was withdrawn within 3 months after TAE in 9 patients and within 6 months in 12 additional patients. The mean reduction in volume was 42% at 3 months (p = 0.01) and 54% at 6 months (p = 0.001). One patient required a cyst sclerosis to reach the objective. The absence of sufficient volume reduction was due to an excessive basal renal volume, a missed accessory artery and/or renal artery revascularization. Embolization of enlarged polycystic kidneys appears to be an advantageous alternative to nephrectomy before renal transplantation.

▶ Autosomal dominant polycystic kidney disease (ADPCKD) is the primary cause of kidney failure in approximately 10% of patients listed for renal transplantation. The need for and timing of native nephrectomy in these patients remains a controversial topic. Patients who have markedly enlarged kidneys that prohibit placement of a renal allograft and those with recurrent symptoms, such as pain, cyst infection, and bleeding, may need native nephrectomy prior to transplantation. Native nephrectomy, done as a separate procedure prior to renal transplantation, carries the risk of a major operation and may delay transplantation. Combining nephrectomy and transplantation in one procedure may subject the transplant procedure to the risks of nephrectomy.

In this article, the authors use transcatheter arterial embolization (TAE) to effect volume reduction of enlarged polycystic kidneys. In a pilot study with 25 patients, volume reduction was sufficient in 21 patients to enable transplantation within

6 months. There were no major complications, and no patients received a blood transfusion. The remaining 4 patients required more invasive procedures to allow for transplantation.

This interesting study nicely demonstrates an alternative to native nephrectomy in patients with ADPCKD. Following TAE, volume reduction of the native kidneys is successfully accomplished in most patients. What is unclear, however, are whether these patients could have proceeded to transplantation without TAE and whether TAE delays transplantation more than nephrectomy. Therefore, the role of TAE in the treatment of patients with ADPCKD will need to be determined by direct comparison to simultaneous and staged nephrectomy. At present, TAE offers a good alternative.

V. Krishnamurthi, MD

Robotic-Assisted Laparoscopic Donor Nephrectomy with Transvaginal Extraction of the Kidney
Pietrabissa A, Abelli M, Spinillo A, et al (Univ of Pavia, Italy)
Am J Transplant 10:2708-2711, 2010

Transvaginal recovery of the kidney has recently been reported, in a donor who had previously undergone a hysterectomy, as a less-invasive approach to perform laparoscopic live-donor nephrectomy. Also, robotic-assisted laparoscopic kidney donation was suggested to enhance the surgeon's skills during renal dissection and to facilitate, in a different setting, the closure of the vaginal wall after a colpotomy. We report here the technique used for the first case of robotic-assisted laparoscopic live-donor nephrectomy with transvaginal extraction of the graft in a patient with the uterus in place. The procedure was carried out by a multidisciplinary team, including a gynecologist. Total operative time was 215 min with a robotic time of 95 min. Warm ischemia time was 3 min and 15 s. The kidney was pre-entrapped in a bag and extracted transvaginally. There was no intra- or postoperative complication. No infection was seen in the donor or in the recipient. The donor did not require postoperative analgesia and was discharged from the hospital 24 h after surgery. Our initial experience with the combination of robotic surgery and transvaginal extraction of the donated kidney appears to open a new opportunity to further minimize the trauma to selected donors.

▶ This article demonstrates another advance in live donor nephrectomy surgery. Specifically, both groups show that vaginal extraction of a live-donor allograft can be safely performed with both a laparoscopic approach and a robotic-assisted laparoscopic approach. From both reports, minimal morbidity was encountered by the kidney donors, and both grafts functioned well. Of note, the second group expanded the applicability of vaginal extraction by performing the procedure in a patient with a uterus in place.

These authors are to be commended on advancing the field by demonstrating a new technique. What remains in doubt, however, is the widespread applicability of this new approach. For a new technique to become an equivalent standard of care, it must have a complication rate equal to that of the current technique. At present, laparoscopic donor nephrectomy has a very low complication rate, with most donors being discharged within 48 hours and approaching baseline status by 2 weeks. It is difficult to envision vaginal extraction substantially improving upon this already high standard. Additionally, the infectious risks to the recipient, following allograft extraction from the vagina, are not well delineated and will require focused and lengthy follow-up.

The significance of these articles is in their demonstration of technical feasibility and potential applicability to a, as of now undefined, specific patient population.

V. Krishnamurthi, MD

4   Female Urology

Diagnostics

Differences in continence system between community-dwelling black and white women with and without urinary incontinence in the EPI study
DeLancey JOL, Fenner DE, Guire K, et al (Univ of Michigan, Ann Arbor; et al)
Am J Obstet Gynecol 202:584.e1-584.e12, 2010

Objective.—We sought to compare continence system function of black and white women in a population-based sample.

Study Design.—As part of a cross-sectional population-based study, black and white women ages 35-64 years were invited to have pelvic floor testing to achieve prespecified groups of women with and without urinary incontinence. We analyzed data collected from 335 women classified as continent (n = 137) and stress (n = 102) and urge (n = 96) incontinent based on full bladder stress test and symptoms. Continence system functions were compared across racial and continence groups.

Results.—Comparing black to white women, maximal urethral closure pressure (MUCP) was 22% higher in blacks than whites (68.0 vs 55.8 cm H_2O, $P < .0001$). White and black women with stress incontinence had MUCP 19% and 23% lower than continent women. MUCP in urge incontinent white women was as low as stress incontinent whites, but blacks with urge had normal urethral function.

Conclusion.—Black women have higher urethral closure pressures than white women. White women with urge incontinence, but not black women, have reduced MUCP.

▶ The authors were able to recruit 335 women from the community to travel to a urology clinic to have urodynamic testing performed. This is a notable accomplishment. Half of the women were white, and half were black. Approximately one-third had stress urinary incontinence (SUI), one-third had urge urinary incontinence (UUI), and one-third were continent. Maximum urethral closure pressure (MUCP) measurements were used as an indicator of urethral function. In women with SUI, the MUCP values were lower than those of the continent women in both races. In women with UUI, the MUCP values were low in white women but normal in black women. The use of MUCP as a measure of urethral function could be debated. However, these findings suggest that the etiology of urge incontinence symptoms may be different in white versus black women. If this is true, it implies that treatment outcomes for UUI may differ between the races.

J. Q. Clemens, MD

A Randomized, Controlled Trial Comparing an Innovative Single Incision Sling With an Established Transobturator Sling to Treat Female Stress Urinary Incontinence
Hinoul P, Vervest HAM, den Boon J, et al (Ziekenhuis Oost-Limburg, Genk, Belgium; Sint Elisabeth Ziekenhuis, Tilburg, The Netherlands; Isala Ziekenhuis, Zwolle, The Netherlands; et al)
J Urol 185:1356-1362, 2011

Purpose.—Mid urethral sling procedures have become the surgical treatment of choice for female stress urinary incontinence. Innovative modifications of mid urethral sling procedures were recently introduced with the claim of offering similar efficacy and decreased morbidity. We compared the efficacy and morbidity of an innovative single incision mid urethral tape and an established transobturator procedure.

Materials and Methods.—We performed a prospective, randomized, controlled trial in 6 teaching hospitals in Belgium and The Netherlands between 2007 and 2009. A total of 96 patients received a TVT Secur™ single incision sling and 98 received a TVT™ Obturator System. We collected data on patient characteristics, surgery related parameters, adverse events, clinical followup, Urogenital Distress Inventory and SF-36® scores, validated questionnaires on daily life activities and visual analog scores objectifying pain. Followup was 1 year.

Results.—One-year followup was available for 75 single incision sling and 85 obturator system cases. Stress urinary incontinence could be objectified in 16.4% of the patients with a single incision sling and in 2.4% with an obturator system (p <0.05). Stress urinary incontinence was subjectively reported by 24% of single incision sling and 8% of obturator system patients (p <0.05). One year after surgery the mean ± SD UDI incontinence domain score in the single incision sling and obturator system groups was 21 ± 24 and 13 ± 21, respectively (p <0.01). Patients with a single incision sling experienced significantly less pain during the first 2 weeks after surgery (p <0.05) and returned significantly earlier to normal daily activity. The OR of re-intervention for stress urinary incontinence 1 year after receiving a single incision sling vs an obturator system was 2.3 (95% CI 1.9−2.7).

Conclusions.—The single incision sling procedure is associated with less postoperative pain and a lower objective cure rate than the obturator system procedure.

▶ In this well-done multicenter randomized controlled trial, the TVT Secur was inferior to a TVT transobturator sling as measured by multiple different parameters. This supports the findings of several other studies published over the last

2 years, suggesting that mini slings may not be overall as efficacious as either retropubic slings or transobturator slings. Nevertheless, these minimally invasive procedures are associated with comparably little postoperative pain and a rapid convalescence. However, this study demonstrated numerically higher complications in the TVT Secur procedure as compared with the transobturator TVT, including more perioperative bleeding complications and postoperative complications such as mesh exposure (7 vs 1) and urinary tract infections (6 vs 2). The long-term efficacy of the mini slings remains unknown, and, hopefully, this study and others that had been previously published will take their data out for several more years and report on the long-term durability of this most minimally invasive midurethral sling.

E. S. Rovner, MD

Non-Pharmacologic Therapy

Improving Urinary Incontinence in Overweight and Obese Women Through Modest Weight Loss
Wing RR, for the Program to Reduce Incontinence by Diet and Exercise (PRIDE) (Miriam Hosp, Providence, RI; et al)
Obstet Gynecol 116:284-292, 2010

Objective.—To examine the relationship between magnitude of weight loss and changes in urinary incontinence frequency.

Methods.—Overweight and obese women (N = 338) with 10 or more urinary incontinence episodes per week were assigned randomly to an intensive 6-month behavioral weight loss program followed immediately by a 12-month weight maintenance program (intervention; n = 226) or to a structured education program (control; n = 112). The intervention and control groups were combined to examine the effects of the magnitude of weight loss on changes in urinary incontinence assessed by 7-day voiding diary, pad test, and self-reported satisfaction with change in urinary incontinence.

Results.—Compared with participants who gained weight (reference), those who lost 5% to less than 10% or 10% or more of their body weight had significantly greater percent reductions in urinary incontinence episodes and were more likely to achieve at least a 70% reduction in the frequency of total and urge urinary incontinence episodes at 6, 12, and 18 months. Satisfaction was also related to magnitude of weight loss; approximately 75% of women who lost 5% to less than 10% of their body weight reported being moderately or very satisfied with their changes in urine leakage.

Conclusion.—Weight losses between 5% and 10% of body weight were sufficient for significant urinary incontinence benefits. Thus, weight loss should be considered as initial treatment for incontinence in overweight and obese women.

▶ There is now level I evidence that overweight women with urinary incontinence are likely to experience significant improvement in the symptoms if they are able to lose weight. However, such lifestyle modification may be met with little enthusiasm by patients, as the degree of required weight loss may seem insurmountable. In this analysis, the authors found that a weight reduction of 5% to 10% was sufficient to cause a significant improvement in symptoms. This was true regardless of the baseline weight or the severity of baseline symptoms. Mean weight in the cohort was 202 lb. This means that, on average, a weight loss of 10 to 20 lb would be sufficient. This may seem feasible to many patients.

J. Q. Clemens, MD

Update of AUA Guideline on the Surgical Management of Female Stress Urinary Incontinence

Dmochowski RR, Blaivas JM, Gormley EA, et al (American Urological Association Education and Res, Inc, Linthicum, MD)
J Urol 183:1906-1914, 2010

Purpose.—We updated the 1997 American Urological Association guideline on female stress incontinence.

Materials and Methods.—MEDLINE® searches of English language publications from 1994 and new searches of the literature published between December 2002 and June 2005 were performed using identified MeSH terms. Articles were selected for the index patient defined as the otherwise healthy woman who elected to undergo surgery to correct stress urinary incontinence or the otherwise healthy woman with incontinence and prolapse who elected to undergo treatment for both conditions.

Results.—A total of 436 articles were identified as suitable for inclusion in the meta-analysis, and an additional 155 articles were suitable for complications data only due to insufficient followup of efficacy outcomes in the latter reports. Surgical efficacy was defined using outcomes pre-specified in the primary evidence articles. Urgency (resolution and de novo) was included as an efficacy outcome due to its significant impact on quality of life. The primary efficacy outcome was resolution of stress incontinence measured as completely dry (cured/dry) or improved (cured/improved). Complications were analyzed similarly to the efficacy outcomes. Subjective complications (pain, sexual dysfunction and voiding dysfunction) were also included as a separate category.

Conclusions.—The surgical management of stress urinary incontinence with or without combined prolapse treatment continues to evolve. New technologies have emerged which have impacted surgical treatment algorithms. Cystoscopy has been added as a standard component of the procedure during surgical implantation of slings.

▶ The first American Urological Association (AUA) guidelines on the surgical management of female stress urinary incontinence were published in 1997 and actually represented the very first guidelines document produced by the AUA. This update document represents a further analysis of the published literature through 2005. Importantly, this document did not review or evaluate transobturator slings, as there was not sufficient evidence available in the literature by 2005. At 24 months, 48 months and greater than 48 months, all of the procedures evaluated were felt to be options for the index patient with stress incontinence, although the outcomes for the 5 major types of procedures (injectables, laparoscopic suspensions, midurethral slings, pubovaginal slings, and retropubic suspensions) are not equivalent. This was felt to be because of the fact that each of these procedures offers unique benefits and potential morbidities, which should be discussed with the patient.

Other important conclusions in this document include that it should be a standard that intraoperative cystoscopy be performed in all patients undergoing sling surgery and that the tensioning of any sling procedure being performed concomitantly with vaginal prolapse surgery should only be adjusted after completion of the vaginal prolapse portion of the procedure.

E. S. Rovner, MD

Pelvic Prolapse

Outcomes after anterior vaginal wall repair with mesh: a randomized, controlled trial with a 3 year follow-up

Nieminen K, Hiltunen R, Takala T, et al (Univ of Tampere, Finland; Central Hosp of South Ostrobothnia, Seinäjoki, Finland; Central Hosp of Päijät-Häme, Lahti, Finland; et al)
Am J Obstet Gynecol 203:235.e1-235.e8, 2010

Objective.—The objective of the study was to compare anterior colporrhaphy with and without a mesh.

Study Design.—Two hundred two women with anterior prolapse were assigned to undergo colporrhaphy alone or reinforced with a tailored polypropylene mesh. Before and 2, 12, 24, and 36 months after surgery, the outcome was assessed by examination and standard questions. The primary endpoint was anatomic recurrence of anterior vaginal prolapse. Secondary outcomes were symptom resolution, reoperation, and mesh exposure.

Results.—Recurrences of anterior vaginal prolapse were noted in 40 of the 97 (41%) in the colporrhaphy group and 14 of 105 (13%) in the mesh group ($P < .0001$). The number needed to treat was thus 4. The proportion of symptomatic patients, including those with dyspareunia, did not differ between the groups. The mesh erosion rate was 19%.

Conclusion.—At 3 year follow-up, anterior colporrhaphy with mesh reinforcement significantly reduced anatomic recurrences of anterior vaginal prolapse, but no difference in symptomatic recurrence were noted and the mesh erosion rate was high. The use of mesh was not associated with an increase in dyspareunia.

▶ This is an impressive study with an excellent design and a superb long-term follow-up. Notably, there were very few patients lost to follow-up. This considerably strengthens the conclusions of the study. A significant weakness that the authors acknowledge is that patients with significant apical prolapse requiring vaginal vault suspension were excluded from the analysis. Thus, it is unclear whether the results of this well-done study can be extended to these individuals.

The high mesh erosion rate in this study (19%) is tempered with the knowledge that most of these were asymptomatic and that there was no difference in sexual outcomes between the 2 groups with respect to dyspareunia.

It is clear from this study that the use of mesh for anterior vaginal wall repair reduces anatomical recurrences at 3-year follow-up. However, whether or not this difference in anatomical recurrence is clinically important or relevant is obscured by the fact that there was equivalence between the groups with respect to symptomatic recurrence. In vaginal prolapse surgery, it is likely that a perfect anatomical result is not necessary for resolution of the patients' symptoms.

E. S. Rovner, MD

Trocar-guided mesh repair of vaginal prolapse using partially absorbable mesh: 1 year outcomes
Milani AL, Hinoul P, Gauld JM, et al (Reinier de Graaf Group, Delft, the Netherlands; Evidence-Based Medicine, Paris, France; Evidence-Based Medicine, Livingston, England, UK; et al)
Am J Obstet Gynecol 204:74.e1-74.e8, 2011

Objective.—To evaluate anatomic and functional outcomes at 1-year following trocar-guided transvaginal prolapse repair using a partially absorbable mesh.

Study Design.—Prospective multicentre cohort study at 11 international sites. One hundred twenty-seven patients with pelvic organ prolapse stage ≥ III had surgery and were evaluated at 3 months and 1-year postsurgery compared with baseline. Instruments of measurements: Pelvic Organ Prolapse Quantification, Pelvic Floor Distress Inventory-20, Pelvic Floor Impact Questionnaire-7, Pelvic Organ Prolapse/Urinary Incontinence Sexual Function Questionnaire-12, and Patients Global Impression of Change.

Results.—Anatomic success, defined as prolapse stage ≤ I in the treated vaginal compartments, was 77.4% (95% confidence interval, 69.0–84.4%). Significant improvements in bother, quality of life, and sexual function were detected at 3 months and 1 year compared with baseline. At 1-year after surgery, 86.2% of patients indicated their prolapse situation to be "much better." Mesh exposure rate was 10.2% and rate of de novo dyspareunia 2% at 1 year.

Conclusion.—These results demonstrate improved anatomic support, associated with excellent functional improvements, without apparent safety concerns.

▶ The optimal approach to the repair of vaginal prolapse remains elusive. The rapid uptake of the use of various types of mesh, especially in the form of mesh kits, underscores the lack of physician and patient satisfaction with the current array of nonmesh repairs. Coincident with this rise in the use of mesh has been a rise in the number of mesh-related complications. Whether a partially absorbable mesh would reduce these complications is unclear. In this study of a partially absorbable mesh product, the exposure rate was still in excess of 10%. Although the efficacy in this trial at a relatively short-term interval of 1 year seems to be similar to that of other studies using mesh, longer-term data are necessary before we can declare that partially absorbable mesh is equivalent to nonabsorbable mesh. Furthermore, with longer-term follow-up, mesh exposure and other complications may (or may not) increase as well.

E. S. Rovner, MD

Anterior Colporrhaphy versus Transvaginal Mesh for Pelvic-Organ Prolapse

Altman D, for the Nordic Transvaginal Mesh Group (Karolinska Institutet, Stockholm, Sweden; et al)
N Engl J Med 364:1826-1836, 2011

Background.—The use of standardized mesh kits for repair of pelvic-organ prolapse has spread rapidly in recent years, but it is unclear whether this approach results in better outcomes than traditional colporrhaphy.

Methods.—In this multicenter, parallel-group, randomized, controlled trial, we compared the use of a trocar-guided, transvaginal polypropylene-mesh repair kit with traditional colporrhaphy in women with prolapse of the anterior vaginal wall (cystocele). The primary outcome was a composite of the objective anatomical designation of stage 0 (no prolapse) or 1 (position of the anterior vaginal wall more than 1 cm above the hymen), according to the Pelvic Organ Prolapse Quantification system, and the subjective absence of symptoms of vaginal bulging 12 months after the surgery.

Results.—Of 389 women who were randomly assigned to a study treatment, 200 underwent prolapse repair with the transvaginal mesh kit and 189 underwent traditional colporrhaphy. At 1 year, the primary outcome was significantly more common in the women treated with transvaginal mesh repair (60.8%) than in those who underwent colporrhaphy (34.5%) (absolute difference, 26.3 percentage points; 95% confidence interval, 15.6 to 37.0). The surgery lasted longer and the rates of intraoperative hemorrhage were higher in the mesh-repair group than in the colporrhaphy group ($P<0.001$ for both comparisons). Rates of bladder perforation were 3.5% in the mesh-repair group and 0.5% in the colporrhaphy group ($P=0.07$), and the respective rates of new stress urinary incontinence after surgery were 12.3% and 6.3% ($P=0.05$). Surgical reintervention to correct mesh exposure during follow-up occurred in 3.2% of 186 patients in the mesh-repair group.

Conclusions.—As compared with anterior colporrhaphy, use of a standardized, trocar-guided mesh kit for cystocele repair resulted in higher short-term rates of successful treatment but also in higher rates of surgical complications and postoperative adverse events. (Funded by the Karolinska Institutet and Ethicon; ClinicalTrials.gov number, NCT00566917.)

▶ This is a well-done randomized controlled trial (RCT) to address the issue of mesh in anterior vaginal wall repair. This confirms prior RCTs that have concluded that mesh augments the anatomic result but results in a trade-off of more complications and more bleeding. Whether these results are valid for patients who need concomitant surgery (hysterectomy, posterior repair, anti-incontinence surgery, etc) is unknown because these patients were excluded. Furthermore, only a single type of mesh repair kit was used. It is unclear whether these results would be similar with other mesh repair kits. In addition, no patients with stage 4 pelvic organ prolapse were enrolled. This may bias the findings as well. Finally, these patients will need to be followed for several years to see if these conclusions are valid in the long term.

E. S. Rovner, MD

Pharmacologic Therapy

Efficacy and Tolerability of Fesoterodine in Older and Younger Subjects With Overactive Bladder

Kraus SR, Ruiz-Cerdá JL, Martire D, et al (Univ of Texas Health Science Ctr at San Antonio; La Fe Univ Hosp, Valencia, Spain; Pfizer Incorporated, NY; et al)
Urology 76:1350-1357, 2010

Objectives.—To assess the effect of age on fesoterodine efficacy and tolerability in subjects with an overactive bladder.

Methods.—The data from 2 randomized, 12-week studies of 1681 subjects treated with fesoterodine 4 or 8 mg or placebo were pooled and stratified by age. The subjects completed 3-day bladder diaries at baseline and weeks 2 and 12, the King's Health Questionnaire at baseline and week 12, and the Treatment Benefit Scale at week 12.

Results.—Of the subjects aged <65 years, fesoterodine 4 and 8 mg was associated with statistically significant improvements in the diary variables at week 12 versus placebo. Greater improvement in urgency urinary incontinence was seen with fesoterodine 8 mg versus 4 mg. For those aged ≥65 to <75 years, fesoterodine 4 and 8 mg significantly improved all diary variables, except for the mean voided volume and micturition frequency versus placebo. In subjects aged ≥75 years, fesoterodine 8 mg significantly improved all diary variables, except for mean voided volume, versus placebo. No significant improvements were observed with fesoterodine 4 mg versus placebo. Fesoterodine significantly improved several King's Health Questionnaire domains versus placebo in all age groups. Fesoterodine 4 mg did not significantly improve any domains in subjects aged ≥75 years. In all age groups, the treatment response rates were significantly greater with both fesoterodine doses versus placebo. Dry mouth and constipation occurred more frequently in subjects aged ≥75 years receiving fesoterodine 8 mg than in those receiving fesoterodine 4 mg or placebo, although the discontinuation rates because of dry mouth and constipation were not increased.

Conclusions.—Fesoterodine 4 and 8 mg effectively treated overactive bladder symptoms in subjects aged <75 years. Fesoterodine 8 mg was effective in subjects aged ≥75 years.

▶ With increasing age, overactive bladder (OAB) symptoms become more common and more severe. Antimuscarinic medications are the standard pharmacologic agents used to treat this condition, but these medications could be associated with bothersome or even dangerous anticholinergic side effects in the elderly. For some reason, the risk profile of the common OAB meds have not been well studied in the elderly, and the studies that examined this issue have defined elderly as > 65 years, which is too young in my opinion. Therefore, I was glad to see that this study defined elderly as individuals older than 75 years. This study confirms my clinical impression that many elderly patients require higher doses of the medications to experience improvement in their symptoms. The side effects were quite reasonable and not qualitatively different from those reported in younger subjects. The critical issue, which is not addressed in this article, is quantifying the safety of these agents in elderly individuals with varying degrees of frailty. Although not specified by the authors, I would guess that this group of elderly subjects exhibited very minor degrees of frailty.

J. Q. Clemens, MD

Efficacy and Safety of OnabotulinumtoxinA for Idiopathic Overactive Bladder: A Double-Blind, Placebo Controlled, Randomized, Dose Ranging Trial

Dmochowski R, Chapple C, Nitti VW, et al (Vanderbilt Univ, Nashville, TN; Royal Hallamshire Hosp, Sheffield, UK; New York Univ School of Medicine; et al)

J Urol 184:2416-2422, 2010

Purpose.—Treatment options for patients with overactive bladder refractory to anticholinergics are limited. We assessed the dose response across a range of doses of onabotulinumtoxinA (BOTOX®) in patients with idiopathic overactive bladder and urinary urgency incontinence whose symptoms were not adequately managed with anticholinergics.

Materials and Methods.—In a phase 2, multicenter, randomized, double-blind study, 313 patients with idiopathic overactive bladder and urinary urgency incontinence experiencing 8 or more urinary urgency incontinence episodes a week and 8 or more micturitions daily at baseline received 50, 100, 150, 200 or 300 U intradetrusor onabotulinumtoxinA, or placebo. Symptoms were recorded using a 7-day bladder diary. The primary efficacy variable was weekly urinary urgency incontinence episodes and the primary end point was week 12.

Results.—Demographics and baseline characteristics were balanced across the treatment groups. Durable efficacy was observed for all onabotulinumtoxinA dose groups of 100 U or greater for primary and secondary efficacy measures, including the proportion of incontinence-free patients. When the dose response curves were analyzed, doses greater than 150 U contributed minimal additional or clinically relevant improvement in symptoms. This finding was also reflected in health related quality of life assessments. Dose dependent changes in post-void residual urine volume were observed and the use of clean intermittent catheterization was also dose dependent. The only adverse events significantly greater with onabotulinumtoxinA than with placebo were urinary tract infection and urinary retention.

Conclusions.—OnabotulinumtoxinA at doses of 100 U or greater demonstrated durable efficacy in the management of idiopathic overactive bladder and urinary urgency incontinence. A dose of 100 U may be the dose that appropriately balances the symptom benefits with the post-void residual urine volume related safety profile.

▶ The optimal dose for the treatment of lower urinary tract dysfunction with onabotulinumtoxinA will likely be different in neurogenic patients as compared with idiopathic patients. In this large, multicenter, dose ranging trial, a 100-unit dose of this agent provided satisfactory efficacy with a reasonably good adverse event profile. Prior studies in idiopathic overactive bladder used higher doses of this agent with resultant relatively higher rates of postinjection urinary retention and increased postvoid residuals. This study validates these prior studies in that doses higher than 100 units may simply be an excessive dose.

There remain many aspects of this therapy that need to be defined: the optimal number of injections, the optimal dilution of the agent, the optimal injection template, the optimal delivery vehicle, as well as the optimal interval for redosing. These data gaps exist for both the idiopathic as well as the neurogenic populations. There are many ongoing trials with onabotulinumtoxinA in idiopathic as well as neurogenic overactive bladders that may provide answers to some of these issues.

E. S. Rovner, MD

Tapes and Slings

Midterm Prospective Evaluation of TVT-Secur Reveals High Failure Rate
Cornu J-N, Sèbe P, Peyrat L, et al (Univ Paris VI, France)
Eur Urol 58:157-161, 2010

Background.—TVT-Secur has been described as a new minimally invasive sling for women's stress urinary incontinence (SUI) management, showing promising results in short-term studies.

Objective.—Our goal was to evaluate the outcome of this procedure after a midterm follow-up.

Design, Setting, and Participants.—A prospective evaluation involved 45 consecutive patients presenting SUI associated with urethral hypermobility. Fourteen patients preoperatively reported overactive bladder (OAB) symptoms, but none had objective detrusor overactivity. Eight patients had low maximal urethral closure pressure (MUCP). Four patients had pelvic organ prolapse (POP).

Intervention.—Patients with POP were treated under general anesthesia by Prolift and TVT-Secur procedure. The 41 other patients received TVT-Secur under local anesthesia on an outpatient basis. All interventions were made by the same surgeon.

Measurements.—Postoperative assessment included pad count, bladder diary, clinical examination with stress test, evaluation of satisfaction with the Patient Global Impression of Improvement (PGI-I) scale, and evaluation of side effects. Patients were classified as cured if they used no pads, had no leakage, and had a PGI-I score ≤2; as improved in case of reduction of SUI symptoms >50% and PGI-I score ≤3; and as failure otherwise.

Results and Limitations.—Mean postoperative follow-up was 30.2 ± 9.8 mo (range: 11−40 mo). Short-term evaluation showed a 93.5% success rate, but, at last follow-up, only 18 (40%) patients were cured, while 8 (18%) were improved, and 19 (42%) failed. Twelve patients underwent implantation of TVT or transobturator tape during follow-up. Age, MUCP, or OAB were not associated with failure. Side effects were limited to five cases of de novo OAB and three cases of urinary tract infection. This work is limited by the absence of a comparison group.

Conclusions.—Our experience shows that despite its good short-term efficacy, TVT-Secur is associated with a high recurrence rate of SUI. Therefore, TVT-Secur does not seem appropriate for SUI first-line management in women.

▶ There is a small but emerging body of evidence suggesting that some types and configurations of mini slings are less efficacious than originally thought. Much of these data represent small case series with imperfect follow-up. However, these and other data may hint that the advantages of such a minimally invasive approach that these procedures provide may not be the optimal procedures for the surgical treatment of stress urinary incontinence in women. Is this suboptimal efficacy because of a so-called learning curve effect? These are, after all, relatively new procedures. Until the data mature, and these procedures are subjected to the rigors of multiple randomized and controlled trials in a multicenter fashion, the overall enthusiasm for these procedures should be tempered.

E. S. Rovner, MD

Randomized Trial of Tension-Free Vaginal Tape and Tension-Free Vaginal Tape-Obturator for Urodynamic Stress Incontinence in Women

Teo R, Moran P, Mayne C, et al (Leicester Royal Infirmary, Worcester, UK; Leister and Worcestershire Royal Hosp, Worcester, UK; Leicester General Hosp, Worcester, UK; et al)

J Urol 185:1350-1355, 2011

Purpose.—We compared the efficacy and complications of tension-free vaginal tape and tension-free vaginal tape-obturator.

Materials and Methods.—Women with pure urodynamic stress incontinence undergoing only primary continence surgery were randomized to tension-free vaginal tape or tension-free vaginal tape-obturator at 2 centers between March 2005 and March 2007. Primary outcome was objective cure rate at 6 months, defined by a 24-hour pad test of less than 5 gm. Secondary outcomes were the subjective cure rate on the Patient Global Impression of Improvement, quality of life on the King's Healthcare Questionnaire and symptom severity scores on the International Consultation on Incontinence Questionnaire.

Results.—A total of 127 women were recruited. The study was stopped early due to excess leg pain in the tension-free vaginal tape-obturator group. Of the women 66 were randomized to tension-free vaginal tape and 61 were randomized to tension-free vaginal tape-obturator. Analysis was done by intent to treat. The objective and subjective cure rate at 6 months for tension-free vaginal tape vs tension-free vaginal tape-obturator was 69.7% vs 72.1% and 72.7% vs 67.2% (p = 0.76 and 0.49, respectively). Cure rates at 1 year were similar but loss to followup was high. Objective and subjective cure rates at 1 year for tension-free vaginal tape vs tension-free vaginal tape-obturator were 50% vs 41% and 53% vs 42.6% (p = 0.31 and 0.24, respectively). More women complained of leg pain after receiving a tension-free vaginal tape-obturator (26.4% vs 1.7%, p = 0.0001). The incidence of perioperative complications was low and similar between the groups. Time to discharge home and time to normal activity were not significantly different.

Conclusions.—Short-term cure rates at 6 months were similar. Tension-free vaginal tape-obturator caused more transient leg pain. Each procedure achieved a high cure rate and a low complication rate.

▶ In yet another randomized controlled trial between a retropubic and transobturator approach for the surgical treatment of stress urinary incontinence, equivalence between the 2 procedures was found. This is a small study with only a short-term follow-up of 6 months. Importantly, the results in this study are similar to those from many other studies, including the Trial Of Mid-Urethral Slings, a large National Institutes of Health—sponsored trial. However, the glaring difference between this study and many other randomized control studies looking at transobturator tape for the surgical treatment of stress urinary incontinence is the significant incidence of postoperative leg pain following transobturator sling placement. The incidence of leg pain in this study

(26.4%) is significantly higher than that reported in the literature in either single-surgeon case series or randomized control trials. Notably, the leg pain resolved in all patients in this study by 3 months except in 1 patient who required oral pharmacotherapy for treatment of chronic leg pain. In this regard, these data are somewhat reassuring in that this most debilitating complication spontaneously resolves in most affected individuals. The authors speculate that the high incidence of leg pain reported in the study is because of technical considerations, specifically that the transobturator tape approach used in this study was that of an inside out versus most other studies which used an outside in approach. Although an interesting hypothesis, other studies comparing inside-out with outside-in time over threshold techniques have not reported such findings.

E. S. Rovner, MD

A randomised controlled trial comparing TVT, Pelvicol and autologous fascial slings for the treatment of stress urinary incontinence in women
Guerrero KL, Emery SJ, Wareham K, et al (Southern General Hosp, Glasgow, UK)
BJOG 117:1493-1502, 2010

Objective.—To compare TVT(TM) , Pelvicol(TM) and autologous fascial slings (AFSs).

Design.—A multicentre randomised control trial.

Setting.—Four units in the UK.

Population.—Women requiring primary surgery for stress urinary incontinence (SUI).

Methods.—A total of 201 women with urodynamically proven stress incontinence were randomised into three groups and assessed at baseline, 6 weeks, 6 months and 1 year.

Main Outcome Measure.—The primary outcome was patient-reported improvement rates. Secondary outcomes included operative complications/time, intermittent self-catheterisation (ISC) and re-operation rates. The quality-of-life tools used were the Bristol Female Lower Urinary Tract Symptoms (BFLUTS) and EuroQoL.

Results.—Fifty women had a Pelvicol(TM) sling, 79 had AFSs and 72 had TVT(TM). At 6 months the Pelvicol(TM) arm had poorer improvement rates (73%) than TVT(TM) (92%)/AFS (95%); P=0.003. At 1 year only 61% of the Pelvicol(TM) slings remained as improved, versus 93% of TVTs and 90% of AFSs (P<0.001). Pelvicol(TM) has poorer dry rates (22%) than TVT(TM) (55%)/AFS (48%) (P=0.001) at 1 year; hence, the Pelvicol(TM) arm was suspended following interim analysis. There is no difference in the success rates between TVT(TM) and AFS. One in five women in the Pelvicol(TM) arm had further surgery for SUI by 1 year, but none required further surgery in the other arms. AFS took longer to do (54 minutes versus 35 minutes for TVT(TM) /36 minutes for Pelvicol(TM) and had higher ISC rates (9.9 versus 0% Pelvicol(TM) /TVT(TM) 1.5%).

Hospital stay was shortest for TVT(TM) (2 days). Most BFLUTS domains showed improvement in all three arms. The improvement for women in the Pelvicol(TM) arm, however, was less than for women in the other arms in several key domains.

Conclusions.—Pelvicol(TM) cannot be recommended for the management of SUI. TVT(TM) does not have greater efficacy than AFS, but does utilise fewer resources.

▶ This is an interesting 3-armed trial looking at 3 different interventions for stress urinary incontinence. This is a well-done randomized control trial. It is notable that all of the patients entered into this trial were uncomplicated individuals with stress urinary incontinence. There were no redo cases. Equivalence was found between tension-free vaginal tape (TVT) and autologous pubovaginal fascial sling for the treatment of uncomplicated stress urinary incontinence. Pelvicol was found to be inferior. In fact, the Pelvicol arm had such poor results that the Pelvicol arm was suspended following an interim analysis. Follow-up in this study was relatively short at 1 year. Hopefully, these authors will continue to follow these patients to provide long-term data for these surgical interventions.

The primary outcome measure in this study was a 3-point scale, and the patients categorized themselves as either dry, improved, or wet. Dry rates between the TVT and autologous pubovaginal sling were not statistically significant (TVT 53%, dry vs fascial sling 41% dry). Complications and morbidity were minimal in this trial, with only 1 patient requiring urethrolysis for long-term urinary retention, and this was in the fascial sling group. Bladder injury was slightly higher in the TVT group versus the fascial sling group (4 vs 2).

E. S. Rovner, MD

Retropubic versus Transobturator Midurethral Slings for Stress Incontinence

Richter HE, for the Urinary Incontinence Treatment Network (Univ of Alabama at Birmingham; et al)

N Engl J Med 362:2066-2076, 2010

Background.—Midurethral slings are increasingly used for the treatment of stress incontinence, but there are limited data comparing types of slings and associated complications.

Methods.—We performed a multicenter, randomized equivalence trial comparing outcomes with retropubic and transobturator midurethral slings in women with stress incontinence. The primary outcome was treatment success at 12 months according to both objective criteria (a negative stress test, a negative pad test, and no retreatment) and subjective criteria (self-reported absence of symptoms, no leakage episodes recorded, and no retreatment). The predetermined equivalence margin was ± 12 percentage points.

Results.—A total of 597 women were randomly assigned to a study group; 565 (94.6%) completed the 12-month assessment. The rates of objectively assessed treatment success were 80.8% in the retropubic-sling group and 77.7% in the transobturator-sling group (3.0 percentage-point difference; 95% confidence interval [CI], −3.6 to 9.6). The rates of subjectively assessed success were 62.2% and 55.8%, respectively (6.4 percentage-point difference; 95% CI, −1.6 to 14.3). The rates of voiding dysfunction requiring surgery were 2.7% in those who received retropubic slings and 0% in those who received transobturator slings (P = 0.004), and the respective rates of neurologic symptoms were 4.0% and 9.4% (P = 0.01). There were no significant differences between groups in postoperative urge incontinence, satisfaction with the results of the procedure, or quality of life.

Conclusions.—The 12-month rates of objectively assessed success of treatment for stress incontinence with the retropubic and transobturator approaches met the prespecified criteria for equivalence; the rates of subjectively assessed success were similar between groups but did not meet the criteria for equivalence. Differences in the complications associated with the two procedures should be discussed with patients who are considering surgical treatment for incontinence. (ClinicalTrials.gov number, NCT00325039.)

▶ In this well-funded, multicenter, National Institutes of Health—sponsored trial, retropubic slings were found to have equivalent efficacy to transobturator slings. Although this finding is not particularly surprising, adverse events were numerically greater in the retropubic-sling group as compared with the transobturator-sling group, specifically vascular and/or hematologic adverse events and postoperative voiding dysfunction. The only adverse events that were significantly greater in the transobturator arm of the study were vaginal epithelial perforations and neurological symptoms postoperatively, such as leg weakness.

It is interesting that although there was therapeutic equivalence between these 2 interventions based on prespecified criteria, failure rates were quite variable depending on the measuring tool used to assess efficacy. For example, surgical success at 12 months as measured by a 3-day voiding diary was between 30% and 40%, whereas if measured simply by the need for retreatment, failure rates in both groups were less than 5%. This underscores the importance of the appropriate application of outcome measures in determining actual success rates.

E. S. Rovner, MD

Retropubic versus Transobturator Midurethral Slings for Stress Incontinence
Richter HE, for the Urinary Incontinence Treatment Network (Univ of Alabama at Birmingham; et al)
N Engl J Med 362:2066-2076, 2010

Background.—Midurethral slings are increasingly used for the treatment of stress incontinence, but there are limited data comparing types of slings and associated complications.

Methods.—We performed a multicenter, randomized equivalence trial comparing outcomes with retropubic and transobturator midurethral slings in women with stress incontinence. The primary outcome was treatment success at 12 months according to both objective criteria (a negative stress test, a negative pad test, and no retreatment) and subjective criteria (self-reported absence of symptoms, no leakage episodes recorded, and no retreatment). The predetermined equivalence margin was ±12 percentage points.

Results.—A total of 597 women were randomly assigned to a study group; 565 (94.6%) completed the 12-month assessment. The rates of objectively assessed treatment success were 80.8% in the retropubic-sling group and 77.7% in the transobturator-sling group (3.0 percentage-point difference; 95% confidence interval [CI], −3.6 to 9.6). The rates of subjectively assessed success were 62.2% and 55.8%, respectively (6.4 percentage-point difference; 95% CI, −1.6 to 14.3). The rates of voiding dysfunction requiring surgery were 2.7% in those who received retropubic slings and 0% in those who received transobturator slings (P = 0.004), and the respective rates of neurologic symptoms were 4.0% and 9.4% (P = 0.01). There were no significant differences between groups in postoperative urge incontinence, satisfaction with the results of the procedure, or quality of life.

Conclusions.—The 12-month rates of objectively assessed success of treatment for stress incontinence with the retropubic and transobturator approaches met the prespecified criteria for equivalence; the rates of subjectively assessed success were similar between groups but did not meet the criteria for equivalence. Differences in the complications associated with the two procedures should be discussed with patients who are considering surgical treatment for incontinence. (ClinicalTrials.gov number, NCT00325039.)

▶ This is a large National Institutes of Health—funded comparative effectiveness trial of 2 existing minimally invasive treatments for stress incontinence (transvaginal tape vs transobturator tape). At 12 months, the success rates for the 2 techniques were essentially equivalent. The transvaginal tape was associated with slightly more voiding dysfunction, while the transobturator technique was associated with more episodes of pain and numbness, especially in the inner thigh region. At baseline, the patients exhibited a moderate degree of incontinence on average. Therefore, these results cannot necessarily be extrapolated to all women with stress incontinence. It is important to understand that 12-month outcomes are equivalent for most surgical treatments of stress urinary incontinence, and it is often not until 24 months or later where we see differences in outcomes. Fortunately, the authors have extended the trial, and they do plan to report outcomes at 24 months as well.

J. Q. Clemens, MD

Risk of Infection After Midurethral Synthetic Sling Surgery: Are Postoperative Antibiotics Necessary?

Swartz M, Ching C, Gill B, et al (The Cleveland Clinic, OH)
Urology 75:1305-1308, 2010

Objectives.—To review our postoperative infections using single-dose preoperative antibiotics. Midurethral synthetic sling surgery is commonly performed. Postoperative antibiotics are often prescribed and may have some risk of adverse events (AEs). We are unaware of data suggesting decreased risk of infection with this practice.

Methods.—We reviewed all midurethral synthetic sling surgery charts from 2004 to 2008 performed by 1 surgeon who uses only single-dose preoperative antibiotics (controls), and 2 who also use postoperative antibiotics (cases). A telephone survey was administered, which included questions regarding postoperative infections and AEs related to antibiotic use. Our primary and secondary outcomes were urinary tract infections (UTIs) and AEs related to antibiotic use, respectively. Patients were excluded for bladder injuries, postoperative catheters, and concomitant prolapse surgery.

Results.—We identified 103 cases and 116 controls, and the telephone survey response rate was 81.3%. At baseline, groups had similar characteristics. There was no significant difference in UTIs between cases (6.8%) and controls (9.5%). There were no skin infections. AEs related to antibiotic use were more common among those that received postoperative antibiotics (7.8% vs 0.9%, $P = .03$). There were 5 (63%) yeast infections, 1 (12.5%) rash, 1 (12.5%) case of nausea, and 1 (12.5%) patient with colitis among cases and 1 yeast infection among controls.

Conclusions.—UTI is common after sling surgery, but other infections are rare. The occurrence of UTI does not appear to be lower when postoperative antibiotics are prescribed. However, AEs associated with antibiotic use are increased. These findings do not support the use of postoperative antibiotics.

▶ The overuse of perioperative antibiotics has been a target of numerous contemporary quality improvement initiatives, including the Surgical Care Improvement Project and the Physician Quality Reporting Initiative. In most surgical specialties, standard recommendations exist for discontinuation of antibiotics postoperatively. Urology has been excluded from these guidelines because of a lack of data and the frequent use of urinary catheterization (and consequent bacteriuria) following many urologic surgeries. This single-site retrospective cohort study compared outcomes in women who underwent midurethral synthetic sling surgery for stress urinary incontinence. One group received single-dose perioperative antibiotic prophylaxis (n = 116), while the other received single-dose perioperative prophylaxis followed by 3 days of postoperative antibiotics (n = 103). The infection rate was similar in the 2 groups, but antibiotic-associated complications occurred more commonly in the group that received 3 days of postoperative antibiotics. Importantly, the analysis was limited to women who did not have concomitant surgery and who also did not require any type of postoperative catheterization. The authors acknowledge that a large prospective randomized trial is needed to provide more definitive evidence, but these results do suggest that single-dose prophylaxis is sufficient for uncomplicated sling placement.

J. Q. Clemens, MD

5   Renal Tumors

Diagnosis and Prognosis

Natural History of Renal Cortical Neoplasms During Active Surveillance With Follow-up Longer Than 5 Years

Haramis G, Mues AC, Rosales JC, et al (Columbia Univ Med Ctr, NY)
Urology 77:787-791, 2011

Objectives.—To present our experience with patients who elected active surveillance for renal cortical neoplasms (RCNs) with ≥5 years of follow-up. Few data are available regarding the long-term natural history of RCNs during surveillance.

Methods.—We retrospectively reviewed our urologic oncology database and identified 44 patients with 51 RCNs who had received active surveillance for >5 years of follow-up. The patient and tumor characteristics and tumor growth rate and overall survival data were evaluated.

Results.—The median patient age was 71.7 years (range 55-92), with 32 patients (72.7%) having a Charlson comorbidity index of ≥2. The median tumor size was 2.67 cm (range 0.9-8.6) at diagnosis. Biopsy was performed in 17 patients (38.6%). Of these 17 patients, clear cell renal cell carcinoma was diagnosed in 15 and papillary renal cell carcinoma in 2 patients. The median follow-up was 77.1 months (range 60-137), and the median growth rate was 0.15 cm/y. Of these patients, 2 (4.5%) required delayed intervention. One underwent laparoscopic radical nephrectomy because of a high tumor growth rate, and one elected to withdraw from active surveillance because of personal anxiety, despite having a stable tumor size for 72 months. The latter patient underwent laparoscopic renal cryoablation. Histopathologic examination revealed clear cell renal cell carcinoma in both cases. No metastases or cancer-related deaths occurred in our cohort; 1 patient died of cardiovascular disease.

Conclusions.—Most RCNs undergoing surveillance for >5 years grew slowly. The metastatic potential appeared minimal in patients who demonstrated low or absent tumor growth for a long period.

▶ Active surveillance is one accepted modality for the management of small renal masses. Although there may be significant anxiety associated with monitoring renal lesions, this study corroborates other analyses that show that observation can be a safe method of management, posing minimal risk to selected patients in terms of compromise of oncologic outcomes. In this study of 44 patients, 17 of whom had confirmed renal cell carcinoma, observation at over 5-year follow-up demonstrated no incidence of metastasis or cancer-related death. Growth rates were minimal, although 1 patient was treated for accelerated growth. This study further supports the safety and efficacy of active surveillance in select patients with small renal masses. However, it is unfortunate that surveillance relies on expensive radiographic follow-up, given the absence of any reliable biomarkers for renal disease.

B. M. Benway, MD

Minimally Invasive Approaches

Irreversible Electroporation of Renal Cell Carcinoma: A First-in-Man Phase I Clinical Study

Pech M, Janitzky A, Wendler JJ, et al (Univ of Magdeburg, Germany)
Cardiovasc Intervent Radiol 34:132-138, 2011

Purpose.—Irreversible electroporation (IRE) is a newly developed nonthermal tissue-ablation technique in which high-voltage electrical pulses of microsecond duration are applied to induce irreversible permeabilisation of the cell membrane, presumably through nanoscale defects in the lipid bilayer, leading to apoptosis. The purpose of this study was to assess the feasibility and safety of ablating renal cell carcinoma (RCC) tissue by IRE.

Methods.—Six patients scheduled for curative resection of RCC were included. IRE was performed during anaesthesia immediately before the resection with electrographic synchronisation. Central haemodynamics were recorded before and 5 min after electroporation. Five-channel electrocardiography (ECG) was used for detailed analysis of ST waveforms. Blood sampling and 12-lead ECG were performed before, during, and at scheduled intervals after the intervention.

Results.—Analysis of ST waveforms and axis deviations showed no relevant changes during the entire study period. No changes in central haemodynamics were seen 5 min after IRE. Similarly, haematological, serum biochemical, and ECG variables showed no relevant differences during the investigation period. No changes in cardiac function after IRE therapy were found. One case of supraventricular extrasystole was encountered. Initial histopathologic examination showed no immediate adverse effects of IRE (observation of delayed effects will require a different study design).

Conclusion.—IRE seems to offer a feasible and safe technique by which to treat patients with kidney tumours and could offer some potential advantages over current thermal ablative techniques.

▶ Ablative therapy is a valuable addition to the armamentarium for treatment of localized renal cell carcinoma. Cryoablation and radiofrequency ablation have been used routinely, demonstrating reasonable results. The authors describe the first human implementation of a new form of ablative therapy, which uses electrical pulses to increase cell permeability, leading to apoptosis. This is merely a safety evaluation in human subjects. Aside from 1 patient who experienced some aberrancy on electrocardiogram, the technology appears to be safe to implement. While this is promising, further study is critically needed to determine this technology's ability to provide reliable cell kill with easy monitoring and adjustment of the ablation zone. This technology's effects on immune modulation must also be studied. And most importantly, intermediate- and long-term functional and oncologic outcomes must be determined before this technology can be embraced with confidence.

B. M. Benway, MD

Initial Series of Robotic Radical Nephrectomy with Vena Caval Tumor Thrombectomy
Abaza R (Ohio State Univ Med Ctr & James Cancer Hosp, Columbus)
Eur Urol 59:652-656, 2011

Laparoscopy has become a standard modality for most renal tumors but not as yet for renal cell carcinoma (RCC) involving the inferior vena cava (IVC). Robotic technology may facilitate such complex procedures. We report the first series of robotic nephrectomy with IVC tumor thrombectomy including the first cases requiring cross-clamping of the IVC in a minimally invasive fashion. Five patients underwent robotic nephrectomy with IVC tumor thrombectomy including one patient having two renal veins, each with an IVC thrombus, for a total of six IVC thrombi. The IVC was opened in all patients, and tumor thrombi were delivered intact, followed by sutured closure. The mean patient age was 64 yr (53–70 yr) with a mean body mass index of 36.6 kg/m² (22–43 kg/m²). Thrombi protruded 1 cm, 2 cm, 4 cm, and 5 cm into the IVC in five patients and 3 cm and 2 cm in the patient with two thrombi. The mean estimated blood loss was 170 ml (50–400 ml). Mean operative time was 327 min (240–411 min). Mean length of stay was 1.2 d. There were no complications, transfusions, or readmissions. This early series represents a limited experience by a single surgeon with a new procedure and may not be reproducible in larger numbers or by all surgeons. Further experience is necessary to validate this application.

▶ Traditionally, the surgical management of renal tumors with thrombi that extend into the inferior vena cava (IVC) has been relegated to the domain of open surgery. In this very ambitious initial series from Dr Abaza, he outlines his experience with robot-assisted radical nephrectomy and IVC thrombectomy in 5 patients with infrahepatic tumor thrombus. The IVC could be clamped using a Satinsky clamp in most patients, and in 1 patient who did not tolerate clamping, the thrombus could be milked back into the renal vein using robotic instrumentation.

Quite impressively, intraoperative blood loss was extremely low, averaging only 170 mL, and the length of hospital stay was only 1.2 days. At just over a year of follow-up, no patients have experienced disease recurrence.

This report is quite remarkable in that it further expands the reach of robotic renal surgery to a domain previously believed to be off limits to a minimally invasive approach. However, it remains to be seen if this method remains safe and reproducible in the hands of other surgeons.

B. M. Benway, MD

Nephrectomy

Chronic Kidney Disease Before and After Partial Nephrectomy
Clark MA, Shikanov S, Raman JD, et al (Univ of Chicago, IL; Penn State Milton S. Hershey Med Ctr, PA; et al)
J Urol 185:43-48, 2011

Purpose.—We performed a multi-institutional retrospective cohort study to evaluate baseline renal function of patients who underwent partial nephrectomy for renal tumors, and determined rates of progression to higher stages of chronic kidney disease.

Materials and Methods.—The Modification of Diet in Renal Disease study equation was used to estimate glomerular filtration rate. Preoperative and postoperative serum creatinine values were obtained from patients who underwent partial nephrectomy at 6 institutions with a normal contralateral kidney, and had baseline chronic kidney disease stage I (estimated glomerular filtration rate greater than 90 ml/minute/1.73 m^2), II (estimated glomerular filtration rate 60 to 89 ml/minute/1.73 m^2) or III (estimated glomerular filtration rate 30 to 59 ml/minute/1.73 m^2). The end point was change in chronic kidney disease stage at long-term followup (3 to 18 months). Multivariate logistic and Cox regression models tested the association of newly acquired chronic kidney disease stage III or greater with pertinent demographic, tumor and surgical factors.

Results.—For 1,228 patients with followup creatinine data at least 3 months after partial nephrectomy median baseline glomerular filtration rate was 74 ml/minute/1.73 m^2. At baseline 19%, 59% and 22% of patients had chronic kidney disease stage I, II and III, respectively. At long-term followup for patients with baseline chronic kidney disease stage I or II median postoperative glomerular filtration rate was 67 ml/minute/1.73 m^2 with 29% having progression to chronic kidney disease stage III or greater. Increasing age, female gender, increasing tumor size, clamping of the renal artery and vein, and lower preoperative estimated glomerular filtration rate were independently associated with newly acquired chronic kidney disease stage III or greater. The presence of comorbid conditions such as coronary artery disease, diabetes mellitus or hypertension did not independently predict an increased risk of higher chronic kidney disease stage.

Conclusions.—Chronic kidney disease stage III or greater will develop postoperatively in approximately a third of patients with an estimated glomerular filtration rate greater than 60 ml/minute/1.73 m², and this progression is associated with definable demographic, tumor and surgical factors.

▶ The fact that renal function decreases after a partial nephrectomy should not be surprising in the least. Resection of surrounding normal renal parenchyma and clamping of the renal artery for even a nominal amount of time clearly adversely affect renal function, particularly in the elderly. I think what is surprising about this article is that even patients who have reasonable glomerular filtration (defined as greater than 60 mL/min/1.73 m²), approximately a third progress to chronic kidney stage III disease. The presence of comorbid conditions that would be associated with an increased risk of tissue ischemia, such as coronary artery disease, diabetes mellitus, or hypertension, actually did not appear to increase the risk of developing chronic renal disease. It was primarily associated with age, female gender, larger tumor size, clamping of both the artery and the vein, and lower preoperative glomerular filtration rate.

How is this going to alter practice? Of all the associated factors, only clamping the artery and vein is modifiable by the surgeon. In the vast majority of partial nephrectomies, the vein does not need to be clamped. In addition, off-clamp partials for selected exophytic lesions make sense. In addition, I think that a close monitoring of patients' renal function after a partial nephrectomy is prudent. We are already following these patients because of concerns of recurrence in the remaining renal parenchyma. Even with a small bump in creatinine level, I would have a low threshold for referring patients to a nephrologist for preventive measures to decrease the likelihood that they develop chronic renal insufficiency.

A. S. Kibel, MD

The Impact of Cytoreductive Nephrectomy on Survival of Patients With Metastatic Renal Cell Carcinoma Receiving Vascular Endothelial Growth Factor Targeted Therapy

Choueiri TK, Xie W, Kollmannsberger C, et al (Dana Farber Cancer Inst, Boston, MA; British Columbia Cancer Agency, Vancouver, Canada; et al)
J Urol 185:60-66, 2011

Purpose.—Vascular endothelial growth factor targeted therapy is a standard of care in patients with metastatic renal cell carcinoma. The role of cytoreductive nephrectomy in the era of novel agents remains poorly defined.

Materials and Methods.—We retrospectively reviewed baseline characteristics and outcomes of 314 patients with anti-vascular endothelial growth factor therapy naïve, metastatic renal cell carcinoma from United States and Canadian cancer centers to study the impact of cytoreductive nephrectomy on overall survival.

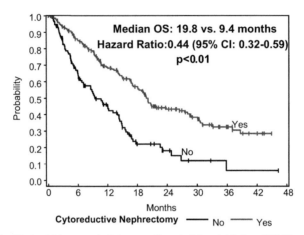

FIGURE 1.—Kaplan-Meier curve depicting overall survival from initiation of VEGF targeted therapy for 314 patients who did or did not receive cytoreductive nephrectomy. (Reprinted from Choueiri TK, Xie W, Kollmannsberger C, et al. The impact of cytoreductive nephrectomy on survival of patients with metastatic renal cell carcinoma receiving vascular endothelial growth factor targeted therapy. *J Urol.* 2011;185:60-66, Copyright 2011, with permission from American Urological Association.)

Results.—Patients who underwent cytoreductive nephrectomy (201) were younger (p <0.01), and more likely to have a better Karnofsky performance status (p <0.01), more than 1 site of metastasis (p = 0.04) and lower corrected calcium levels (p <0.01) compared to those who did not undergo cytoreductive nephrectomy (113). On univariable analysis cytoreductive nephrectomy was associated with a median overall survival of 19.8 months compared to 9.4 months for patients who did not undergo cytoreductive nephrectomy (HR 0.44; 95% CI 0.32, 0.59; p <0.01). On multivariable analysis and adjusting for established prognostic risk factors the overall survival difference persisted (adjusted HR 0.68; 95% CI 0.46, 0.99; p = 0.04) in favor of the cytoreductive nephrectomy group. In subgroup analyses stratified for favorable/intermediate/poor risk criteria, patients in the poor risk group had a marginal benefit (p = 0.06). Similarly patients with Karnofsky performance status less than 80% also had a marginal survival benefit (p = 0.08).

Conclusions.—In this retrospective study cytoreductive nephrectomy was independently associated with a prolonged overall survival of patients with metastatic renal cell carcinoma treated with vascular endothelial growth factor targeted agents, although the benefit is marginal in those patients with poor risk features (Fig 1).

▶ Landmark studies demonstrated that cytoreductive nephrectomy improved patients' overall survival prior to the immunotherapy era.[1] Since the introduction of tyrosine kinase and mammalian target of rapamycin (mTOR) inhibitors, questions have been raised as to whether we should abandon cytoreductive nephrectomy or at least modify our approach to give systemic therapy prior to cytoreductive nephrectomy. Choueiri et al demonstrate that there is a clear survival advantage in patients who undergo cytoreductive nephrectomy with an adjusted hazard ratio of 0.6 with an improvement in survival from 9.4 months to 19.8 months in the patients who receive a cytoreductive nephrectomy. On multivariate analysis, they demonstrated that the overall survival difference persisted with an adjusted hazard ratio of 0.68 ($P = .04$) (Fig 1).

While this is not a randomized trial, it demonstrates that cytoreductive nephrectomy still appears to confirm overall survival advantage in the tyrosine kinase/mTOR inhibitors era. As a result, I still strongly advocate cytoreductive nephrectomy in patients who (1) have good performance status, (2) understand that the survival benefit is measured in months and not years, and (3) realize that the nephrectomy, while contributing to an improvement in overall survival, is not going to be curative. Once ongoing randomized trials are completed in Europe, we will have a more certain understanding of whether cytoreductive nephrectomy continues to demonstrate a survival advantage. Until then, I believe we have to continue to follow the level 1 evidence, which is that cytoreductive nephrectomy works, and data such as what are presented in this article only reinforce that conclusion.

A. S. Kibel, MD

Reference

1. Flanigan RC, Mickisch G, Sylvester R, Tangen C, Van Poppel H, Crawford ED. Cytoreductive nephrectomy in patients with metastatic renal cancer: a combined analysis. *J Urol.* 2004;171:1071-1076.

A Prospective, Randomised EORTC Intergroup Phase 3 Study Comparing the Oncologic Outcome of Elective Nephron-Sparing Surgery and Radical Nephrectomy for Low-Stage Renal Cell Carcinoma

Van Poppel H, Da Pozzo L, Albrecht W, et al (Univ Hosp Gasthuisberg, Leuven, Belgium; Instituto Scientifico H.S. Raffaele, Milano, Italy; Krankenanstalt Rudolfstiftung, Vienna, Austria; et al)
Eur Urol 59:543-552, 2011

Background.—Nephron-sparing surgery (NSS) can safely be performed with slightly higher complication rates than radical nephrectomy (RN), but proof of oncologic effectiveness is lacking.

Objective.—To compare overall survival (OS) and time to progression.

Design, Setting, and Participants.—From March 1992 to January 2003, when the study was prematurely closed because of poor accrual, 541 patients with small (≤ 5 cm), solitary, T1–T2 N0 M0 (Union Internationale Contre le Cancer [UICC] 1978) tumours suspicious for renal cell carcinoma (RCC) and a normal contralateral kidney were randomised to NSS or RN in European Organisation for Research and Treatment of Cancer Genito-Urinary Group (EORTC-GU) noninferiority phase 3 trial 30904.

Intervention.—Patients were randomised to NSS ($n = 268$) or RN ($n = 273$) together with limited lymph node dissection (LND).

Measurements.—Time to event end points was compared with log-rank test results.

Results and Limitations.—Median follow-up was 9.3 yr. The intention-to-treat (ITT) analysis showed 10-yr OS rates of 81.1% for RN and 75.7% for NSS. With a hazard ratio (HR) of 1.50 (95% confidence interval [CI], 1.03—2.16), the test for noninferiority is not significant ($p = 0.77$), and test for superiority is significant ($p = 0.03$). In RCC patients and clinically and pathologically eligible patients, the difference is less pronounced (HR = 1.43 and HR = 1.34, respectively), and the superiority test is no longer significant ($p = 0.07$ and $p = 0.17$, respectively). Only 12 of 117 deaths were the result of renal cancer (four RN and eight NSS). Twenty-one patients progressed (9 after RN and 12 after NSS). Quality of life and renal function outcomes have not been addressed.

Conclusions.—Both methods provide excellent oncologic results. In the ITT population, NSS seems to be significantly less effective than RN in terms of OS. However, in the targeted population of RCC patients, the trend in favour of RN is no longer significant. The small number of progressions and deaths from renal cancer cannot explain any possible OS differences between treatment types.

▶ The authors should be congratulated for completing this randomized phase 3 trial comparing partial nephrectomy with radical nephrectomy in patients with low-stage nonmetastatic renal cell carcinoma. The patient population targeted (clinical T1 and T2 disease) is exactly the patient population in which we frequently use partial nephrectomy and in which it has become the de facto standard of care. Using an intent-to-treat analysis, they demonstrated that radical nephrectomy was associated with an improved overall survival compared with partial nephrectomy (Fig 2 in the original article). This level 1 evidence is the first head-to-head comparison of these 2 treatment modalities and clearly favors radical nephrectomy. The major caveat to this study is that very few patients actually died of renal cell carcinoma. Of the 541 patients randomized in this trial, only 12 renal cancer deaths occurred—4 in the radical nephrectomy group and 8 in the nephron-sparing group. This either speaks to the low malignant potential of tumors treated or to the oncologic effectiveness of both treatments.

I think many people will dismiss this study and continue to do partial nephrectomies. Clearly, the data are quite strong that partial nephrectomy protects the renal unit and decreases the risk of chronic renal insufficiency. It is particularly important in light of the large number of incidental tumors that are being identified in 2011. With that said, I think this study needs to give us great pause. Have we embraced the technology of partial nephrectomy too rapidly? Will the increasing use of minimally invasive approaches alter the survival of patients undergoing nephron-sparing surgery? Lastly, the million-dollar question is whether we are overtreating many of these renal masses and they do not actually need to be treated. While this study answers none of these questions, I for one will certainly be thinking about this study whenever

I counsel a patient as to whether they should get a partial versus a radical nephrectomy.

A. S. Kibel, MD

Partial Nephrectomy

Laparoscopic Techniques Applied to Open Surgery: Sliding-clip Renorrhaphy

Gorin MA, Ramanathan R, Leveillee RJ (Univ of Miami Miller School of Medicine, FL)

Urology 77:751-753, 2011

Objectives.—To describe our initial experience with the laparoscopic technique of sliding-clip renorrhaphy applied to open surgery for small renal masses.

Methods.—Knotless renorrhaphy with the sliding-clip technique is performed by securing suture with Hem-o-lok clips slid under tension against the renal capsule and locked in place with Lapra-Ty clips. This approach was initially described by laparoscopic surgeons to aid with hemostasis, prevent urine leaks, and shorten warm ischemia time. We evaluated the utility of this technique during open partial nephrectomy.

Results.—From February 2009 to June 2010, 9 patients, with mean age of 54 years, underwent open partial nephrectomy using the sliding-clip technique. Mean ischemia time was <20 minutes, with a mean blood loss of approximately 280 mL. No intraoperative complications were reported. One clinically significant complication of a urinoma was found in the perioperative period. No bleeding complications developed.

Conclusions.—The results of our study have shown that the sliding-clip technique is safe and effective in the open surgical management of small renal masses. We recommend this approach over traditional knot tying for renal reconstruction.

▶ Sliding-clip renorrhaphy is one of several innovations of minimally invasive renal surgery that have reduced the challenge and the learning curve of laparoscopic and robot-assisted partial nephrectomy. In this article, the authors describe their use of sliding-clip renorrhaphy in the setting of open partial nephrectomy. The technique was found to be safe, expeditious, and effective. The authors do comment that this method is substantially more expensive than a traditional tied-suture closure, and without comparative data, it is unclear whether sliding-clip renorrhaphy is particularly advantageous in the open setting, in terms of hastening repair, and providing a more reliable repair than a traditional closure.

B. M. Benway, MD

Intraoperative Conversion From Partial to Radical Nephrectomy at a Single Institution From 2003 to 2008

Galvin DJ, Savage CJ, Adamy A, et al (Memorial Sloan-Kettering Cancer Ctr, NY)
J Urol 185:1204-1209, 2011

Purpose.—Little information exists on conversion from partial to radical nephrectomy. We assessed the intraoperative reasons and predictive factors for conversion in a contemporary series of patients undergoing partial nephrectomy.

Materials and Methods.—We identified all patients at our institution who underwent open or laparoscopic partial nephrectomy with conversion to radical nephrectomy between 2003 and 2008. Renal function was assessed by the glomerular filtration rate using the modification of diet in renal disease equation. We used logistic regression analysis to determine whether tumor site, tumor size, body mass index, American Society of Anesthesiologists score, age or gender was associated with the conversion risk.

Results.—The rate of conversion to radical nephrectomy was 6% (61 of 1,029 patients). In the open partial nephrectomy group 59 of 865 cases (7%, 95% CI 5−9) and in the laparoscopic partial nephrectomy group 2 of 164 (1.2%, 95% CI 0.01−4) were converted. The most common reasons for conversion were invasion of hilar structures, size discrepancy and insufficient residual kidney. Patients with conversion were more likely to have larger tumors (per 1 cm increase OR 1.41, 95% CI 1.24−1.59), a central site (central vs peripheral OR 7.74, 95% CI 3.98−15) and a lower preoperative glomerular filtration rate (per 10 ml/minute/1.73 m^2 OR 0.78, 95% CI 0.67−0.91), and present with symptoms (any vs none OR 2.78, 95% CI 1.54−5.04) than those without conversion. The median postoperative glomerular filtration rate was 46 vs 61 ml/minute/1.73 m^2 in patients with vs without conversion.

Conclusions.—Conversion to radical nephrectomy was rare in patients undergoing partial nephrectomy in this series. Increasing tumor size, central site, lower preoperative glomerular filtration rate and symptoms at presentation were associated with an increased risk of conversion, which increases the likelihood of chronic kidney disease postoperatively.

▶ As demonstrated by another study reviewed in this text, radical nephrectomy appears to be associated with an increased risk of renal insufficiency and failure and an increased rate of nononcologic morbidity. However, nephron-sparing surgery is not always feasible in the setting of localized renal malignancy. The authors present an analysis of factors, which increase the risk of conversion to radical nephrectomy during open and minimally invasive partial nephrectomy. Central or hilar tumors were perhaps unsurprisingly associated with an increased risk of conversion, as were larger tumors. Interestingly, impaired preoperative renal function and symptomatic presentation were also associated with an increased risk of conversion. While not assessed for all patients, a subset analysis using the R.E.N.A.L. (radius, exophytic/endophytic, nearness of tumor deepest portion to the collecting system or sinus, anterior/posterior and location relative to the polar line) nephrometry scoring system found that higher nephrometry score was associated with an increased risk of conversion. These data provide valuable information that may be used in preoperative assessment and counseling of patients undergoing renal surgery, and may help to guide discussion regarding expectations for conversion to radical nephrectomy.

B. M. Benway, MD

Can partial nephrectomy preserve renal function and modify survival in comparison with radical nephrectomy?

Medina-Polo J, Romero-Utero J, Rodriguez-Antolín A, et al (Hospital Universitario 12 de Octubre, Madrid, Spain)
Scand J Urol Nephrol 45:143-150, 2011

Objective.—To investigate whether radical nephrectomy (RN) and nephron-sparing surgery (NSS) for T1 renal cell carcinoma influence renal function, oncological outcome or survival rate.

Material and Methods.—A retrospective study was performed, including 290 nephrectomies for tumours of a diameter of less than 7 cm; 174 radical nephrectomies were compared to 116 nephron-sparing surgeries. Preoperative and pathological data were compared between the two groups. The glomerular filtration rate was estimated using the abbreviated Modification of Diet and Renal Disease (MDRD4) study equation. The evolution of renal function was analysed from 6 months to 4 years after surgery, and the oncological outcomes were evaluated by means of cancer and non-cancer survival curves.

Results.—The results showed a major impairment in renal function in the RN group compared to those who underwent NSS (25 vs 7 ml/min/1.73 m^2, 6 months after surgery), a difference that was maintained over time. Moreover, patients undergoing RN had a greater chance of developing renal failure. Overall, the survival curves showed a higher mortality rate for the RN group ($p = 0.034$), although the cancer-specific mortality rate did not show any statistically significant differences ($p = 0.079$).

Conclusions.—For stage T1 renal cortical tumours, NSS should, whenever possible, be regarded as the primary therapeutic option, given that it obtains similar oncological outcomes to RN and preserves renal function, which seems to translate into a lower overall mortality rate.

▶ Nephron-sparing surgery has arguably become the ideal management strategy for localized renal cell carcinoma, demonstrating excellent oncologic outcomes on par with radical nephrectomy. Another potential advantage of partial nephrectomy is the preservation of the normal unaffected renal tissue, thereby maximizing the preservation of renal functional reserve. In this retrospective analysis, the authors evaluated nearly 300 patients who underwent extirpative therapy for T1 renal masses. They found that those patients undergoing radical nephrectomy demonstrated greater renal impairment and an increased risk of renal failure. Moreover, while cancer-specific survival remained equivalent between the 2 groups, overall mortality was higher in the radical nephrectomy group, indicating that the greater decrement in renal function might lead to a cascade of events that places patients at a greater risk of death from any cause. Although limited by its retrospective nature, this study nevertheless strengthens the argument in favor of performing nephron-sparing surgery whenever possible.

B. M. Benway, MD

6 Urothelial Cancer

Patient-specific risk of undetected malignant disease after investigation for haematuria, based on a 4-year follow-up

Edwards TJ, Dickinson AJ, Gosling J, et al (Derriford Hosp, Plymouth, UK; et al)

BJU Int 107:247-252, 2011

Objectives.—• To estimate the diagnostic accuracy of a guidelines-based haematuria clinic protocol by measuring the incidence of undetected malignancy during a follow-up period.

• To estimate an individual's post-test risk of having undetected malignancy using the protocol likelihood ratio and the population prevalence of disease.

Methods.—• Data were collected prospectively on a cohort of 4020 consecutive patients who were referred to a 'one-stop' haematuria clinic between 1998 and 2003.

• All patients had a plain radiograph taken and underwent ultrasonography and flexible cystoscopy as a part of 'first-line' investigation.

• Intravenous urography was performed where indicated after abnormal first-line tests or in patients with persistent haematuria where no abnormality had been detected.

• Records of the initial 687 participants from the first year of the study were reviewed 4 years after the original consultation. Missed diagnoses of urinary tract malignancy were recorded and sensitivities, likelihood ratios and the post-test probability of missing all disease and upper tract malignancy were calculated.

Results.—• As previously reported, the overall prevalence of malignant disease was 12.1% (18.9% for macroscopic haematuria compared with 4.8% for microscopic haematuria).

• The records of the first year's cohort of patients ($N = 687$) were analysed 4 years after their original consultation and 10 potentially 'missed' tumours were identified.

• The sensitivity of the protocol was 90.9% for the detection of all urinary tract malignancy (95% CI, 82.4 to 95.5) and 71% for upper tract tumours alone (95% CI, 45.4–88.3). The latter improves to 78.6% (95% CI, 52.4–92.4) with the addition of further upper tract testing.

• The probability of missing malignant disease overall was 1.7% (95% CI, 0.95–3.04) but this rose sharply to >4% for males over 60 with macroscopic haematuria.

- For those with non-visible haematuria, the percentage probability of missed malignant disease was less than 1%.

Conclusions.—• The haematuria clinic protocol described is robust but it is not infallible.

- The risk of missing malignant disease in the higher risk groups identified in the study is much greater than previous studies would suggest.

- If additional upper tract testing or interval follow-up were to be recommended, it could be rationally targeted at these groups, given the measurable risk shown here.

▶ The study attempts to identify the true incidence of malignancy in a population with either microscopic or macroscopic hematuria. The authors followed up a population with a previous investigation that excluded malignancy with a goal to ascertain the chance of missing cancer. The probability of missing disease is determined by the prevalence of disease. It is a little bit surprising that urinary cytology was not a component of the original evaluation. Unfortunately, follow-up consisted of a medical record and a radiology review 4 years after the initial evaluation. The cited incidence of malignancy at follow-up may be higher than identified in the study. Ideally, all the patients would have had a final complete radiologic and endoscopic evaluation. In the absence of clinical indications, this is not feasible. It is also possible that the cancers were not missed but that the patients developed a cancer during the 4-year follow-up interval. This study does not help answer the question of timing of a follow-up evaluation of patients with hematuria. Persistent gross hematuria requires further evaluation, while microscopic hematuria with a negative urine cytology result may need less vigilant follow-up.

D. E. Coplen, MD

Contemporary Use of Perioperative Cisplatin-Based Chemotherapy in Patients With Muscle-Invasive Bladder Cancer

Raj GV, Karavadia S, Schlomer B, et al (Univ of Texas Southwestern Med Ctr at Dallas)
Cancer 117:276-282, 2011

Background.—Level I evidence indicates that neoadjuvant cisplatin-based chemotherapy, in combination with radical cystectomy (RC), is associated with a significant survival advantage for patients with muscle-invasive bladder cancer. Despite this, neoadjuvant chemotherapy is not uniformly used. Our objective was to determine the patterns of utilization of neoadjuvant chemotherapy in patients undergoing RC for muscle invasive bladder cancer in a contemporary cohort in a tertiary care center.

Methods.—A retrospective review was performed of patients with bladder cancer who underwent RC between 2003 and 2008 at our institution. Clinical stage, pathologic stage, renal function, and perioperative chemotherapy treatments were tabulated. Primary outcome measures were the type and use of neoadjuvant chemotherapy among eligible patients.

Secondary measures were the utilization patterns of adjuvant chemotherapy, renal function, pathologic outcomes, and disease specific and overall survival. Reasons for nonutilization of chemotherapy were also examined.

Results.—Among 238 patients who underwent RC for bladder cancer, 145 had a preoperative clinical stage ≥T2. Only 17% (25 of 145) of these patients received cisplatin-based neoadjuvant chemotherapy. The renal function was adequate (CrCl >60 ml/min) in 97 (67%) of these patients. Patients who received neoadjuvant chemotherapy had higher p0 rates (29% vs 8%) than patients who did not receive neoadjuvant therapy. Advanced patient age, comorbidities, concerns over toxicity of chemotherapy, and the modest nature of benefit from neoadjuvant chemotherapy may explain why this treatment is not often used.

Conclusions.—Despite level I evidence, neoadjuvant cisplatin-based chemotherapies continue to be underutilized in the management of bladder cancer, even at a high-volume tertiary center. A prospective evaluation of management choices, including the patient and physician factors involved in the use of perioperative cisplatin-based chemotherapy in bladder cancer, is indicated.

▶ This is a single-institution assessment of their utilization of neoadjuvant chemotherapy. The striking fact is that only 17% of their patients received neoadjuvant-based chemotherapy. They were unable to assess in most patients why the patient did not receive neoadjuvant chemotherapy; however, in those they were able to assess, it appeared to be primarily because of comorbidity and with less common reasons being patient preference, toxicity of the chemotherapy, and active bleeding necessitating a more urgent procedure.

Obviously, I think it goes without saying that neoadjuvant chemotherapy should be used in more patients with bladder cancer than are currently using it. I think it is quite striking that in this academic center, which is clearly in favor of neoadjuvant chemotherapy, only a substantial minority of their patients received this treatment. My primary curiosity is whether in the future the utilization will increase because the group is more aware that they are not using it, or if toxicity in patient selection would remain a permanent barrier to its widespread utilization.

A. S. Kibel, MD

Detection and Clinical Outcome of Urinary Bladder Cancer With 5-Aminolevulinic Acid-Induced Fluorescence Cystoscopy: A Multicenter Randomized, Double-Blind, Placebo-Controlled Trial
Stenzl A, Penkoff H, Dajc-Sommerer E, et al (Med Ctr of Eberhard Karls Univ, Tübingen, Germany; Private Clinic Graz-Ragnitz, Graz, Austria; Regional Clinic St Poelten, Austria; et al)
Cancer 117:938-947, 2011

Background.—The medical community lacks results from prospective controlled multicenter studies of the diagnostic efficacy of 5-aminolevulinic acid (5-ALA) cystoscopy on tumor recurrence in patients with superficial bladder tumors.

Methods.—A prospective randomized, double-blind, placebo-controlled study was conducted in 370 patients with nonmuscle-invasive urinary bladder carcinoma who received either 5-ALA (n = 187) or a placebo (n = 183) intravesically before cystoscopy. Each group underwent cystoscopy under visible white light and under fluorescent light followed by transurethral tumor resection. The primary study objective was to evaluate the 12-month recurrence-free survival.

Results.—Slightly more patients with tumors were detected by using 5-ALA than by using the placebo (88.5% vs 84.7%). The mean numbers of tumor specimens per patient were 1.8 (5-ALA) and 1.6 (placebo). Intra-patient comparison of fluorescent light versus white light cystoscopy in patients randomized to receive 5-ALA showed a higher tumor detection rate with fluorescent light than with white light cystoscopy. In patients receiving 5-ALA cystoscopy, the percentage of lesions that would not have been detected in these patients by white light cystoscopy ranged between 10.9% (pT1) and 55.9% (atypia). Progression-free survival was 89.4% (5-ALA) and 89.0% (placebo) ($P = .9101$), and recurrence-free survival 12 months after tumor resection was 64.0% (5-ALA) and 72.8% (placebo) ($P = .2216$).

Conclusions.—In comparison to the placebo, 5-ALA cystoscopy did not increase the rates of recurrence-free or progression-free survival 12 months after tumor resection. Although more tumors per patient were detected in the 5-ALA group, the higher detection rate did not translate into differences in long-term outcome.

▶ This randomized prospective double-blind placebo-controlled study of approximately 370 patients demonstrated that more tumors were detected using the 5-aminolevulinic acid (5-ALA) cystoscopy. This increased detection rate translated to a decrease in recurrence rate of approximately 8% did not achieve statistical significance ($P = .22$). The authors also looked to progression-free survival and found absolutely no benefit with a progression-free survival of approximately 11% on both groups ($P = .91$).

My 3 fundamental goals in treating patients with bladder cancer are the following: (1) decrease the number of times they need to go to the operating room, (2) hang onto their bladder as long as possible, and (3) improve their survival. This diagnostic treatment modality I think will clearly improve number 1. Because 80% of patients with bladder cancer have superficial disease, this has the potential to alter management of most patients with bladder cancer. I doubt whether it will ever have an impact on number 2 or number 3.

I believe that modifications in cystoscopy are inevitable. The only question is whether 5-ALA cystoscopy will be the primary modality or if other novel ways of evaluating the bladder for occult bladder cancer will eventually be found to outperform this particular modality.

A. S. Kibel, MD

7 Prostate Cancer

Screening

PCA3 Molecular Urine Test for Predicting Repeat Prostate Biopsy Outcome in Populations at Risk: Validation in the Placebo Arm of the Dutasteride REDUCE Trial

Aubin SMJ, Reid J, Sarno MJ, et al (Gen-Probe Incorporated, San Diego, CA; et al)

J Urol 184:1947-1952, 2010

Purpose.—We determined the performance of PCA3 alone and in the presence of other covariates as an indicator of contemporaneous and future prostate biopsy results in a population with previous negative biopsy and increased serum prostate specific antigen.

Materials and Methods.—Urine PCA3 scores were determined before year 2 and year 4 biopsies from patients in the placebo arm of the REDUCE trial, a prostate cancer risk reduction study evaluating men with moderately increased serum prostate specific antigen results and negative biopsy at baseline. PCA3, serum prostate specific antigen and percent free prostate specific antigen results were correlated with biopsy outcome via univariate logistic regression and ROC analyses. Multivariate logistic regression was also performed including these biomarkers together with prostate volume, age and family history.

Results.—PCA3 scores were measurable from 1,072 of 1,140 subjects (94% informative rate). PCA3 scores were associated with positive biopsy rate (p <0.0001) and correlated with biopsy Gleason score (p = 0.0017). PCA3 AUC of 0.693 was greater than serum prostate specific antigen (0.612, p = 0.0077 vs PCA3). The multivariate logistic regression model yielded an AUC of 0.753 and exclusion of PCA3 from the model decreased AUC to 0.717 (p = 0.0009). PCA3 at year 2 was a significant predictor of year 4 biopsy outcome (AUC 0.634, p = 0.0002), whereas serum prostate specific antigen and free prostate specific antigen were not predictive (p = 0.3281 and 0.6782, respectively).

Conclusions.—PCA3 clinical performance was validated in the largest repeat biopsy study to date. Increased PCA3 scores indicated increased risk of contemporaneous cancers and predicted future biopsy outcomes.

Use of PCA3 in combination with serum prostate specific antigen and other risk factors significantly increased diagnostic accuracy.

▶ This prostate cancer gene 3 (PCA3) is the latest marker attempting to complement prostate-specific antigen (PSA) in screening. The group of patients that has the potential highest utility at the current time is men who have had a previous negative biopsy and are deciding whether to have a repeat biopsy for an elevated PSA. This is exactly the patient population that was studied in the Reduction by Dutasteride of Prostate Cancer Events (REDUCE) trial. While REDUCE was focused on prostate cancer prevention, the investigators were savvy enough to include prospective analysis of markers: In this case, PCA3. Importantly, all the patients underwent a biopsy, so there is little to no ascertainment bias. The most important finding is that the area under the curve was improved with PCA3. This was true as both a continuous variable and using a cut point of 35. This clearly outperformed not only serum PSA but also percent free PSA.

Does this mean that we should be ordering a PCA3 test on ALL of our patients? I think the answer is still out on that. I would say, however, that data like this encourage me that it could be of significant utility in a patient population that is having difficulty deciding whether or not to proceed with a second biopsy. If the PCA3 is elevated, then there is a strong indication that they have an increased risk of prostate cancer and likely should undergo a biopsy. If the PCA3 is low, then possibly a biopsy could be avoided. It is important to recognize that a negative PCA3 does not indicate there is no possibility of having prostate cancer. It also is important to recognize that an elevated PCA3 does not guarantee there is a diagnosis of prostate cancer. This is a better test than PSA in this patient population but is not perfect.

A. S. Kibel, MD

Comorbidity and Mortality Results From a Randomized Prostate Cancer Screening Trial
Crawford ED, Grubb R III, Black A, et al (Univ of Colorado Health Sciences Ctr, Denver; Washington Univ School of Medicine, St Louis, MO; Natl Cancer Inst, Rockville, MD; et al)
J Clin Oncol 29:355-361, 2011

Purpose.—Estimates of prostate cancer–specific mortality (PCSM) were similar for men randomly assigned to intervention compared with usual care on the Prostate, Lung, Colorectal and Ovarian PC screening study. However, results analyzed by comorbidity strata remain unknown.

Patients and Methods.—Between 1993 and 2001, of 76,693 men who were randomly assigned to usual care or intervention at 10 US centers, 73,378 (96%) completed a questionnaire that inquired about comorbidity and prostate-specific antigen (PSA) testing before random assignment. Fine and Gray's multivariable analysis was performed to assess whether the randomized screening arm was associated with the risk of PCSM in men with no or minimal versus at least one significant comorbidity, adjusting for age and prerandomization PSA testing.

Results.—After 10 years of follow-up, 9,565 deaths occurred, 164 from PC. A significant decrease in the risk of PCSM (22 v 38 deaths; adjusted hazard ratio [AHR], 0.56; 95% CI, 0.33 to 0.95; $P = .03$) was observed in men with no or minimal comorbidity randomly assigned to intervention versus usual care, and the additional number needed to treat to prevent one PC death at 10 years was five. Among men with at least one significant comorbidity, those randomly assigned to intervention versus usual care did not have a decreased risk of PCSM (62 v 42 deaths; AHR, 1.43; 95% CI, 0.96 to 2.11; $P = .08$).

Conclusion.—Selective use of PSA screening for men in good health appears to reduce the risk of PCSM with minimal overtreatment.

▶ The initial publication from the Prostate, Lung, Colorectal and Ovarian (PLCO) screening trial failed to demonstrate an improvement in overall survival or prostate cancer–specific mortality for prostate-specific antigen–based screening. One of the issues raised in all negative trials is if there is a subset of men who actually benefited. Clearly, men who are likely to die of other causes are less likely to benefit from screening than healthy men. This study assesses that critical question. The authors analyzed PLCO patients who had no to minimal comorbidity and demonstrated that screening was associated with an almost 50% reduction in the risk of prostate cancer death (adjusted hazard ratio of 0.56 [95% confidence interval, 0.32-0.95; $P = .03$]).

While not specifically examined in this article, it appears reasonable to guess that patients with significant comorbid disease probably did not benefit from any sort of screening in the PLCO. Patients need to have at least a 10-year life expectancy to benefit from any sort of treatment, and therefore screening for a disease that doesn't need to be cured is unlikely to improve life expectancy. On the other hand, men with long life expectancy are much more likely to benefit from screening and treatment. It is important to point out that the vast majority of the patients in this study died of other causes. In the screened population, almost 10 000 deaths occurred. Yet, it was only approximately 50 that were from prostate cancer. While this may be because of successful treatment of the disease, it is important to recognize that most patients with prostate cancer are going to die of other causes. Reserve screening for the healthy!

A. S. Kibel, MD

An Empirical Evaluation of Guidelines on Prostate-specific Antigen Velocity in Prostate Cancer Detection
Vickers AJ, Till C, Tangen CM, et al (Memorial Sloan-Kettering Cancer Ctr, NY; Fred Hutchinson Cancer Res Ctr, Seattle, WA; et al)
J Natl Cancer Inst 103:1-8, 2011

Background.—The National Comprehensive Cancer Network arid American Urological Association guidelines on early detection of prostate cancer recommend biopsy on the basis of high prostate-specific antigen (PSA) velocity, even in the absence of other indications such as an elevated PSA or a positive digital rectal exam (DRE).

Methods.—To evaluate the current guideline, we compared the area under the curve of a multivariable model for prostate cancer including age, PSA, DRE, family history, and prior biopsy, with and without PSA velocity, in 5519 men undergoing biopsy, regardless of clinical indication, in the control arm of the Prostate Cancer Prevention Trial. We also evaluated the clinical implications of using PSA velocity cut points to determine biopsy in men with low PSA and negative DRE in terms of additional cancers found and unnecessary biopsies conducted. All statistical tests were two-sided.

Results.—Incorporation of PSA velocity led to a very small increase in area under the curve from 0.702 to 0.709. Improvements in predictive accuracy were smaller for the endpoints of high-grade cancer (Gleason score of 7 or greater) and clinically significant cancer (Epstein criteria). Biopsying men with high PSA velocity but no other indication would lead to a large number of additional biopsies, with close to one in seven men being biopsied. PSA cut points with a comparable specificity to PSA velocity cut points had a higher sensitivity (23% vs 19%), particularly for high-grade (41% vs 25%) and clinically significant (32% vs 22%) disease. These findings were robust to the method of calculating PSA velocity.

Conclusions.—We found no evidence to support the recommendation that men with high PSA velocity should be biopsied in the absence of other indications; this measure should not be included in practice guidelines.

▶ The Prostate Cancer Prevention Trial (PCPT) continues to provide a wealth of information for evaluating our diagnostic and treatment paradigms for prostate cancer patients. This rather nice study from Dr Vickers and colleagues asked the very pertinent question—should prostate-specific antigen (PSA) velocity be included in guidelines for the diagnosis and treatment of prostate carcinoma? Their conclusion is no. They did not find evidence to support including PSA velocity. This is an important question that they evaluated in a well-characterized study using sound methodology. However, I disagree with their fundamental conclusions.

The reason that PSA velocity is included in many guidelines (including the National Comprehensive Cancer Network Guidelines) is that it is a marker of prostate cancer lethality. The idea, therefore, is that prostate cancers that are going to potentially lead to death can be detected earlier when they are still treatable by tracking changes in PSA. The velocities incorporated into nomograms have usually been identified from cohorts of cancer patients that were not detected by screening and frequently were not treated. Because screening and treatment presumably alter the natural history of the disease, a treated screened cohort is not as useful to assess PSA velocity. The PCPT cohort is fundamentally different. These are patients who not only were not screen-detected cancers; they were cancers that were detected by biopsies irrespective of the patients' PSA. Therefore, you could describe them accurately as a superscreened cohort. This does not reflect a current screening paradigm and, therefore, has limited applicability to determining whether screening guidelines are actually useful or not. In addition, many of the patients were treated, which hopefully fundamentally alters the natural history of the disease. Lastly and most importantly, the patients have not been followed long enough to determine whether or not a mortality has occurred.

This does not mean I think a critical evaluation of what is included in screening guidelines should be continued. On the contrary, I think articles like this provide additional information, which will slowly modify the guidelines as new knowledge comes forth.

A. S. Kibel, MD

Prediction of Significant Prostate Cancer Diagnosed 20 to 30 Years Later With a Single Measure of Prostate-Specific Antigen at or Before Age 50
Lilja H, Cronin AM, Dahlin A, et al (Memorial Sloan-Kettering Cancer Ctr, NY; Lund Univ, Malmö, Sweden)
Cancer 117:1210-1219, 2011

Background.—We previously reported that a single prostate-specific antigen (PSA) measured at ages 44-50 was highly predictive of subsequent prostate cancer diagnosis in an unscreened population. Here we report an additional 7 years of follow-up. This provides replication using an independent data set and allows estimates of the association between early PSA and subsequent advanced cancer (clinical stage $\geq$T3 or metastases at diagnosis).

Methods.—Blood was collected from 21,277 men in a Swedish city (74% participation rate) during 1974-1986 at ages 33-50. Through 2006, prostate cancer was diagnosed in 1408 participants; we measured PSA in archived plasma for 1312 of these cases (93%) and for 3728 controls.

Results.—At a median follow-up of 23 years, baseline PSA was strongly associated with subsequent prostate cancer (area under the curve, 0.72; 95% CI, 0.70-0.74; for advanced cancer, 0.75; 95% CI, 0.72-0.78). Associations between PSA and prostate cancer were virtually identical for the initial and replication data sets, with 81% of advanced cases (95% CI, 77%-86%) found in men with PSA above the median (0.63 ng/mL at ages 44-50).

Conclusions.—A single PSA at or before age 50 predicts advanced prostate cancer diagnosed up to 30 years later. Use of early PSA to stratify risk would allow a large group of low-risk men to be screened less often but increase frequency of testing on a more limited number of high-risk men. This is likely to improve the ratio of benefit to harm for screening.

▶ The prostate-specific antigen (PSA) gets a notoriously bad rap for identification of prostate cancer. I think that is in large part because multiple other factors, from prostate size to infection, elevated PSA. This fact coupled with the fact that most patients have histologic prostate cancer means that PSA leads to an accidental positive biopsy in many men. However, it is important to recognize that PSA is associated with prostate cancer risk and that it can assist us in early detection of the disease. It may be that our problem with PSA is not so much on PSA as a test but as to who and how we are using it as a screening test. The current National Comprehensive Cancer Network Guidelines actually indicate that screening tests should be obtained early, and a slight elevation in PSA identifies patients who are at increased risk for developing lethal or aggressive prostate cancer later in life and, therefore, would benefit from more aggressive screening. This study by Lilja et al reinforces the utility of that approach. Relatively small elevations in PSA in a younger population (aged between 44 and 50 years) were associated with not just risk of prostate cancer but risk of lethal prostate cancer approximately 30 years later. The assay appeared to work best when focusing on men who had PSAs of either greater than the median (greater than or equal to 0.63 ng/mL) or in the top quartile (greater than 0.95 ng/mL).

Maybe we should be using PSA more like colonoscopy. We would get an initial test at a relatively young age, and if it was at all elevated, those patients we would screen more aggressively over the subsequent decades. In contrast, patients with absolutely no elevation in their PSA in most cases could safely be spared screening for prostate cancer.

A. S. Kibel, MD

Randomised prostate cancer screening trial: 20 year follow-up
Sandblom G, Varenhorst E, Rosell J, et al (Karolinska Inst, Stockholm, Sweden; Linköping Univ Hosp, Sweden; et al)
BMJ 342:d1539, 2011

Objective.—To assess whether screening for prostate cancer reduces prostate cancer specific mortality.

Design.—Population based randomised controlled trial.

Setting.—Department of Urology, Norrköping, and the South-East Region Prostate Cancer Register.

Participants.—All men aged 50-69 in the city of Norrköping, Sweden, identified in 1987 in the National Population Register (n=9026).

Intervention.—From the study population, 1494 men were randomly allocated to be screened by including every sixth man from a list of dates of birth. These men were invited to be screened every third year from 1987 to 1996. On the first two occasions screening was done by digital rectal examination only. From 1993, this was combined with prostate specific antigen testing, with 4 μg/L as cut off. On the fourth occasion (1996), only men aged 69 or under at the time of the investigation were invited.

Main Outcome Measures.—Data on tumour stage, grade, and treatment from the South East Region Prostate Cancer Register. Prostate cancer specific mortality up to 31 December 2008.

Results.—In the four screenings from 1987 to 1996 attendance was 1161/1492 (78%), 957/1363 (70%), 895/1210 (74%), and 446/606 (74%), respectively. There were 85 cases (5.7%) of prostate cancer diagnosed in the screened group and 292 (3.9%) in the control group. The risk ratio for death from prostate cancer in the screening group was 1.16 (95% confidence interval 0.78 to 1.73). In a Cox proportional hazard analysis comparing prostate cancer specific survival in the control group with that in the screened group, the hazard ratio for death from prostate cancer was 1.23 (0.94 to 1.62; P=0.13). After adjustment for age at start of the study, the hazard ratio was 1.58 (1.06 to 2.36; P=0.024).

Conclusion.—After 20 years of follow-up the rate of death from prostate cancer did not differ significantly between men in the screening group and those in the control group.

Trial Registration.—Current Controlled Trials, ISRCTN06342431.

▶ About 20 years ago, multiple groups around the world had the courage and forethought to embark on long-term projects to determine if prostate-specific antigen (PSA)—based screening saved lives. This is a randomized trial of approximately 9000 patients, roughly 1 in 6 randomized to receive screening for prostate cancer. The strength of this trial is the long follow-up, almost 20 years, with excellent compliance. The primary end point was prostate cancer—specific survival. The authors found no benefit with a *P* value of .065. However, when they did a multivariate analysis adjusting for age at the time of enrollment, they found that the *P* value actually became statistically significant with a hazard ratio of 1.58 (*P* = .024).

While this study was not powered to examine overall survival, they did examine this end point and found no improvement (*P* = .14).

Like most large studies, the devil is in the details, and I do not believe that this study has any relevance for our current screening and treatment paradigm in the United States. The first thing that needs to be recognized is that these patients were screened initially from 1987 to 1996, and only in the last 2 screening rounds was PSA included. So, at least initially the patients were being screened by digital rectal examination alone. This clearly has implications as to whether this is applicable in 2011 when PSA screening is so widespread.

The second thing is that while overall survival was not statistically significant, if you look at Fig 1 in the original article, you can see that the curves did separate and then come back together. What this indicates is simply that over a 20-year period, if you are looking at an elderly population, you are going to find that the majority of these patients die. Is this relevant for prostate cancer screening and treatment? Absolutely yes. It is the reason why we should not be screening and treating elderly patients. However, for a younger population, this has less of an impact.

Third of all, if you look at the treatment these patients received, the vast majority did not receive treatment with curative intent. In the nonscreened arm, 50% were treated with hormone therapy and roughly 30% were treated with watchful waiting. In the screening cohort, roughly 43% were treated with watchful waiting and 31% were treated with hormone therapy. So, it appears that only between 15% and 20% of the patients in each arm were actually treated with curative intent. Whether you are a fan of screening or not, I think it is apparent that if you screen patients for cancer and then you do not attempt to cure them of the disease, it is unlikely that the screening will reduce mortality.

I believe this study will add more fuel to the fire for people who are against screening for prostate cancer; however, I think it bears absolutely no relevance to our current diagnosis and treatment paradigm in 2011.

A. S. Kibel, MD

Mortality results from the Göteborg randomised population-based prostate-cancer screening trial
Hugosson J, Carlsson S, Aus G, et al (Sahlgrenska Academy at Univ of Göteborg, Sweden; et al)
Lancet Oncol 11:725-732, 2010

Background.—Prostate cancer is one of the leading causes of death from malignant disease among men in the developed world. One strategy to decrease the risk of death from this disease is screening with prostate-specific antigen (PSA); however, the extent of benefit and harm with such screening is under continuous debate.

Methods.—In December, 1994, 20 000 men born between 1930 and 1944, randomly sampled from the population register, were randomised by computer in a 1:1 ratio to either a screening group invited for PSA testing every 2 years (n=10 000) or to a control group not invited (n=10 000). Men in the screening group were invited up to the upper age limit (median 69, range 67−71 years) and only men with raised PSA concentrations were offered additional tests such as digital rectal examination and prostate biopsies. The primary endpoint was prostate-cancer specific mortality, analysed according to the intention-to-screen principle. The study is ongoing, with men who have not reached the upper age limit invited for PSA testing. This is the first planned report on cumulative prostate-cancer incidence and mortality calculated up to Dec 31, 2008. This study is registered as an International Standard Randomised Controlled Trial ISRCTN54449243.

Findings.—In each group, 48 men were excluded from the analysis because of death or emigration before the randomisation date, or prevalent prostate cancer. In men randomised to screening, 7578 (76%) of 9952 attended at least once. During a median follow-up of 14 years, 1138 men in the screening group and 718 in the control group were diagnosed with prostate cancer, resulting in a cumulative prostate-cancer incidence of 12·7% in the screening group and 8·2% in the control group (hazard ratio 1·64; 95% CI 1·50−1·80; p<0·0001). The absolute cumulative risk reduction of death from prostate cancer at 14 years was 0·40% (95% CI 0·17−0·64), from 0·90% in the control group to 0·50% in the screening group. The rate ratio for death from prostate cancer was 0·56

(95% CI 0·39—0·82; p=0·002) in the screening compared with the control group. The rate ratio of death from prostate cancer for attendees compared with the control group was 0·44 (95% CI 0·28—0·68; p=0·0002). Overall, 293 (95% CI 177—799) men needed to be invited for screening and 12 to be diagnosed to prevent one prostate cancer death.

Interpretation.—This study shows that prostate cancer mortality was reduced almost by half over 14 years. However, the risk of over-diagnosis is substantial and the number needed to treat is at least as high as in breast-cancer screening programmes. The benefit of prostate-cancer screening compares favourably to other cancer screening programs.

▶ Two randomized trials recently published in the *New England Journal of Medicine*,[1,2] continue to create controversy as to whether or not screening for prostate cancer saves lives. The Prostate, Lung, Colorectal, and Ovarian Cancer trial demonstrated no survival advantage, whereas the European Randomized Study of Screening for Prostate Cancer (ERSPC) demonstrated survival advantage. However, in the ERSPC trial, a rather large number of patients needed to be screened, roughly 1500, to identify and treat 48 cancers and, therefore, to save 1 life. Concerns were raised that even if prostate-specific antigen (PSA) screening did save lives, the overtreatment would be significant. This is a third trial that has been followed for slightly longer (14 years) and demonstrates a benefit, which is more reasonable. They demonstrated that 293 patients would need to be screened to diagnose and treat 12 cancers and, therefore, to save 1 life. This is much more in keeping with a screening program, which is efficacious and reasonable in a large population. Studies like this with longer follow-up are going to demonstrate that PSA screening does actually save lives.

Is this study going to put PSA screening to rest? Absolutely not. This will continue to be controversial. Clearly, we are overdiagnosing patients with prostate cancer, and many of these patients are being overtreated and therefore not benefitting from the initial diagnosis. They unfortunately suffer the morbidity associated with these treatments without any benefit. The question will always remain: how many cancers are we treating unnecessarily to save a life? I am not sure exactly where to draw the line, but I know that 12 is much better than 48.

A. S. Kibel, MD

References

1. Andriole GL, Crawford ED, Grubb RL 3rd, et al. Mortality results from a randomized prostate-cancer screening trial. *N Engl J Med.* 2009;360:1310-1319.
2. Schröder FH, Hugosson J, Roobol MJ, et al. Screening and prostate-cancer mortality in a randomized European study. *N Engl J Med.* 2009;360:1320-1328.

Risk

Effects of Prostate-Specific Antigen Testing on Familial Prostate Cancer Risk Estimates

Bratt O, Garmo H, Adolfsson J, et al (Lund Univ, Helsingborg, Sweden; Regional Oncological Centre, Uppsala, Sweden; Karolinska Inst, Stockholm, Sweden; et al)

J Natl Cancer Inst 102:1336-1343, 2010

Background.—Family history is a strong risk factor for prostate cancer. The aim of this study was to investigate whether increased diagnostic activity is related to the incidence of prostate cancer among brothers of men with prostate cancer.

Methods.—Data were from the nationwide population-based Prostate Cancer Database Sweden (PCBaSe Sweden), which includes data from the National Prostate Cancer Register, the Swedish Cancer Register, the Register of the Total Population, the Multi-Generation Register, and the Census database. We investigated the relationship of tumor characteristics, time from diagnosis of the index patient (ie, prostate cancer patients in the National Prostate Cancer Register for whom at least one brother and their father could be identified), calendar period, geographic factors, and socio-economic status to standardized incidence ratios (SIRs) for prostate cancer among 22 511 brothers of 13 975 index patients in PCBaSe Sweden.

Results.—Brothers of index patients with prostate cancer were at increased risk for a diagnosis of prostate cancer (SIR = 3.1, 95% confidence interval [CI] = 2.9 to 3.3). Risk was higher for T1c tumors (SIR = 3.4, 95% CI = 3.2 to 3.8) than for metastatic tumors (SIR = 2.0, 95% CI = 1.5 to 2.6), and risk of T1c tumors was especially high during the first year after the diagnosis of the index patient (SIR = 4.3, 95% CI = 3.8 to 4.9), compared with the following years (SIR range = 2.8–3.3), and for brothers of index patients who had a higher socioeconomic status (SIR = 4.2, 95% CI = 3.7 to 4.7), compared with brothers of index patients with lower socioeconomic status (SIR = 2.8, 95% CI = 2.4 to 3.2).

Conclusions.—Increased diagnostic activity among men with a family history of prostate cancer appears to contribute to their increased risk of prostate cancer and to lead to detection bias in epidemiological and genetic studies of familial prostate cancer.

▶ Patients who have a family history of prostate cancer are at substantially higher risk of developing the disease. Is this because of a genetic predisposition or simply that family members of cancer patients are more likely to be screened and treated? This study examined the nationwide population-based Prostate Cancer Database Sweden, which included multiple different registries, to determine the risk of disease in the population at large. They found an increased risk of brothers being diagnosed with prostate cancer, with an increased risk of approximately 3 times that of the general population. It was quite striking that there was a substantially higher risk of being diagnosed with T1c prostate cancer in the year following a relative's diagnosis, and this seemed to be particularly related to higher socioeconomic status. What this tells me is that men who are reasonably well off are much more likely to go and be screened and, therefore, be diagnosed with prostate cancer if they have a brother who has recently been diagnosed with the disease. I'm not dismissing the genetic predisposition, but this indicates that some of the association may simply be because of ascertainment bias. The authors also found an increased risk of metastatic tumors in patients with a brother diagnosed with the disease. Because metastatic disease is clearly unambiguously clinically significant prostate cancer, this would indicate that hidden in the ascertainment bias is a real and substantial genetic predisposition to aggressive prostate cancer in first-degree relatives. I think both of these epidemiologic facts need to be kept in mind when evaluating the siblings and family members of patients with prostate cancer. Clearly, a family predisposition to prostate cancer may simply be the fact that the disease has been aggressively sought within a family in which the disease has recently been diagnosed. With that said, a family member who has a family history of prostate cancer, particularly lethal prostate cancer, needs to be taken quite seriously and should be aggressively screened for the disease.

A. S. Kibel, MD

Coffee Consumption and Prostate Cancer Risk and Progression in the Health Professionals Follow-up Study
Wilson KM, Kasperzyk JL, Rider JR, et al (Harvard School of Public Health, Boston, MA; Brigham and Women's Hosp, Boston, MA)
J Natl Cancer Inst 103:1-9, 2011

Background.—Coffee contains many biologically active compounds, including caffeine and phenolic acids, that have potent antioxidant activity and can affect glucose metabolism and sex hormone levels. Because of these biological activities, coffee may be associated with a reduced risk of prostate cancer.

Methods.—We conducted a prospective analysis of 47 911 men in the Health Professionals Follow-up Study who reported intake of regular and decaffeinated coffee in 1986 and every 4 years thereafter. From 1986 to 2006, 5035 patients with prostate cancer were identified, including 642 patients with lethal prostate cancers, defined as fatal or metastatic. We used Cox proportional hazards models to assess the association between coffee and prostate cancer, adjusting for potential confounding by smoking, obesity, and other variables. All *P* values were from two-sided tests.

Results.—The average intake of coffee in 1986 was 1.9 cups per day. Men who consumed six or more cups per day had a lower adjusted relative risk for overall prostate cancer compared with nondrinkers (RR = 0.82, 95% confidence interval [CI] = 0.68 to 0.98, P_{trend} = .10). The association was stronger for lethal prostate cancer (consumers of more than six cups of coffee per day: RR = 0.40, 95% CI = 0.22 to 0.75, P_{trend} = .03). Coffee consumption was not associated with the risk of nonadvanced or low-grade cancers and was only weakly inversely associated with high-grade cancer. The inverse association with lethal cancer was similar for regular and decaffeinated coffee (each one cup per day increment: RR = 0.94, 95% CI = 0.88 to 1.01, P = .08 for regular coffee and RR = 0.91, 95% CI = 0.83 to 1.00, P = .05 for decaffeinated coffee). The age-adjusted incidence rates for men who had the highest (≥6 cups per day) and lowest (no coffee) coffee consumption were 425 and 519 total prostate cancers, respectively, per 100 000 person-years and 34 and 79 lethal prostate cancers, respectively, per 100 000 person-years.

Conclusions.—We observed a strong inverse association between coffee consumption and risk of lethal prostate cancer. The association appears to be related to non-caffeine components of coffee.

▶ The headlines read "Coffee Consumption Decreases Prostate Cancer Risk." This analysis of the Health Professionals Follow-up Study of almost 50 000 patients demonstrates that coffee consumption was associated with decreased risk of prostate cancer that approached statistical significance (P = .10) and a stronger association with a decreased risk of lethal prostate carcinoma that was statistically significant (P = .03). What is particularly striking in this article data is that the decreased risk really appeared to have a dose effect for multiple different parameters that would be associated with more aggressive prostate cancer. Lethal prostate cancer, defined as the subset of advanced prostate cancer who died of their disease, was associated with a decreased risk when you drank more coffee. Advanced prostate cancer, defined as the category of patients with stage T3b, T4, N1, or M1 prostate cancer at the time of diagnosis, with metastatic disease, or who died of prostate cancer, was associated with a decreased risk. Lastly, high-grade cancer was associated with a decreased risk. The benefit was not clear until they drank 6 or more cups per day. Interestingly, there did not appear to be a clear dose effect with nonadvanced prostate cancer and with low-grade prostate cancer. This would indicate that this appears to be protective for the type of cancer that we most want to prevent. Does this mean that patients should be encouraged to drink more than 6 cups of coffee a day? I would hesitate to go that far at this point in time. We have seen multiple epidemiologic studies that have shown very strong effects but when translated to the clinical environment have not actually had any impact on the disease. In addition, I am sure that drinking more than 6 cups of coffee a day will be associated with significant side effects, possibly clinically significant. With that said, I think these are intriguing data and a story that I think will continue to develop and evolve over time. If the nutrient in the coffee that decreases the risks could be identified, then this potentially could be a preventive measure in the future. However, we are not there yet.

A. S. Kibel, MD

Active Surveillance Compared With Initial Treatment for Men With Low-Risk Prostate Cancer: A Decision Analysis

Hayes JH, Ollendorf DA, Pearson SD, et al (Harvard Med School, Boston, MA; et al)
JAMA 304:2373-2380, 2010

Context.—In the United States, 192 000 men were diagnosed as having prostate cancer in 2009, the majority with low-risk, clinically localized disease. Treatment of these cancers is associated with substantial morbidity. Active surveillance is an alternative to initial treatment, but long-term outcomes and effect on quality of life have not been well characterized.

Objective.—To examine the quality-of-life benefits and risks of active surveillance compared with initial treatment for men with low-risk, clinically localized prostate cancer.

Design and Setting.—Decision analysis using a simulation model was performed: men were treated at diagnosis with brachytherapy, intensity-modulated radiation therapy (IMRT), or radical prostatectomy or followed up by active surveillance (a strategy of close monitoring of newly diagnosed patients with serial prostate-specific antigen measurements, digital rectal examinations, and biopsies, with treatment at disease progression or patient choice). Probabilities and utilities were derived from previous studies and literature review. In the base case, the relative risk of prostate cancer—specific death for initial treatment vs active surveillance was assumed to be 0.83. Men incurred short- and long-term adverse effects of treatment.

Patients.—Hypothetical cohorts of 65-year-old men newly diagnosed as having clinically localized, low-risk prostate cancer (prostate-specific antigen level <10 ng/mL, stage ≤T2a disease, and Gleason score <6).

Main Outcome Measure.—Quality-adjusted life expectancy (QALE).

Results.—Active surveillance was associated with the greatest QALE (11.07 quality-adjusted life-years [QALYs]), followed by brachytherapy (10.57 QALYs), IMRT (10.51 QALYs), and radical prostatectomy (10.23 QALYs). Active surveillance remained associated with the highest QALE even if the relative risk of prostate cancer—specific death for initial treatment vs active surveillance was as low as 0.6. However, the QALE gains and the optimal strategy were highly dependent on individual preferences for living under active surveillance and for having been treated.

Conclusions.—Under a wide range of assumptions, for a 65-year-old man, active surveillance is a reasonable approach to low-risk prostate cancer based on QALE compared with initial treatment. However, individual preferences play a central role in the decision whether to treat or to pursue active surveillance.

▶ The authors should be congratulated on performing a novel assessment of the trade-offs in the management of low-risk prostate cancer. We have all been faced with the difficult problem of counseling patients as to the best treatment for low-risk prostate cancer. Balancing the significant morbidity of treatment against the small but real risk of progression if the treatment is delayed is difficult. Clearly, the vast majority of low-risk prostate cancer patients aren't harmed by active surveillance. However, the uncertainty and anxiety stem from the less than ideal prediction of the rare events of progression and mortality while on active surveillance. There are several important strengths in this article. First is the authors' concerted effort to obtain model probabilities through a systematic review of the literature. However, some chosen inputs may unduly implicate adverse events with specific treatment. For example, the long-term probability of erectile dysfunction after nerve-sparing prostatectomy is 45.3% compared with 6.4% after radiation. This estimate is substantially higher than that reported in contemporary surgical series. A second strong point of this decision model is the ability to manipulate parameters and evaluate the response via sensitivity analysis. Not surprisingly, the values assigned to outcomes clearly influenced the model. Treatment is better than active surveillance if a patient perceived surveillance as burdensome or placed a high value on receiving curative treatment without complications. The most critical aspect of the analysis is that it does not demonstrate that active surveillance is better than treatment because the confidence intervals for each treatment option widely overlap. The intricacy of the model reflects and highlights the complexity of patient choice. The volume of information needed by the patient is massive, and the task of education is daunting. This article provided evidence that active surveillance is a reasonable option if an individual patient is willing to trade a certain amount of cure for a potentially higher quality of life.

A. S. Kibel, MD

Diagnostics

Prevalence and Significance of Fluoroquinolone Resistant Escherichia coli in Patients Undergoing Transrectal Ultrasound Guided Prostate Needle Biopsy

Liss MA, Chang A, Santos R, et al (Univ of California-Irvine; et al)
J Urol 185:1283-1288, 2011

Purpose.—We estimated the prevalence of fluoroquinolone resistant Escherichia coli in patients undergoing repeat transrectal ultrasound guided prostate needle biopsy and identified high risk groups.

Materials and Methods.—From January 2009 to March 2010 rectal swabs of 136 men from 3 institutions undergoing transrectal ultrasound guided prostate needle biopsy were obtained. There were 33 men with no previous biopsy who served as the controls. Participants completed questionnaires and rectal swab culture was obtained just before performing the prostate biopsy. Selective media was used to specifically isolate fluoroquinolone resistant E. coli and sensitivities were obtained. The patients were contacted via telephone 7 days after the procedure for a followup questionnaire.

Results.—A total of 30 patients had cultures positive for fluoroquinolone resistant bacteria for an overall rate of 22% (95% CI 15, 29). Patients with diabetes and Asian ethnicity had higher risks of resistant rectal flora

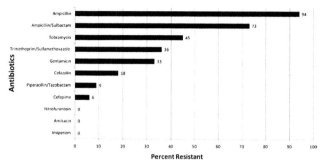

FIGURE.—Resistance pattern for fluoroquinolone resistant E. coli. (Reprinted from Liss MA, Chang A, Santos R, et al. Prevalence and significance of fluoroquinolone resistant Escherichia coli in patients undergoing transrectal ultrasound guided prostate needle biopsy. *J Urol.* 2011;185:1283-1288, Copyright 2011, with permission from American Urological Association.)

colonization (OR 2.3 and 2.8, respectively). However, differences did not reach statistical significance (p = 0.09 and p = 0.08, respectively). Patients with no prior biopsy had a positive rate of 15% (5 of 33) compared to 24% (25 of 103) in those with 1 or more prior biopsies (OR 1.8, p = 0.27). Five patients (3.6%) had post-biopsy fever while only 1 of those patients had a positive rectal swab.

Conclusions.—Using selective media to isolate fluoroquinolone resistant E. coli from the rectum before transrectal ultrasound guided prostate biopsy, we isolated organisms in 22% of patients with a wide resistance pattern. This protocol may be used to provide information regarding targeted antibiotic prophylaxis before transrectal prostate biopsies (Fig).

▶ Infection after transrectal prostatic biopsy is an increasingly frequent complication. With more patients on active surveillance, the number of biopsies will only increase. American Urological Association guidelines recommend antibiotic prophylaxis with quinolones. The authors estimate the rates of fluoroquinolone resistance in men undergoing prostate biopsy. A total of 5/125 (4%) evaluable patients had a postbiopsy fever. The vast majority of men with quinolone resistance did not develop fevers after biopsy. Is the quinolone efficacious in those situations, or are those men simply not at risk for developing an infection? Certainly based on randomized trials, prophylaxis is indicated. The pattern of antibiotic resistance in men with quinolone resistance is shown in the figure. Subset analysis did not reveal a group of men at higher risk for quinolone resistance. As can be seen, amikacin resistance was nonexistent in this study. A switch to aminoglycoside would be more time intensive and expensive. The additional cost would need to be balanced against a potential reduction in hospital admissions and the cost thereof. The incidence of infections needs to be monitored and will direct potential change in prophylaxis.

D. E. Coplen, MD

Immediate Risk of Suicide and Cardiovascular Death After a Prostate Cancer Diagnosis: Cohort Study in the United States

Fang F, Keating NL, Mucci LA, et al (Brigham and Women's Hosp, Boston, MA; Harvard Med School, Boston, MA; et al)

J Natl Cancer Inst 102:307-314, 2010

Background.—Receiving a cancer diagnosis is a stressful event that may increase risks of suicide and cardiovascular death, especially soon after diagnosis.

Methods.—We conducted a cohort study of 342 497 patients diagnosed with prostate cancer from January 1, 1979, through December 31, 2004, in the Surveillance, Epidemiology, and End Results Program. Follow-up started from the date of prostate cancer diagnosis to the end of first 12 calendar months after diagnosis. The relative risks of suicide and cardiovascular death were calculated as standardized mortality ratios (SMRs) comparing corresponding incidences among prostate cancer patients with those of the general US male population, with adjustment for age, calendar period, and state of residence. We compared risks in the first year and months after a prostate cancer diagnosis. The analyses were further stratified by calendar period at diagnosis, tumor characteristics, and other variables.

Results.—During follow-up, 148 men died of suicide (mortality rate = 0.5 per 1000 person-years) and 6845 died of cardiovascular diseases (mortality rate = 21.8 per 1000 person-years). Patients with prostate cancer were at increased risk of suicide during the first year (SMR = 1.4, 95% confidence interval [CI] = 1.2 to 1.6), especially during the first 3 months (SMR = 1.9, 95% CI = 1.4 to 2.6), after diagnosis. The elevated risk was apparent in pre–prostate-specific antigen (PSA) (1979–1986) and peri–PSA (1987–1992) eras but not since PSA testing has been widespread (1993–2004). The risk of cardiovascular death was slightly elevated during the first year (SMR = 1.09, 95% CI = 1.06 to 1.12), with the highest risk in the first month (SMR = 2.05, 95% CI = 1.89 to 2.22), after diagnosis. The first-month risk was statistically significantly elevated during the entire study period, and the risk was higher for patients with metastatic tumors (SMR = 3.22, 95% CI = 2.68 to 3.84) than for those with local or regional tumors (SMR = 1.57, 95% CI = 1.42 to 1.74).

Conclusion.—A diagnosis of prostate cancer may increase the immediate risks of suicide and cardiovascular death.

▶ This study examined 342 497 patients with newly diagnosed prostate cancer and identified 148 men who committed suicide and 6845 men who died of a cardiovascular event. While it is important to recognize that absolute risk of suicide and even cardiovascular deaths in patients with newly diagnosed prostate cancer is relatively low and that some of the deaths may be attributed simply to chance, this clearly raises concerns that some of the deaths were because of the stress of the recent diagnosis of prostate cancer. I think this is one of the clear unfortunate outcomes of our hypervigilance for prostate cancer in the United States. Many patients hear cancer with a capital C, imagining a short life expectancy with significant disease and treatment-associated morbidity. For this reason, I think it is critical that we do everything in our power to decrease the stress associated with the diagnosis. Reinforce to the patients that while this is a real disease and that in many cases aggressive treatment is warranted, prostate cancer is unlikely to cause them any harm in the short run and that they have plenty of time to decide how to manage the disease. Obviously, this needs to be balanced against the risks that patients will ignore the disease diagnosis, particularly those who are at high risk for progression and dying of the disease. However, this article demonstrates that undue anxiety clearly has the potential to cause great harm.

A. S. Kibel, MD

The genomic complexity of primary human prostate cancer
Berger MF, Lawrence MS, Demichelis F, et al (The Broad Inst of Harvard and MIT, Cambridge, MA; Weill Cornell Med College, NY; et al)
Nature 470:214-220, 2011

Prostate cancer is the second most common cause of male cancer deaths in the United States. However, the full range of prostate cancer genomic alterations is incompletely characterized. Here we present the complete sequence of seven primary human prostate cancers and their paired normal counterparts. Several tumours contained complex chains of balanced (that is, 'copyneutral') rearrangements that occurred within or adjacent to known cancer genes. Rearrangement breakpoints were enriched near open chromatin, androgen receptor and ERG DNA binding sites in the setting of the ETS gene fusion *TMPRSS2-ERG*, but inversely correlated with these regions in tumours lacking ETS fusions. This observation suggests a link between chromatin or transcriptional regulation and the genesis of genomic aberrations. Three tumours contained rearrangements that disrupted *CADM2*, and four harboured events disrupting either *PTEN* (unbalanced events), a prostate tumour suppressor, or *MAGI2* (balanced events), a PTEN interacting protein not previously implicated in prostate tumorigenesis. Thus, genomic rearrangements may arise from transcriptional or chromatin aberrancies and engage prostate tumorigenic mechanisms.

▶ This group from Harvard sequenced the entire genome from 7 prostate tumors. In doing so, they identified novel genetic rearrangements and mutations in prostate cancer. The details of which genes in what pathway are not as important, neither is the fact that it was done. We now have the capability to sequence every last base pair in tumors. As the cost comes down, this will be possible in every patient we treat. As a clinician, this should be both exciting and alarming. What are we going to do with all the information? This is going to rapidly progress from a novelty to routine clinical practice. Be prepared!

A. S. Kibel, MD

Natural History/Outcomes

Comparative Effectiveness of Prostate Cancer Treatments: Evaluating Statistical Adjustments for Confounding in Observational Data

Hadley J, Yabroff KR, Barrett MJ, et al (George Mason Univ, Fairfax, VA; Natl Cancer Inst, Bethesda, MD; Information Management Services, Inc, Rockville, MD; et al)

J Natl Cancer Inst 102:1780-1793, 2010

Background.—Using observational data to assess the relative effectiveness of alternative cancer treatments is limited by patient selection into treatment, which often biases interpretation of outcomes. We evaluated methods for addressing confounding in treatment and survival of patients with early-stage prostate cancer in observational data and compared findings with those from a benchmark randomized clinical trial.

Methods.—We selected 14302 early-stage prostate cancer patients who were aged 66–74 years and had been treated with radical prostatectomy or conservative management from linked Surveillance, Epidemiology, and End Results-Medicare data from January 1, 1995, through December 31, 2003. Eligibility criteria were similar to those from a clinical trial used to benchmark our analyses. Survival was measured through December 31, 2007, by use of Cox proportional hazards models. We compared results from the benchmark trial with results from models with observational data by use of traditional multivariable survival analysis, propensity score adjustment, and instrumental variable analysis.

Results.—Prostate cancer patients receiving conservative management were more likely to be older, nonwhite, and single and to have more advanced disease than patients receiving radical prostatectomy. In a multivariable survival analysis, conservative management was associated with greater risk of prostate cancer-specific mortality (hazard ratio [HR] = 1.59, 95% confidence interval [CI] = 1.27 to 2.00) and all-cause mortality (HR = 1.47, 95% CI = 1.35 to 1.59) than radical prostatectomy. Propensity score adjustments resulted in similar patient characteristics across treatment groups, although survival results were similar to traditional multivariable survival analyses. Results for the same comparison from the instrumental variable approach, which theoretically equalizes both observed and unobserved patient characteristics across treatment groups, differed from the traditional multivariable and propensity score results but were consistent with findings from the subset of elderly patient with early-stage disease in the trial (ie, conservative management vs radical prostatectomy: for prostate cancer-specific mortality, HR = 0.73, 95% CI = 0.08 to 6.73; for all-cause mortality, HR = 1.09, 95% CI = 0.46 to 2.59).

Conclusion.—Instrumental variable analysis may be a useful technique in comparative effectiveness studies of cancer treatments if an acceptable instrument can be identified.

▶ In evaluating any study, it is important to recognize that the type of statistical analysis used influences the results. This rather nice article analyzed Surveillance, Epidemiology, and End Results—Medicare data to determine if radical prostatectomy is better than watchful waiting. Depending on which analysis you believe, radical prostatectomy is either much better or no better than observation in a population of men older than 65 years. The authors do a fantastic job of outlining the different statistical methods and their strengths and weaknesses, but at the end of the day, we are left with the same question: How do you treat the patient in front of you? The randomized data have clearly demonstrated that the benefit in a population of patients for radical prostatectomy is low. This article reinforces that finding. However, there clearly are older patients who need aggressive treatment, because of either their potential longevity or a more aggressive phenotype. Future studies are needed to help us identify those patients. Until then, we will have to sort through the retrospective data with a critical eye on the analysis performed.

A. S. Kibel, MD

Radiation Therapy

Comparative Risk-Adjusted Mortality Outcomes After Primary Surgery, Radiotherapy, or Androgen-Deprivation Therapy for Localized Prostate Cancer

Cooperberg MR, for the Cancer of the Prostate Strategic Urologic Research Endeavor (CaPSURE) Investigators (Univ of California at San Francisco Helen Diller Family Comprehensive Cancer Ctr; et al)
Cancer 116:5226-5234, 2010

Background.—Because no adequate randomized trials have compared active treatment modalities for localized prostate cancer, the authors analyzed risk-adjusted, cancer-specific mortality outcomes among men who underwent radical prostatectomy, men who received external-beam radiation therapy, and men who received primary androgen-deprivation therapy.

Methods.—The Cancer of the Prostate Strategic Urologic Research Endeavor (CaPSURE) registry comprises men from 40 urologic practice sites who are followed prospectively under uniform protocols, regardless of treatment. In the current study, 7538 men with localized disease were analyzed. Prostate cancer risk was assessed using the Kattan preoperative nomogram and the Cancer of the Prostate Risk Assessment (CAPRA) score, both well validated instruments that are calculated from clinical data at the time of diagnosis. A parametric survival model was constructed to compare outcomes across treatments adjusting for risk and age.

Results.—In total, 266 men died of prostate cancer during follow-up. Adjusting for age and risk, the hazard ratio for cancer-specific mortality relative to prostatectomy was 2.21 (95% confidence interval [CI], 1.50-3.24) for radiation therapy and 3.22 (95% CI, 2.16-4.81) for androgen deprivation. Absolute differences between prostatectomy and radiation therapy were small for men at low risk but increased substantially for men at intermediate and high risk. These results were robust to a variety of different analytic techniques, including competing risks regression analysis, adjustment by CAPRA score rather than Kattan score, and examination of overall survival as the endpoint.

Conclusions.—Prostatectomy for localized prostate cancer was associated with a significant and substantial reduction in mortality relative to radiation therapy and androgen-deprivation monotherapy. Although this was not a randomized study, given the multiple adjustments and sensitivity analyses, it is unlikely that unmeasured confounding would account for the large observed differences in survival (Fig 1).

▶ One of the hardest discussions in urology is advising a man on the best treatment for his localized prostate carcinoma. We have to balance the distant risk of death from disease, with the immediate risk of complications. While surgeons, radiation therapists, and medical oncologists all have their views on the best treatment, ultimately we know that there are no randomized data that prove that one treatment is better than the next. Studies such as this one by Cooperberg et al provide the best available evidence that surgery cures more patients.

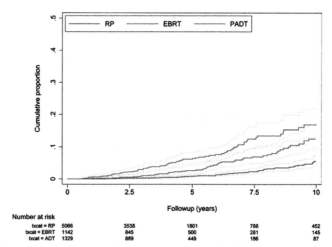

FIGURE 1.—These unadjusted Kaplan-Meier curves illustrate the likelihood of prostate cancer-specific mortality according to primary treatment. The 95% confidence intervals are given as dashed lines for each treatment. RP indicates radical prostatectomy; EBRT, external-beam radiotherapy; PADT, primary androgen-deprivation therapy; txcat, treatment category. (Reprinted from Cooperberg MR, for the Cancer of the Prostate Strategic Urologic Research Endeavor (CaPSURE) Investigators. Comparative risk-adjusted mortality outcomes after primary surgery, radiotherapy, or androgen-deprivation therapy for localized prostate cancer. *Cancer.* 2010;116:5226-5234. Copyright 2010 American Cancer Society. This material is reproduced with permission of Wiley-Liss, Inc., a subsidiary of John Wiley & Sons, Inc.)

Adjusting for age and aggressiveness of the cancer, cancer-specific mortality was roughly twice as high for radiation therapy and 3 times as high for androgen deprivation, compared with radical prostatectomy. The absolute benefit was not as striking with a benefit of approximately 5% at 10 years (Fig 1). This lack of absolute benefit should not be surprising because only 3% of the entire cohort died of prostate cancer.

The real strengths of this study are the large number of patients (approximately 8000) being treated in the community environment. Therefore, it likely reflects what are the true results for the treatment of prostate cancer. The main problem rests on the fact that it is not a randomized trial. Radiation therapists will correctly point out that there are differences in who gets referred for radiation therapy—older sicker patients with more aggressive disease. This does not mean that these results are not accurate; radiation therapy is associated with worse outcome. The question remains—is it because of the therapy or the patient selection? As additional studies with similar results are published, my guess is that both will be true—there is an increased cure rate, but it is not as dramatic as outlined in this article.

A. S. Kibel, MD

Analysis of Pathologic Extent of Disease for Clinically Localized Prostate Cancer After Radical Prostatectomy and Subsequent Use of Adjuvant Radiation in a National Cohort

Schreiber D, Rineer J, Yu JB, et al (State Univ of New York Downstate Med Ctr, Brooklyn; The Univ of Texas M D Anderson Cancer Ctr, Houston; Yale School of Medicine, New Haven, CT)
Cancer 116:5757-5766, 2010

Background.—The Surveillance, Epidemiology, and End Results database was analyzed to explore the pathologic extent of disease for clinically localized prostate cancer after radical prostatectomy as well as the use of adjuvant radiation in this population.

Methods.—Identified were patients from 2004 to 2006 with clinically staged T1c-2cNx-0M0 prostate adenocarcinoma who underwent radical prostatectomy. All patients had complete clinical and pathologic data. The use of postoperative radiation was recorded. Logistic regression analysis was performed to identify unadjusted and adjusted predictors for extraprostatic disease or positive surgical margins and for adjuvant radiation use.

Results.—A total of 35,642 patients were identified. For those patients with Gleason 7 (4 + 3) and a prostate-specific antigen (PSA) level of ≥10.1 ng/mL or Gleason 8 to 10 with any PSA level, the rate of organ-confined disease with negative surgical margins was found to be <50%. Of those with indications for adjuvant radiation, 11.1% received the treatment.

Conclusions.—This large population-based study detailed the risk of extraprostatic extension and positive surgical margins in a broad setting across multiple regions and communities, as well as the use of adjuvant radiation for these patients. As of 2006, 11.1% of patients who had indications for adjuvant radiation received this treatment, providing a useful baseline for future patterns of care studies.

▶ The take-home message of this article is that only 11% of patients with the clinical/pathologic characteristics that would make them ideal candidates for adjuvant radiation therapy are getting it. Why? The most obvious answer is that the data obtained were prior to the widespread dissemination of the randomized trials demonstrating an advantage. However, I don't think the results are much different today. The management of locally advanced prostate cancer remains a dilemma despite the fact that we have 3 randomized trials that demonstrate a clear benefit. I think adjuvant radiation therapy has not been embraced for several reasons: (1) The perception that it increases the complication rate exists. (2) The Southwest Oncology Group trial, which demonstrated an improvement in overall survival, was in the pre—prostate-specific antigen (PSA) or early PSA era. (3) Most patients with positive margins or pT3 disease with negative margins are unlikely to fail. (4) Salvage radiation therapy is curative in 50% of patients if delivered when the PSA level is low. As a result, there is a belief that treatment at the time of PSA relapse will provide the same level of cure. This is not based on level 1 evidence but on interpretation of the data. I personally offer my patients both options. Most choose observation with delayed salvage radiation therapy. However, if I had a patient with Gleason 8 positive margin, there is no doubt that I'd work to convince him to be treated immediately.

A. S. Kibel, MD

Treatment Comparison

Radical Prostatectomy versus Watchful Waiting in Early Prostate Cancer
Bill-Axelson A, for the SPCG-4 Investigators (Univ Hosp, Uppsala, Sweden: et al)
N Engl J Med 364:1708-1717, 2011

Background.—In 2008, we reported that radical prostatectomy, as compared with watchful waiting, reduces the rate of death from prostate cancer. After an additional 3 years of follow-up, we now report estimated 15-year results.

Methods.—From October 1989 through February 1999, we randomly assigned 695 men with early prostate cancer to watchful waiting or radical prostatectomy. Follow-up was complete through December 2009, with histopathological review of biopsy and radical-prostatectomy specimens and blinded evaluation of causes of death. Relative risks, with 95% confidence intervals, were estimated with the use of a Cox proportional-hazards model.

Results.—During a median of 12.8 years, 166 of the 347 men in the radical-prostatectomy group and 201 of the 348 in the watchful-waiting group died (P = 0.007). In the case of 55 men assigned to surgery and 81 men assigned to watchful waiting, death was due to prostate cancer. This yielded a cumulative incidence of death from prostate cancer at 15 years of 14.6% and 20.7%, respectively (a difference of 6.1 percentage points; 95% confidence interval [CI], 0.2 to 12.0), and a relative risk with surgery of 0.62 (95% CI, 0.44 to 0.87; P = 0.01). The survival benefit was similar before and after 9 years of follow-up, was observed also among men with low-risk prostate cancer, and was confined to men younger than 65 years of age. The number needed to treat to avert one death was 15 overall and 7 for men younger than 65 years of age. Among men who underwent radical prostatectomy, those with extracapsular tumor growth had a risk of death from prostate cancer that was 7 times that of men without extracapsular tumor growth (relative risk, 6.9; 95% CI, 2.6 to 18.4).

Conclusions.—Radical prostatectomy was associated with a reduction in the rate of death from prostate cancer. Men with extracapsular tumor growth may benefit from adjuvant local or systemic treatment. (Funded by the Swedish Cancer Society and the National Institutes of Health.)

▶ This update of Swedish Randomized Trial provides 15-year data on the outcomes of patients undergoing radical prostatectomy compared with patients who underwent a watchful waiting approach. The 15-year data reinforce some of the messages from earlier articles. For the entire cohort, there is an improvement in overall survival, prostate cancer mortality, and metastasis-free survival favoring radical prostatectomy. Subset analysis confirms the prior findings that the benefit seems to be predominately in patients under the age of 65 years. This is in large part because of the fact that in the older population, an extremely high percentage (~50%) of these patients have died of other causes. This highlights one of the key issues in treating an elderly population, which is that they are highly likely to die of other causes before they can benefit from the treatment.

The new twist on this article is an analysis of patients with lower risk disease, defined as prostate-specific antigen of less than 10 and a Gleason score of 6 or below. The authors found a benefit for the group as a whole in terms of overall survival with a relative risk of 0.62 (95% confidence interval [CI], 0.42-0.92, P = .02). They looked at the risk of death from prostate cancer in this cohort. It did not achieve statistical significance, relative risk equals 0.53 (95% CI, 0.24-1.14, P = .14). However, there was a benefit for distant metastases, relative risk equals 0.43 (95% CI, 0.23-0.79, P = .008). As depicted in Fig 2 in the original article, you can see a clear benefit in terms of metastasis-free survival. However, while there is a trend for decreased risk from death of prostate cancer, this did not achieve statistical significance.

I think this supports what we all know intuitively. A subset of patients with low-risk disease are at risk for progressing to metastatic disease and dying of their cancer. This benefit should be predominately in patients who are younger because they have a longer life expectancy for which the disease could potentially progress. With that said, older patients with low-risk disease probably do not benefit from any sort of intervention because of the fact that they are going to die of other causes. What this article leaves unanswered is whether or not patients with high-risk disease, who are older, would benefit from some sort of intervention. I often see patients who are in their late 60s and early 70s with Gleason 7, 8, 9, and 10 score. It is my belief that these patients have disease that is biologically aggressive and capable of metastasizing and killing the patient within their lifetime. This study does not answer whether these patients benefit from an aggressive intervention.

A. S. Kibel, MD

Denosumab versus zoledronic acid for treatment of bone metastases in men with castration-resistant prostate cancer: A randomised, double-blind study
Fizazi K, Carducci M, Smith M, et al (Univ of Paris Sud, Villejuif, France; Johns Hopkins Univ, Baltimore, MD; Massachusetts General Hosp Cancer Ctr, Boston; et al)
Lancet 377:813-822, 2011

Background.—Bone metastases are a major burden in men with advanced prostate cancer. We compared denosumab, a human monoclonal antibody against RANKL, with zoledronic acid for prevention of skeletal-related events in men with bone metastases from castration-resistant prostate cancer.

Methods.—In this phase 3 study, men with castration-resistant prostate cancer and no previous exposure to intravenous bisphosphonate were enrolled from 342 centres in 39 countries. An interactive voice response system was used to assign patients (1:1 ratio), according to a computer-generated randomisation sequence, to receive 120 mg subcutaneous denosumab plus intravenous placebo, or 4 mg intravenous zoledronic acid plus subcutaneous placebo, every 4 weeks until the primary analysis cutoff date. Randomisation was stratified by previous skeletal-related event, prostate-specific antigen concentration, and chemotherapy for prostate cancer within 6 weeks before randomisation. Supplemental calcium and vitamin D were strongly recommended. Patients, study staff, and investigators were masked to treatment assignment. The primary endpoint was time to first on-study skeletal-related event (pathological fracture, radiation therapy, surgery to bone, or spinal cord compression), and was assessed for non-inferiority. The same outcome was further assessed for superiority as a secondary endpoint. Efficacy analysis was by intention to treat. This study is registered with ClinicalTrials.gov, number NCT00321620, and has been completed.

Findings.—1904 patients were randomised, of whom 950 assigned to denosumab and 951 assigned to receive zoledronic acid were eligible for the efficacy analysis. Median duration on study at primary analysis cutoff date was 12·2 months (IQR 5·9—18·5) for patients on denosumab and 11·2 months (IQR 5·6—17·4) for those on zoledronic acid. Median time to first on-study skeletal-related event was 20·7 months (95% CI

18·8—24·9) with denosumab compared with 17·1 months (15·0—19·4) with zoledronic acid (hazard ratio 0·82, 95% CI 0·71—0·95; p=0·0002 for non-inferiority; p=0·008 for superiority). Adverse events were recorded in 916 patients (97%) on denosumab and 918 patients (97%) on zoledronic acid, and serious adverse events were recorded in 594 patients (63%) on denosumab and 568 patients (60%) on zoledronic acid. More events of hypocalcaemia occurred in the denosumab group (121 [13%]) than in the zoledronic acid group (55 [6%]; p<0·0001). Osteonecrosis of the jaw occurred infrequently (22 [2%] *vs* 12 [1%]; p=0·09).

Interpretation.—Denosumab was better than zoledronic acid for prevention of skeletal-related events, and potentially represents a novel treatment option in men with bone metastases from castration-resistant prostate cancer.

▶ This is a randomized phase III trial that compares denosumab with zoledronic acid for the prevention of skeletal-related events. Denosumab is a monoclonal antibody to receptor activator of nuclear factor-κB (RANK) ligand, which is a key activator of osteoblastic bone resorption, and therefore denosumab stabilizes bone. Previous work has demonstrated that zoledronic acid is better than placebo at preventing skeletal-related events and demonstrated that denosumab does a better job than zoledronic acid at preventing osteoporosis. This, however, is the first study to examine specifically which is better at decreasing the likelihood of skeletal-related events. The take-home message is that denosumab does a better job decreasing the time until skeletal-related events by approximately 3 months. While the overall adverse effect profile appeared to be very similar between the 2, it is important to note that denosumab was associated with a higher rate of hypocalcemia. Also, while osteonecrosis of the jaw was not different statistically between the 2 treatments and was relatively low at approximately 1% to 2%, denosumab did approximately double the risk of osteonecrosis in a nonstatistically significant manner ($P = .09$).

The clear advantages of denosumab are ease of administration (sub q) and the fact that you do not have to alter the dose in the face of renal insufficiency. RANK ligand has no effect on renal function, and there is no need for renal monitoring. Both of these I think are substantial improvements over the bisphosphonates. In addition, it now proves to be more efficacious. While clearly a fracture is important, it is important to recognize that these studies generally use composite end points in the risk of a clinical fracture. Skeletal-related events were defined as a pathologic fracture, radiation therapy to the bone, or surgery to the bone. These patients were heavily monitored with skeletal surveys that were done every 12 weeks, which clearly unmasked many fractures that might not have become clinically significant until a later date.

A. S. Kibel, MD

Active Surveillance Program for Prostate Cancer: An Update of the Johns Hopkins Experience

Tosoian JJ, Trock BJ, Landis P, et al (The Johns Hopkins Univ School of Medicine, Baltimore, MD)
J Clin Oncol 29:2185-2190, 2011

Purpose.—We assessed outcomes of men with prostate cancer enrolled in active surveillance.

Patients and Methods.—Since 1995, a total of 769 men diagnosed with prostate cancer have been followed prospectively (median follow-up, 2.7 years; range, 0.01 to 15.0 years) on active surveillance. Enrollment criteria were for very-low-risk cancers, defined by clinical stage (T1c), prostate-specific antigen density < 0.15 ng/mL, and prostate biopsy findings (Gleason score ≤ 6, two or fewer cores with cancer, and ≤ 50% cancer involvement of any core). Curative intervention was recommended on disease reclassification on the basis of biopsy criteria. The primary outcome was survival free of intervention, and secondary outcomes were rates of disease reclassification and exit from the program. Outcomes were compared between men who did and did not meet very-low-risk criteria.

Results.—The median survival free of intervention was 6.5 years (range, 0.0 to 15.0 years) after diagnosis, and the proportions of men remaining free of intervention after 2, 5, and 10 years of follow-up were 81%, 59%, and 41%, respectively. Overall, 255 men (33.2%) underwent intervention at a median of 2.2 years (range, 0.6 to 10.2 years) after diagnosis; 188 men (73.7%) underwent intervention on the basis of disease reclassification on biopsy. The proportions of men who underwent curative intervention ($P =$ .026) or had biopsy reclassification ($P < .001$) were significantly lower in men who met enrollment criteria than in those who did not. There were no prostate cancer deaths.

Conclusion.—For carefully selected men, active surveillance with curative intent appears to be a safe alternative to immediate intervention. Limiting surveillance to very-low-risk patients may reduce the frequency of adverse outcomes.

▶ Dr Carter's Johns Hopkins' active surveillance series is one of the longest continuous programs, with its inception back in 1995. Close to 800 patients with a diagnosis of prostate cancer have been followed prospectively. The group believes quite strongly in using grade progression as a sign of disease aggressiveness and therefore repeats the biopsies yearly. Interestingly, they believe equally strongly that prostate-specific antigen kinetics in general is not a useful marker to trigger intervention. Of the 769 patients in the data set, 96 withdrew or died of other causes, 439 had no biopsy reclassification of which 67 still opted for some form of treatment because of patient anxiety, and 235 underwent biopsy reclassification of which 188 underwent a form of treatment (Fig 1 in the original article).

The important finding of this article is that the number of patients who required intervention gradually increased with time. At 10-year follow-up, approximately 59% of the patients have required some form of intervention. This does not mean that the 59% undergoing active surveillance who progressed did not benefit because a prolonged period of observation frees the patient from the side effects during that period of time. The key fact is whether these patients were more likely to die of their disease as a result of the delay. Of the patients who underwent an intervention, roughly 5% of the patients who underwent surgery and 15% of the patients who underwent radiation therapy suffered a biochemical recurrence. To date, no men in the cohort developed metastatic disease or died as a result of their prostate cancer. I think this speaks volumes about the safety of this approach, while at the same time it is important for patients to recognize that no management strategy works 100% of the time.

What is the take-home message for patients? Extremely low-risk disease can be safely managed with an active surveillance approach. It seems like the risk of developing metastatic disease or dying of prostate cancer is extremely low in this closely followed population but is not 0%. However, patients need to understand that there is a small risk that they could progress, and it is likely that they will require intervention at a future point in time.

A. S. Kibel, MD

Outcomes in Localized Prostate Cancer: National Prostate Cancer Register of Sweden Follow-up Study
Stattin P, on behalf of the National Prostate Cancer Register (NPCR) of Sweden (Umeå Univ Hosp, Sweden; et al)
J Natl Cancer Inst 102:950-958, 2010

Background.—Treatment for localized prostate cancer remains controversial. To our knowledge, there are no outcome studies from contemporary population-based cohorts that include data on stage, Gleason score, and serum levels of prostate-specific antigen (PSA).

Methods.—In the National Prostate Cancer Register of Sweden Follow-up Study, a nationwide cohort, we identified 6849 patients aged 70 years or younger. Inclusion criteria were diagnosis with local clinical stage T1-2 prostate cancer from January 1, 1997, through December 31, 2002, a Gleason score of 7 or less, a serum PSA level of less than 20 ng/mL, and treatment with surveillance (including active surveillance and watchful waiting, n = 2021) or curative intent (including radical prostatectomy, n = 3399, and radiation therapy, n = 1429). Among the 6849 patients, 2686 had low-risk prostate cancer (ie, clinical stage T1, Gleason score 2-6, and serum PSA level of <10 ng/mL). The study cohort was linked to the Cause of Death Register, and cumulative incidence of death from prostate cancer and competing causes was calculated.

Results.—For the combination of low- and intermediate-risk prostate cancers, calculated cumulative 10-year prostate cancer—specific mortality was 3.6% (95% confidence interval [CI] = 2.7% to 4.8%) in the surveillance group and 2.7% (95% CI = 2.1% to 3.45) in the curative intent group. For those with low-risk disease, the corresponding values were

2.4% (95% CI = 1.2% to 4.1%) among the 1085 patients in the surveillance group and 0.7% (95% CI = 0.3% to 1.4%) among the 1601 patients in the curative intent group. The 10-year risk of dying from competing causes was 19.2% (95% CI = 17.2% to 21.3%) in the surveillance group and 10.2% (95% CI = 9.0% to 11.4%) in the curative intent group.

Conclusion.—A 10-year prostate cancer–specific mortality of 2.4% among patients with low-risk prostate cancer in the surveillance group indicates that surveillance may be a suitable treatment option for many patients with low-risk disease.

▶ In evaluating studies comparing treatment alternatives for prostate cancer, the devil is always in the details. The key criticism of this study is simply that the follow-up is relatively short. As we all know, the benefit for treatment of prostate cancer is limited to patients who have at least a 10-year life expectancy. As a result, one would not expect to see a benefit in this study. Therefore, it is quite striking that hidden in the text of the article is that after adjusting for risk category, comorbidity, and socioeconomic status they actually found that prostate cancer–specific survival was better in men undergoing radical prostatectomy compared with the surveillance group (relative risk, 0.49; 95% confidence interval [CI], 0.34-0.71). The same benefit was seen for patients who received radiation therapy; however, it was not statistically significant (relative risk, 0.72; 95% CI, 0.47-1.11).

The important message delivered from the authors is that the risk of dying of prostate cancer for patients with low-risk disease is incredibly low at 10 years. A 2.4% prostate cancer mortality among patients with untreated low-risk prostate cancer at 10 years demonstrates how indolent some forms of this disease are. This is going to be particularly important as we evaluate less-invasive treatment modalities such as CyberKnife, proton beam radiation therapy, and focal ablation. All these modalities are going to be focused very much on patients with low-risk disease, and there will be claims that they are highly efficacious when in fact they are treating disease with a low risk of contributing to patient mortality. Studies that have a large number of patients with indolent disease and claim great benefit from the treatment are probably because of the biology of the disease and not because of the intervention.

A. S. Kibel, MD

Watchful Waiting/Outcomes

Prognostic value of an RNA expression signature derived from cell cycle proliferation genes in patients with prostate cancer: a retrospective study
Cuzick J, on behalf of the Transatlantic Prostate Group (Queen Mary Univ of London, UK; et al)
Lancet Oncol 12:245-255, 2011

Background.—Optimum management of clinically localised prostate cancer presents unique challenges because of the highly variable and often indolent natural history of the disease. To predict disease aggressiveness, clinicians combine clinical variables to create prognostic models, but the models have limited accuracy. We assessed the prognostic value of a predefined cell cycle progression (CCP) score in two cohorts of patients with prostate cancer.

Methods.—We measured the expression of 31 genes involved in CCP with quantitative RT-PCR on RNA extracted from formalin-fixed paraffin-embedded tumour samples, and created a predefined score and assessed its usefulness in the prediction of disease outcome. The signature was assessed retrospectively in a cohort of patients from the USA who had undergone radical prostatectomy, and in a cohort of randomly selected men with clinically localised prostate cancer diagnosed by use of a transurethral resection of the prostate (TURP) in the UK who were managed conservatively. The primary endpoint was time to biochemical recurrence for the cohort of patients who had radical prostatectomy, and time to death from prostate cancer for the TURP cohort.

Findings.—After prostatectomy, the CCP score was useful for predicting biochemical recurrence in the univariate analysis (hazard ratio for a 1-unit change [doubling] in CCP $1 \cdot 89$; 95% CI $1 \cdot 54 - 2 \cdot 31$; $p = 5 \cdot 6 \times 10^{-9}$) and the best multivariate analysis ($1 \cdot 77$, $1 \cdot 40 - 2 \cdot 22$; $p = 4 \cdot 3 \times 10^{-6}$). In the best predictive model (final multivariate analysis), the CCP score and prostate-specific antigen (PSA) concentration were the most important variables and were more significant than any other clinical variable. In the TURP cohort, the CCP score was the most important variable for prediction of time to death from prostate cancer in both univariate analysis ($2 \cdot 92$, $2 \cdot 38 - 3 \cdot 57$, $p = 6 \cdot 1 \times 10^{-22}$) and the final multivariate analysis ($2 \cdot 57$, $1 \cdot 93 - 3 \cdot 43$; $p = 8 \cdot 2 \times 10^{-11}$), and was stronger than all other prognostic factors, although PSA concentration also added useful information. Heterogeneity in the hazard ratio for the CCP score was not noted in any case for any clinical variables.

Interpretation.—The results of this study provide strong evidence that the CCP score is a robust prognostic marker, which, after additional validation, could have an essential role in determining the appropriate treatment for patients with prostate cancer.

▶ We need better tools to identify who has prostate cancer that is potentially going to cause loss of life and who has prostate cancer that can be safely observed. This is becoming increasingly important, as we are aware of overtreatment concerns, and, therefore, more patients are placed on active surveillance protocols. Because some of the patients on active surveillance progress, tools to identify who were at risk would be incredibly useful. At the same time, in many patients who are undergoing radical prostatectomy or radiation therapy that has all the morbidity associated with the intervention, however, the cancer would not have progressed if they had not been treated.

This 31-gene model, which has been developed by Myriad Genetics, provides an opportunity to better counsel our patients as to their risk of progression. They examined 2 sets of patients. The first was a cohort of patients with clinically localized prostate cancer diagnosed with transurethral resection.

This demonstrated that the cell cycle progression signature was strongly associated with death from prostate cancer on both univariate and multivariate analyses, with a hazard ratio of 2.97 ($P = 8.2 \times 10^{-11}$). A second cohort of radical prostatectomy specimens demonstrated an association with risk of biochemical recurrence, which was also statistically significant on both univariate and multivariate analyses, with a hazard ratio of 1.77 ($P = 4.3 \times 10^{-6}$).

Obviously, there are issues with both the cohorts studied. The radical prostatectomy cohort clearly had already undergone a surgical intervention. It would be better to know the risk of progression prior to undergoing radical surgery. More importantly, the end point was biochemical recurrence, which does not uniformly progress to prostate cancer mortality. The problem with the transurethral resection of prostate cohort is that this is not how tumors are commonly diagnosed in 2011 and, therefore, potentially may not extrapolate. In addition, the tumors analyzed were from the transition zone, and this is not commonly the area of the prostate gland where cancers are diagnosed in 2011.

With these caveats, I believe this is exactly the direction that our diagnostic testing should go in prostate cancer. It will be interesting to see whether or not this signature proves to have utility in additional cohorts and gains traction in our clinics.

A. S. Kibel, MD

Radical Prostatectomy Outcomes

Recovery of Erectile Function After Nerve Sparing Radical Prostatectomy and Penile Rehabilitation With Nightly Intraurethral Alprostadil Versus Sildenafil Citrate

McCullough AR, Hellstrom WG, Wang R, et al (New York Univ School of Medicine; Univ of Texas-Houston; Texas A & M Univ, Temple; et al)
J Urol 183:2451-2456, 2010

Purpose.—To our knowledge we report the first large, randomized, prospective penile rehabilitation clinical trial to compare the effectiveness of nightly intraurethral alprostadil vs sildenafil citrate after nerve sparing prostatectomy.

Materials and Methods.—We performed a prospective, randomized, open label, multicenter American study in men with normal erectile function who underwent bilateral nerve sparing radical prostatectomy. The International Index of Erectile Function erectile function domain was the primary end point. Subjects initiated nightly treatment within 1 month of surgery with intraurethral alprostadil or oral sildenafil citrate (50 mg) for 9 months. After 1-month washout and before sexual activity subjects self-administered sildenafil citrate (100 mg) for a total of 6 attempts in 1 month. Secondary end points were the global assessment question, sexual encounter profile, Erectile Dysfunction Inventory of Treatment Satisfaction and measured stretched penile length.

Results.—Of 139 men who started intraurethral alprostadil and 73 who started sildenafil citrate, 97 and 59, respectively, completed the trial. There were no statistically significant differences in International Index of Erectile Function erectile function domain and intercourse success rates to intraurethral alprostadil. The global assessment question was significantly better only at 6 months for intraurethral alprostadil (p <0.028). At completion there were no differences between treatments for any of the end points.

Conclusions.—This is the first study to directly compare the ability of alprostadil and a phosphodiesterase-5 inhibitor to enhance penile recovery subsequent to bilateral nerve sparing radical prostatectomy. The use of nightly subtherapeutic intraurethral alprostadil is well tolerated after radical prostatectomy. The benefit to return of erectile function of nightly sildenafil citrate and subtherapeutic intraurethral alprostadil appears to be comparable within the first year of surgery.

▶ In this open-label randomized study, men who had undergone bilateral nerve sparing prostatectomy were allocated to treatment with nightly intraurethral alprostadil suppositories on a dose-escalation protocol or sildenafil 50 mg for 9 months, starting 1 month after surgery. After a 1-month washout period, men were instructed to attempt intercourse at least 6 times in 1 month using 100 mg sildenafil on demand. One hundred fifty-six men completed the trial. Both the mean International Index of Erectile Function score and the percentage of men reporting recovery of erectile function improved over the course of the study. It was determined that there was no significant difference in outcome between the 2 treatment arms other than a slightly higher rate of positive response to the question, "Has the treatment you have been taking during this study improved your erection?" in the suppository group at the 6-month time point.

The dropout rate was higher in the prostaglandin group (30% vs 19% in the sildenafil group), with pain the most common reason for drop out. Of greater concern is the lack of a placebo control group, a difficult thing to facilitate in a study such as this where an oral medication is being compared with a suppository. It may be argued that intraurethral prostaglandin is not inferior to sildenafil based on these results, and therefore, men who wish to be on some form of rehabilitation protocol but have trouble tolerating phosphodiesterase type 5 inhibitors might consider this intervention as an alternative. However, whether or not penile rehabilitation after radical prostatectomy is in itself a useful intervention remains to be determined by large-scale and better-controlled studies.

A. Shindel, MD

Annual Surgical Caseload and Open Radical Prostatectomy Outcomes: Improving Temporal Trends
Budäus L, Abdollah F, Sun M, et al (Prostate Cancer Ctr Univ Hosp Hamburg-Eppendorf, Germany; Univ of Montreal Health Centre, Quebec, Canada; et al)
J Urol 184:2285-2290, 2010

Purpose.—Radical prostatectomy is the standard of care for localized prostate cancer. Numerous previous reports show the relationship between surgical experience and various outcomes. We examined the effect of surgical experience on complications and transfusion rates, and determined individual surgeon annual caseload trends in a contemporary radical prostatectomy cohort.

Materials and Methods.—We analyzed annual caseload temporal trends in 34,803 patients who underwent surgery between 1999 and 2008 in Florida. Logistic regression models controlled for clustering among surgeons addressed the relationship of surgical experience, defined as the number of radical prostatectomies done since January 1, 1999 until each radical prostatectomy, with complications and transfusions.

Results.—During the study period the proportion of surgeons in the high annual caseload tertile (24 radical prostatectomies or greater yearly) and the proportion of patients treated by those surgeons increased from 5% to 10% and from 20% to 55%, respectively. Conversely complication and transfusion rates decreased from 14.3% to 9.2% and 12.6% to 6.9%, respectively. Radical prostatectomies done by surgeons in the high surgical experience tertile (86 or greater radical prostatectomies) decreased the risk of any complication by 33% and of any transfusion by 30% vs those in patients operated on by surgeons in the low surgical experience tertile (27 or fewer radical prostatectomies).

Conclusions.—The proportion of surgeons in the high annual caseload tertile and the proportion of patients treated by these surgeons steadily increased during the last decade. Complication and transfusion rates decreased with time. The implications of these encouraging findings may result in improved outcomes in patients with surgically managed prostate cancer.

▶ More is often not better, but it appears for prostatectomy that more cases translate into better outcomes. We are seeing specific surgeons and specific centers consolidating all the radical prostatectomies. Budäus et al examined Florida cancer data and found that specific surgeons are performing more radical prostatectomies and that this increased volume appears to translate to a lower complication rate. The first question is one of causation. While the implication is that practice makes perfect, it is also possible that a surgeon with low complication rate is more likely to get referrals and build a larger practice. The second question is if practice does make perfect, then how does one get from being a low-volume surgeon to a high-volume surgeon? The idea that only experienced surgeons should operate is flawed. After all, where will the new, experienced surgeons come from? What is clear is that if you have no desire to perform many of these cases, and only see a few patients a year, it is in the patients' best interest to refer these patients to physicians who frequently perform these procedures.

A. S. Kibel, MD

Androgen Deprivation

Coronary Revascularization and Mortality in Men With Congestive Heart Failure or Prior Myocardial Infarction Who Receive Androgen Deprivation

Nguyen PL, Chen MH, Goldhaber SZ, et al (Brigham and Women's Hosp, Boston, MA; Univ of Connecticut, Storrs; Harvard Med School, Boston; et al)
Cancer 117:406-413, 2011

Background.—A study was undertaken to determine the impact of prior coronary revascularization (angioplasty, stent, or coronary artery bypass graft) on the risk of all-cause mortality after neoadjuvant hormonal therapy (HT) for prostate cancer (PC) in men with a history of coronary artery disease (CAD)-induced congestive heart failure (CHF) or myocardial infarction (MI).

Methods.—Among 7839 men who received radiation with or without a median of 4 months of HT for PC from 1991 to 2006, 495 (6.3%) had CAD-induced CHF or MI and formed the study cohort. Of these men, 250 (50.5%) had been revascularized before treatment for PC. Cox regression was used to determine whether HT increased the risk of all-cause mortality, and whether revascularization altered this risk, after adjusting for known PC prognostic factors and a propensity score for revascularization.

Results.—Median follow-up was 4.1 years. Neoadjuvant HT was associated with an increased risk of all-cause mortality (28.9% vs 15.7% at 5 years; adjusted hazard ratio [HR], 1.73; 95% confidence interval [CI], 1.13-2.64; $P = .01$). Men who received HT without revascularization had the highest risk of all-cause mortality (33.3%; adjusted HR, 1.48; 95% CI, 1.01-2.18; $P = .047$), whereas men who were revascularized and did not receive HT had the lowest risk of all-cause mortality (9.4%; adjusted HR, 0.51; 95% CI, 0.28-0.93; $P = .028$). The reference group had an intermediate risk of all-cause mortality (23.4%) and was comprised of men in whom HT use and revascularization were either both given or both withheld.

Conclusions.—In men with a history of CAD-induced CHF or MI, neoadjuvant HT is associated with an excess risk of mortality, which appears to be reduced but not eliminated by prior revascularization.

▶ The debate as to the potential cardiovascular risks associated with androgen deprivation therapy continues to rage. I think most clinicians recognize that while the studies are imperfect, there is clear evidence that androgen deprivation therapy does increase the risk of a cardiovascular event. The question that always remains is whether this risk can be ameliorated by judicial evaluation of these patients prior to instituting androgen deprivation therapy. This is particularly important in patients who are receiving androgen deprivation therapy in combination with external beam radiation therapy. Many radiation oncologists evaluate these patients and then have the cardiovascular disease treated prior to instituting androgen deprivation therapy. This study would indicate that prior revascularization will decrease but not entirely eliminate this risk. Data like these reinforce to my mind that this is a real phenomenon. Clearly, revascularization will not completely improve the heart's vascular supply or function. Therefore, I think the fact that there continues to be residual effect is in keeping with the fact that androgen deprivation therapy does cause cardiac toxicity.

The clinical implications are clear. (1) Only institute androgen deprivation therapy if the patient is going to benefit, and (2) every effort should be made to evaluate and treat any evidence of ischemia prior to instituting androgen deprivation therapy in those who appear to warrant this treatment.

A. S. Kibel, MD

Antitumour activity of MDV3100 in castration-resistant prostate cancer: a phase 1–2 study
Scher HI, the Prostate Cancer Foundation/Department of Defense Prostate Cancer Clinical Trials Consortium (Memorial Sloan-Kettering Cancer Ctr, NY; et al)
Lancet 375:1437-1446, 2010

Background.—MDV3100 is an androgen-receptor antagonist that blocks androgens from binding to the androgen receptor and prevents nuclear translocation and co-activator recruitment of the ligand-receptor complex. It also induces tumour cell apoptosis, and has no agonist activity. Because growth of castration-resistant prostate cancer is dependent on continued androgen-receptor signalling, we assessed the antitumour activity and safety of MDV3100 in men with this disease.

Methods.—This phase 1–2 study was undertaken in five US centres in 140 patients. Patients with progressive, metastatic, castration-resistant prostate cancer were enrolled in dose-escalation cohorts of three to six patients and given an oral daily starting dose of MDV3100 30 mg. The final daily doses studied were 30 mg (n=3), 60 mg (27), 150 mg (28), 240 mg (29), 360 mg (28), 480 mg (22), and 600 mg (3). The primary objective was to identify the safety and tolerability profile of MDV3100 and to establish the maximum tolerated dose. The trial is registered with ClinicalTrials.gov, number NCT00510718.

Findings.—We noted antitumour effects at all doses, including decreases in serum prostate-specific antigen of 50% or more in 78 (56%) patients, responses in soft tissue in 13 (22%) of 59 patients, stabilised bone disease in 61 (56%) of 109 patients, and conversion from unfavourable to favourable circulating tumour cell counts in 25 (49%) of the 51 patients. PET imaging of 22 patients to assess androgen-receptor blockade showed decreased ^{18}F-fluoro-5α-dihydrotestosterone binding at doses from 60 mg to 480 mg per day (range 20–100%). The median time to progression was 47 weeks (95% CI 34–not reached) for radiological progression. The maximum tolerated dose for sustained treatment (>28 days) was

240 mg. The most common grade 3—4 adverse event was dose-dependent fatigue (16 [11%] patients), which generally resolved after dose reduction. *Interpretation.*—We recorded encouraging antitumour activity with MDV3100 in patients with castration-resistant prostate cancer. The results of this phase 1—2 trial validate in man preclinical studies implicating sustained androgen-receptor signalling as a driver in this disease.

▶ Our understanding of the role of androgen signaling in metastatic prostate cancer has grown by leaps and bounds over the past 5 years. The change from androgen-resistant prostate cancer to castration-resistant prostate cancer is not simply a superficial change in nomenclature; it reflects a profound transformation in our understanding of the disease. In the past, androgen was produced in the testicles and to a lesser extent in the adrenal glands. It was then transported though the circulation to the prostate cancer cell where it had its effect. Therefore, by decreasing the blood levels of androgen, the tumor's growth was inhibited. We now know that the tumor and the surrounding stroma actually produce androgen from cholesterol and, therefore, can use the androgen axis to grow even when serum levels of testosterone are castrate. This paradigm shift offers an opportunity to better treat the patient by focusing less on decreasing serum androgen levels and more on decreasing androgen activity within the tumor.

MDV3100 fits into this paradigm perfectly. This antiandrogen binds to the androgen receptor much more tightly than previous antiandrogens and, as a result, has a much stronger effect on the tumor growth. This phase I/II study demonstrates the potential for this drug in castration-resistant prostate cancer. There are several striking features. The first is that a decrease in the prostate-specific antigen (PSA) of 50% or more was seen in 56% of the patients. There were soft tissue responses in 22% of the patients. Circulating tumor cell counts decreased in 49% of the patients, and, lastly, positron emission tomographic imaging of the androgen receptor actually showed decreased binding of androgens to the receptor in 20% to 100% of the patients. The Forest Plot (Fig 2 in the original article) clearly demonstrates that the vast majority of the patients had a substantial decrease in their PSA level.

On the basis of this elegant study, phase III trials are moving forward testing this drug in late-stage disease at the 240-mg dose. I believe that all urologists who treat prostate cancer should be aware of these changes in the way we are thinking about castration-resistant prostate cancer and that these drugs will likely soon be available. We are going to be the ones who advise patients on novel antiandrogen therapy and likely prescribe these medications.

A. S. Kibel, MD

Risk of colorectal cancer in men on long-term androgen deprivation therapy for prostate cancer

Gillessen S, Templeton A, Marra G, et al (Kantonsspital, St Gallen, Switzerland; Univ of Zurich, Switzerland; et al)
J Natl Cancer Inst 102:1760-1770, 2010

Background.—Androgen deprivation with gonadotropin-releasing hormone (GnRH) agonists or orchiectomy is a common but controversial treatment for prostate cancer. Uncertainties remain about its use, particularly with increasing recognition of serious side effects. In animal studies, androgens protect against colonic carcinogenesis, suggesting that androgen deprivation may increase the risk of colorectal cancer.

Methods.—We identified 107 859 men in the linked Surveillance, Epidemiology, and End Results (SEER)—Medicare database who were diagnosed with prostate cancer in 1993 through 2002, with follow-up available through 2004. The primary outcome was development of colorectal cancer, determined from SEER files on second primary cancers. Cox proportional hazards regression was used to assess the influence of androgen deprivation on the outcome, adjusted for patient and prostate cancer characteristics. All statistical tests were two-sided.

Results.—Men who had orchiectomies had the highest unadjusted incidence rate of colorectal cancer (6.3 per 1000 person-years; 95% confidence interval [CI] = 5.3 to 7.5), followed by men who had GnRH agonist therapy (4.4 per 1000 person-years; 95% CI = 4.0 to 4.9), and men who had no androgen deprivation (3.7 per 1000 person-years; 95% CI = 3.5 to 3.9). After adjustment for patient and prostate cancer characteristics, there was a statistically significant dose—response effect (P_{trend} = .010) with an increasing risk of colorectal cancer associated with increasing duration of androgen deprivation. Compared with the absence of these treatments, there was an increased risk of colorectal cancer associated with use of GnRH agonist therapy for 25 months or longer (hazard ratio [HR] = 1.31, 95% CI = 1.12 to 1.53) or with orchiectomy (HR = 1.37, 95% CI = 1.14 to 1.66).

Conclusion.—Long-term androgen deprivation therapy for prostate cancer is associated with an increased risk of colorectal cancer.

▶ This study examined 107 859 men in the linked Surveillance, Epidemiology, and End Results—Medicare database who were diagnosed with prostate cancer in 1993 through 2002. They clearly demonstrated that androgen deprivation is associated with increased risk of colorectal carcinoma. There is a clear dose response with men undergoing orchiectomy and longer periods of gonadotropin-releasing hormone agonist therapy being more likely to have disease. Importantly, there was concern that this may simply be because of the use of pelvic radiation therapy in conjunction with androgen deprivation. However, subset analysis of patients who did not receive radiation therapy demonstrated essentially the same finding.

This is just another example of how androgen deprivation is associated with an increased risk of long-term adverse events. Add colorectal carcinoma to osteoporosis, diabetes, and, possibly, cardiovascular events. While men in this age group should already be undergoing routine screening, I believe that urologists should be reinforcing this message with all our patients.

A. S. Kibel, MD

Advanced Disease

Sipuleucel-T Immunotherapy for Castration-Resistant Prostate Cancer

Kantoff PW, for the IMPACT Study Investigators (Harvard Med School, Boston, MA; et al)

N Engl J Med 363:411-422, 2010

Background.—Sipuleucel-T, an autologous active cellular immunotherapy, has shown evidence of efficacy in reducing the risk of death among men with metastatic castration-resistant prostate cancer.

Methods.—In this double-blind, placebo-controlled, multicenter phase 3 trial, we randomly assigned 512 patients in a 2:1 ratio to receive either sipuleucel-T (341 patients) or placebo (171 patients) administered intravenously every 2 weeks, for a total of three infusions. The primary end point was overall survival, analyzed by means of a stratified Cox regression model adjusted for baseline levels of serum prostate-specific antigen (PSA) and lactate dehydrogenase.

Results.—In the sipuleucel-T group, there was a relative reduction of 22% in the risk of death as compared with the placebo group (hazard ratio, 0.78; 95% confidence interval [CI], 0.61 to 0.98; $P = 0.03$). This reduction represented a 4.1-month improvement in median survival (25.8 months in the sipuleucel-T group vs. 21.7 months in the placebo group). The 36-month survival probability was 31.7% in the sipuleucel-T group versus 23.0% in the placebo group. The treatment effect was also observed with the use of an unadjusted Cox model and a log-rank test (hazard ratio, 0.77; 95% CI, 0.61 to 0.97; $P = 0.02$) and after adjustment for use of docetaxel after the study therapy (hazard ratio, 0.78; 95% CI, 0.62 to 0.98; $P = 0.03$). The time to objective disease progression was similar in the two study groups. Immune responses to the immunizing antigen were observed in patients who received sipuleucel-T. Adverse events that were more frequently reported in the sipuleucel-T group than in the placebo group included chills, fever, and headache.

Conclusions.—The use of sipuleucel-T prolonged overall survival among men with metastatic castration-resistant prostate cancer. No effect on the time to disease progression was observed. (Funded by Dendreon; ClinicalTrials.gov number, NCT00065442.)

▶ A few years ago we were desperate for new treatments for advanced prostate cancer. Now, overnight we have multiple new options. This randomized trial demonstrated that immunotherapy improves survival in patients with castration-resistant prostate carcinoma. The findings in this study are consistent with prior underpowered studies that demonstrated an overall survival advantage for sipuleucel-T. Interestingly, this prior work did not demonstrate an improvement in progression-free survival. This most recent study was large enough to finally put this question to rest. There clearly was an overall survival advantage and, once again, no improvement in progression-free survival. The hazard ratio demonstrated an improvement of approximately 22%, which was statistically significant. This translated to just over a 4-month improvement in survival.

This is not a curative therapy. As can be seen from Fig 2 in the original article, most of these patients eventually died. However, it is hard to argue with the results. Overall survival is the ultimate end point of any clinical trial. The poor survival in both arms of the trial reflects the fact that these are patients who have received prior therapies and have progressed through them and reached the end stage of their disease. I think it would be interesting to see how this drug performs earlier in the disease progression when the immune system is more robust. I think the most encouraging thing is that this treatment, along with others, heralds a new age in the treatment of metastatic prostate cancer and gives hope to our patients that we will eventually provide a substantial improvement in both their quantity and quality of life.

A. S. Kibel, MD

Antiandrogen monotherapy in patients with localized or locally advanced prostate cancer: final results from the bicalutamide Early Prostate Cancer programme at a median follow-up of 9.7 years
Iversen P, on behalf of the Casodex Early Prostate Cancer Trialists' Group (Rigshospitalet, Copenhagen, Denmark; et al)
BJU Int 105:1074-1081, 2010

Objective.—To evaluate the efficacy and tolerability of bicalutamide 150 mg once-daily as immediate hormonal therapy in patients with prostate cancer or as adjuvant to radical prostatectomy or radiotherapy.

Patients and Methods.—In all, 8113 patients with localized (T1-2, N0/Nx) or locally advanced (T3-4, any N; or any T, N+) prostate cancer (all M0) were enrolled in three complementary, double-blind, placebo-controlled trials. Patients were randomized to receive standard care plus either oral bicalutamide 150 mg once-daily or oral placebo. Primary endpoints were progression-free survival (PFS) and overall survival (OS). Data were collated from individual trials and evaluated in a combined analysis.

Results.—Overall, at a median follow-up of 9.7 years, bicalutamide significantly improved PFS (hazard ratio 0.85, 95% confidence interval 0.79–0.91; $P = 0.001$). Compared with placebo there was no difference in OS (hazard ratio 1.01, $P = 0.77$). Patients who derived benefit from bicalutamide in terms of PFS were those with locally advanced disease, with OS significantly favouring bicalutamide in patients with locally advanced disease undergoing radiotherapy ($P = 0.031$). Patients with localized disease showed no clinically or statistically significant improvements in PFS; there was a survival trend in favour of placebo in patients with localized disease undergoing watchful waiting ($P = 0.054$). The overall tolerability of bicalutamide was consistent with previous analyses, with breast pain (73.7%) and gynaecomastia (68.8%) the most frequently reported adverse events in patients randomized to bicalutamide.

Conclusions.—Bicalutamide 150 mg, either as monotherapy or adjuvant to standard care, improved PFS in patients with locally advanced prostate cancer, but not in patients with localized disease. A pre-planned subset analysis showed a benefit for OS in patients with locally advanced disease undergoing radiotherapy. Bicalutamide 150 mg might represent an alternative for patients with locally advanced prostate cancer considering androgen-deprivation therapy.

▶ We are constantly searching for a less toxic method of androgen deprivation. This group began an ambitious study 10 years ago to determine if high-dose bicalutamide improves survival. Over 8000 men from all stages were enrolled. Unfortunately, the long-term results demonstrate absolutely no improvement in overall survival for the entire cohort with a hazard ratio of 1.01. The progression-free survival did favor bicalutamide with a hazard ratio of 0.85 ($P = .001$); however, subset analysis demonstrated no advantage in localized disease and only a slight advantage in patients with locally advanced disease. Patients who underwent radiation therapy appeared to benefit. These results are in keeping with the known benefit for androgen deprivation in advanced disease and the known synergy between hormone therapy and radiation therapy.

This does not mean that less toxic treatment doesn't have a role. With the increasing use of intermittent androgen deprivation therapy, I think less aggressive approaches continue to be attractive. However, this article should serve as an important reminder that less aggressive therapy may not provide as good a cure in unselected patients.

A. S. Kibel, MD

Other

The Impact of Prostate Biopsy and Periprostatic Nerve Block on Erectile and Voiding Function: A Prospective Study
Klein T, Palisaar RJ, Holz A, et al (Ruhr-Univ-Bochum, Herne, Germany)
J Urol 184:1447-1452, 2010

Purpose.—We evaluated the effect of multiple core prostate biopsy and periprostatic nerve block on voiding and erectile function.

Materials and Methods.—A total of 198 patients in whom prostate cancer was suspected were randomly assigned to undergo 10-core prostate biopsy with (71) or without (74) periprostatic nerve block. The 53 men with a history of negative prostate biopsy underwent 20-core saturation prostate biopsy with periprostatic nerve block. The International Prostate Symptom Score and International Index of Erectile Function were completed before, and 1, 4 and 12 weeks after biopsy to measure changes in voiding and erectile function, and quality of life. Upon prostate cancer diagnosis patients were excluded from further analysis.

Results.—The International Prostate Symptom Score was significantly increased in all patients at week 1, which persisted at weeks 4 and 12 after saturation biopsy (p = 0.007 and 0.035, respectively). After 10-core prostate biopsy with periprostatic nerve block patients had a higher International Prostate Symptom Score at weeks 4 and 12 but this was not statistically significant (p >0.05). Quality of life was significantly affected at all times after saturation prostate biopsy (p = 0.001, 0.003 and 0.010, respectively). International Index of Erectile Function scores decreased significantly in all groups at week 1 (p <0.05). The decrease persisted at week 4 in each 10-core prostate biopsy group.

Conclusions.—Prostate biopsy causes impaired voiding. Saturation prostate biopsy and periprostatic nerve block seem to have a lasting impact on voiding function. Erectile function is transiently affected by prostate biopsy regardless of periprostatic nerve block and the number of cores. Patients who undergo prostate biopsy must be informed about these side effects.

▶ The impact of prostate biopsy on erectile function has been a topic of concern, as more patients with prostate cancer elect active surveillance programs with multiple repeat biopsies planned. Previous reports have suggested that there is a transient decline in erectile function after a single prostate biopsy; other studies have suggested that multiple biopsies are a risk factor for subsequent development of erectile dysfunction (ED).

In this study, there was a transient decline in erectile function (as assessed by mean International Index of Erectile Function-Erectile Function [IIEF-EF] domain score) at 1 and 4 weeks postprocedure in men who underwent 10-core prostate biopsy and did not have evidence of cancer on the pathology specimen; this resolved itself after 12 weeks in men who had periprostatic nerve block, but had not resolved at 12 weeks in men who did not receive the block. Interestingly, men who underwent saturation biopsy did not have a significant decline in their IIEF-EF score postprocedure at any time point. Degree of pain was associated with erectile function score, suggesting that pain might be the factor driving poorer erectile function in these men.

While the mean IIEF-EF score was lower at the specified time points, there was no significant difference in the number of men with no, mild, mild-moderate, moderate, and severe ED at any time point after 1 week when domain scores were stratified by validated cutoff points. This suggests that the decline in erectile function after a single prostate biopsy is a generally subtle one that may not be clinically apparent to the individual patient. The potentially complex influence of periprostatic nerve block on erectile function merits further study.

A. Shindel, MD

8 Testicular Cancer

Randomized Trials in 2466 Patients With Stage I Seminoma: Patterns of Relapse and Follow-up

Mead GM, for the MRC/EORTC seminoma trial collaborators (Southampton General Hosp, UK; et al)
J Natl Cancer Inst 103:241-249, 2011

Background.—From July 1, 1989, through March 31, 2001, 2466 patients with stage I seminoma were evaluated in three randomized non-inferiority trials: the TE10, TE18, and TE19 trials. We analyzed mature results of these studies.

Methods.—The TE10 trial randomly assigned 478 patients to para-aortic and ipsilateral iliac lymph node (dogleg field) or para-aortic only radiation therapy (total dose = 30 Gy). The TE18 trial randomly assigned 1094 patients to a total dose of 30 or 20 Gy of radiation therapy, predominantly to a para-aortic field. The TE19 trial randomly assigned 1477 patients to radiation therapy or a single injection of carboplatin at a dose of seven times the area under the curve. Time to relapse was determined from Kaplan—Meier curves, and such data were compared by use of Cox regression models. Noninferiority in TE18 and TE19 required the upper limit of the 90% confidence intervals (CIs) (reflecting the one-sided test for noninferiority at a 5% statistical significance level) to exclude a hazard ratio (HR) of greater than 2.0 and a doubling of the 5-year relapse rates observed in the control arm. The TE10 trial was not powered to exclude clinically relevant differences in overall relapse rates but was assessed against the same criteria.

Results.—Median follow-up times were 6.4—12 years in the three trials. We identified the noninferiority of the following treatments: 20 Gy of radiation therapy in the TE18 trial (HR of relapse = 0.63, 90% CI = 0.38 to 1.04) and carboplatin in the TE19 trial (HR of relapse = 1.25, 90% CI = 0.83 to 1.89). Para-aortic radiation therapy in the TE10 trial was associated with a hazard ratio of relapse of 1.15 (90% CI = 0.54 to 2.44). Relapse occurred after 3 years in only four (0.2%) of all 2466 patients. Computed tomography scans had little impact on the detection of relapse after radiation therapy; seven of the 904 patients allocated radiation therapy in TE19 had a relapse detected by this method.

Conclusion.—This large and mature dataset from three randomized trials has provided support for the use of either radiation therapy or carboplatin therapy as adjuvant treatment for stage I seminoma.

▶ This is a pooled analysis of 2466 patients with stage I seminoma treated in 2 randomized trials. The pooled analysis is not designed to prove which is best but to examine patterns of recurrence. There are several take-home messages. The first is that recurrence is rare for all treatments. The condition recurred in only 98 patients. Of these, recurrence occurred in only 4 patients after 3 years (50, 61, 64, and 91 months). The pattern of recurrence was clearly dependent on the treatment, with radiation therapy recurrences occurring outside the field of radiation and chemotherapy recurrences occurring predominantly in the abdomen. Importantly, only 4 patients died of disease, for a crude cancer-specific survival of 99.8% (95% confidence interval, 99.6%-99.9%). The authors recommend no additional imaging after 3 years and that routine follow-up may not be needed.

The treatment alternative that is missing from this analysis is surveillance. While this has been widely utilized for nonseminomatous tumors, it has not been embraced for seminomas. The underlying concern is that treatment results in a very high durable cure rate with minimal complications. This pooled analysis not only provides information on where and when to look for recurrence, but it also provides a standard by which observation can be judged.

A. S. Kibel, MD

9 Sexual Function

Long-Term Infection Outcomes After Original Antibiotic Impregnated Inflatable Penile Prosthesis Implants: Up to 7.7 Years of Followup
Carson CC III, Mulcahy JJ, Harsch MR (Univ of North Carolina at Chapel Hill; Univ of Arizona, Tuscon; American Med Systems, Minnetonka, MN)
J Urol 185:614-618, 2011

Purpose.—Although some studies suggest that most infections associated with inflatable penile prosthesis implantation develop within year 1 after surgery, device related infections have been reported 5 years after implantation or later and the infection risk with time is not well characterized. We previously reported a statistically significantly lower infection rate for original inflatable penile prostheses impregnated with antibiotic treatment with minocycline and rifampin vs nonimpregnated inflatable penile prostheses at 1-year followup. Long-term data are now available on infection revision after initial implantation of antibiotic impregnated vs nonimpregnated prostheses.

Materials and Methods.—We retrospectively reviewed patient information forms voluntarily filed with the manufacturer after the initial implantation of more than 39,000 inflatable penile prostheses to compare the revision rate due to infection for antibiotic impregnated vs nonimpregnated implants between May 1, 2001 and December 31, 2008. Life table analysis was used to evaluate device survival from revision surgery.

Results.—On life table survival analysis initial revision events due to infection were significantly less common in the impregnated vs the nonimpregnated group (log rank p <0.0001). At up to 7.7 years of followup 1.1% of 35,737 vs 2.5% of 3,268 men with impregnated vs nonimpregnated implants underwent initial revision due to infection.

Conclusions.—To our knowledge this long-term outcome analysis provides the first substantial clinical evidence of a decrease in costly infection related revision using an antibiotic impregnated inflatable penile prosthesis.

► The authors use a manufacturer's database to assess infectious complications requiring penile implant removal. The incidence of infection is likely an underestimate in both groups because of the voluntary nature of the data reporting and collection. Follow-up is shorter in the impregnated group because the 2 groups are not contemporary. It is impossible to know if the perioperative management (antibiotics, skin preparation, etc) is comparable in the 2 groups. There is a higher revision rate in the nonimpregnated group (Fig in the original article), and the discrepancy increases over time. Some of the noninfectious revisions may be simply related to device age. Implantation of antibiotic impregnated penile prostheses is recommended to decrease the morbidity and cost of revision or explantation.

D. E. Coplen, MD

Identification of Late-Onset Hypogonadism in Middle-Aged and Elderly Men
Wu FCW, for the EMAS Group (Univ of Manchester, UK; et al)
N Engl J Med 363:123-135, 2010

Background.—The association between aging-related testosterone deficiency and late-onset hypogonadism in men remains a controversial concept. We sought evidence-based criteria for identifying late-onset hypogonadism in the general population on the basis of an association between symptoms and a low testosterone level.

Methods.—We surveyed a random population sample of 3369 men between the ages of 40 and 79 years at eight European centers. Using questionnaires, we collected data with regard to the subjects' general, sexual, physical, and psychological health. Levels of total testosterone were measured in morning blood samples by mass spectrometry, and free testosterone levels were calculated with the use of Vermeulen's formula. Data were randomly split into separate training and validation sets for confirmatory analyses.

Results.—In the training set, symptoms of poor morning erection, low sexual desire, erectile dysfunction, inability to perform vigorous activity, depression, and fatigue were significantly related to the testosterone level. Increased probabilities of the three sexual symptoms and limited physical vigor were discernible with decreased testosterone levels (ranges, 8.0 to 13.0 nmol per liter [2.3 to 3.7 ng per milliliter] for total testosterone and 160 to 280 pmol per liter [46 to 81 pg per milliliter] for free testosterone). However, only the three sexual symptoms had a syndromic association with decreased testosterone levels. An inverse relationship between an increasing number of sexual symptoms and a decreasing testosterone level was observed. These relationships were independently confirmed in the validation set, in which the strengths of the association between symptoms and low testosterone levels determined the minimum criteria necessary to identify late-onset hypogonadism.

Conclusions.—Late-onset hypogonadism can be defined by the presence of at least three sexual symptoms associated with a total testosterone level of less than 11 nmol per liter (3.2 ng per milliliter) and a free testosterone level of less than 220 pmol per liter (64 pg per milliliter).

▶ Linear regression analysis was used to analyze this population sample of over 3000 men in Europe to determine which symptoms classically associated with hypogonadism are genuinely predictive of low testosterone level in a nonclinic population of men between the ages of 40 and 79 years. It was concluded that sexual symptoms, specifically decreased sexual thoughts, loss of AM erections, and erectile dysfunction, were significantly associated with total testosterone levels less than 3.2 ng/mL and a free testosterone level of 64 pg/mL. Threshold values were calculated for each of these 3 variables individually; the risk of decreased morning erection was most pronounced at total testosterone levels of 319 ng/dL (11 nmol/L), for low sexual thoughts at 232 ng/dL (8 nmol/L), and for erectile dysfunction at 247 ng/dL (8.5 nmol/L). Free testosterone threshold levels were approximately 160 pmol/L for low frequency of sexual thoughts and 280 pmol/L for both decreased morning erections and erectile dysfunction; however, addition of free testosterone data did little to change classification of patients, and the authors advised that free testosterone is typically not necessary for the diagnosis, except in borderline cases.

In addition to these 3 sexual symptoms, inability to engage in vigorous physical activity, inability to walk more than a kilometer, inability to bend/stoop/kneel, loss of energy, sadness, and fatigue were also significantly more likely in men with lower testosterone levels. Interestingly, based on the criteria of low serum testosterone levels and symptoms, just 2% of this population met criteria for the diagnosis of late-onset hypogonadism.

Testosterone has been widely hailed as a panacea by many men looking to restore youthful vigor, and there is little doubt that testosterone may play a very important role for select men with bothersome symptoms. Unfortunately, there has been a great deal of controversy of what constitutes a genuinely low testosterone level; reference ranges vary wildly between laboratories. It is also likely that many men have been and continue to be treated with testosterone supplementation for symptoms that do not necessarily meet criteria for true hypogonadism. Objective population-based data such as these provide much needed clarity with respect to what constitutes a testosterone level that is likely to be associated with clinically meaningful symptoms. Future studies on testosterone therapy for symptoms should use evidence-based criteria such as these rather than arbitrary serum testosterone level cut points for enrollment criteria.

A. Shindel, MD

The Dopamine Transporter Gene (*DAT1*) Polymorphism is Associated with Premature Ejaculation
Santtila P, Jern P, Westberg L, et al (Åbo Akademi Univ, Turku, Finland; Univ of Gothenburg, Sweden; et al)
J Sex Med 7:1538-1546, 2010

Introduction.—Previous research has suggested brain dopamine (DA) neurotransmission to be involved in the control of ejaculation. Furthermore, previous studies indicate a partly hereditary background to premature ejaculation.

Aim.—To investigate whether the dopamine transporter gene (*DAT1*) polymorphism is associated with premature ejaculation.

Methods.—Retrospective self-reports of four indicators reflecting ejaculatory function—anteportal ejaculation, number of penile thrusts, ejaculation latency time, and feeling of control over ejaculation—and saliva samples for DNA analysis were obtained from 1,290 men (M = 26.9, standard deviation = 4.7 years; range 18—45) with sexual experience.

Main Outcome Measures.—Calculations of allelic effects were computed using the Generalized Estimating Equations module of SPSS 17.

Results.—Carriers of the 10R10R genotype had scores indicating a lower threshold to ejaculate on each of the indicators compared to the combined 9R9R/9R10R carrier group. The differences were significant both for the composite score and for anteportal ejaculation, number of thrusts, and feeling of control over ejaculation, but not for ejaculation latency time. The effect of the polymorphism remained significant after controlling for age, homosexual experience, having a regular sexual partner, level of sexual desire, and frequency of sexual activity, hence suggesting that it is not secondary to an association between the studied polymorphism and some other aspect of sexual behavior, but due to a specific influence of DA on ejaculation.

Conclusions.—The findings of the present study support results of previous studies indicating involvement of dopaminergic neurotransmission in ejaculation.

▶ Long conceived of as a psychological disorder, the biological underpinnings of an early or a premature ejaculation (PE) continue to be elucidated. It is interesting to observe the evolution in our concept of PE; our understanding of the disorder seems to be developing in much the same way that erectile dysfunction changed from a primarily psychogenic to a primarily organic disorder.

Dopamine is known to have proerectile and proejaculatory actions as shown in many previous studies in both humans and animals. In this study, polymorphisms of the dopamine transporter gene (*DAT1*) were investigated in 1290 Scandinavian men. The protein product of *DAT1* is responsible for reuptake of dopamine from the synaptic cleft. The alleles of interest in this study are classified as 9-repeat (9R) and 10-repeat (10R); the 9R allele has been associated with greater dopaminergic activity in the brain. Men were queried using recall on various parameters germane to ejaculatory function.

When compared with men who were heterozygous for the alleles of interest or homozygous for the 9R polymorphism, men homozygous for the 10R genotype were significantly more likely to have anteportal ejaculation, a lower number of thrusts after penetration and prior to ejaculation, and a lack of control over ejaculation. The frequency of sexual activity and having a regular partner were associated with lower odds of PE. After multivariate adjustment for sexual characteristics and behaviors, including sexual desire and erectile function, men homozygous for the 10R allele still had a significantly greater risk of PE.

These data are somewhat counterintuitive as they suggest more rapid dopamine reuptake (as occurs with the 10R allele) is associated with more rapid ejaculation. This conflicts with previous research, underscoring the complexity of central neurotransmission. These data will hopefully spur greater interest in central regulation of ejaculation, particularly when taken in conjunction with previous reports suggesting that polymorphisms in the gene responsible for synthesis of the serotonin transporter also influence ejaculation latency.

A. Shindel, MD

Effect of Angiotensin II and its Receptor Antagonists on Human Corpus Cavernous Contractility and Oxidative Stress: Modulation of Nitric Oxide Mediated Relaxation

Ertemi H, Mumtaz FH, Howie AJ, et al (Univ College London Med School, Enfield, UK; Chase Farm Hosp, Enfield, UK)
J Urol 185:2414-2420, 2011

Purpose.—To our knowledge the interaction between angiotensin II and nitric oxide in the control of human corpus cavernous function has not been assessed previously. We determined the presence and role of angiotensin II and its receptors in human penile function.

Materials and Methods.—Corpus cavernous tissue was obtained from 35 patients undergoing gender reassignment surgery. Immunohistochemical analysis was done to determine angiotensin II peptide tissue distribution. Organ bath studies were done to determine the angiotensin II/nitric oxide interaction on corpus cavernous smooth muscle function. The role of oxidative stress in the angiotensin II response was also examined using the nicotinamide adenine dinucleotide phosphate oxidase inhibitor apocynin.

Results.—Angiotensin II was distributed in arteriolar endothelium, endothelium lining sinusoids and smooth muscle cells, and caused dose dependent contraction of human corpus cavernous smooth muscle strips that was inhibited by the angiotensin type 1 receptor antagonist losartan. Relaxation of corpus cavernous smooth muscle induced by the nitric oxide donor sodium nitroprusside or electrical field stimulation was potentiated by losartan. Apocynin decreased angiotensin II induced corpus cavernous contraction.

Conclusions.—Angiotensin II and nitric oxide interact to modulate human cavernous function since losartan potentiated sodium nitroprusside and electrical field stimulation mediated corpus cavernous smooth muscle relaxation. The angiotensin II response involves the production of superoxide and the development of oxidative stress. These findings support the role of angiotensin II in the regulation of human penile smooth muscle tone and suggest that angiotensin type 1 receptor inhibition may be a therapeutic approach to erectile dysfunction.

▶ In this study corporal tissue obtained during gender reassignment surgery in male to female transgendered persons was subjected to organ bath experiments to determine the role the vasoconstrictor angiotensin II in erectile physiology. All subjects had been treated with estrogens for at least 2 years, but therapy had been discontinued 2 months prior to tissue procurement.

The angiotensin II peptide was expressed diffusely throughout the corporal tissue. Treatment of the tissue fragments with angiotensin II led to marked smooth muscular contraction, which was inhibited by action of the angiotensin receptor blocker (ARB) losartan as well as by treatment with the nicotinamide adenine dinucleotide phosphate oxidase inhibitor apocynin, a known inhibitor of oxidative stress. It is implied from these data that angiotensin II exerts constrictive effects on penile smooth muscle at least in part by enhancing oxidative stress.

Data such as these suggest a novel therapeutic target for management of erectile dysfunction. Perhaps more importantly, these data give some credence to the use of ARB agents in the management of hypertension. Sexual dysfunction is a common side effect of many medications including β-blockers and thiazide diuretics; the rate of erectile dysfunction during ARB therapy appears to be less, and data such as these might explain this relationship.

A. Shindel, MD

Hypercholesterolemia-Induced Erectile Dysfunction: Endothelial Nitric Oxide Synthase (eNOS) Uncoupling in the Mouse Penis by NAD(P)H Oxidase

Musicki B, Liu T, Lagoda GA, et al (Johns Hopkins Univ, Baltimore, MD)
J Sex Med 2010 [Epub ahead of print]

Introduction.—Hypercholesterolemia induces erectile dysfunction (ED) mostly by increasing oxidative stress and impairing endothelial function in the penis, but the mechanisms regulating reactive oxygen species (ROS) production in the penis are not understood.

Aims.—We evaluated whether hypercholesterolemia activates nicotinamide adenine dinucleotide phosphate (NAD[P]H) oxidase in the penis, providing an initial source of ROS to induce endothelial nitric oxide synthase (eNOS) uncoupling and endothelial dysfunction resulting in ED.

Methods.—Low-density-lipoprotein receptor (LDLR)–null mice were fed Western diet for 4 weeks to induce early-stage hyperlipidemia. Wild type (WT) mice fed regular chow served as controls. Mice received NAD(P)H oxidase inhibitor apocynin (10 mM in drinking water) or vehicle. Erectile function was assessed in response to cavernous nerve electrical stimulation. Markers of endothelial function (phospho [P]-vasodilator-stimulated-protein [VASP]-Ser-239), oxidative stress (4-hydroxy-2-nonenal [HNE]), sources of ROS (eNOS uncoupling and NAD[P]H oxidase subunits $p67^{phox}$, $p47^{phox}$, and $gp91^{phox}$), P-eNOS-Ser-1177, and eNOS were measured by Western blot in penes.

Main Outcome Measures.—The main outcome measures are the molecular mechanisms of ROS generation and endothelial dysfunction in hypercholesterolemia-induced ED.

Results.—Erectile response was significantly ($P < 0.05$) reduced in hypercholesterolemic LDLR-null mice compared with WT mice. Relative to WT mice, hypercholesterolemia increased ($P < 0.05$) protein expressions of

NAD(P)H oxidase subunits $p67^{phox}$, $p47^{phox}$ and $gp91^{phox}$, eNOS uncoupling, and 4-HNE-modified proteins, and reduced ($P < 0.05$) P-VASP-Ser-239 expression in the penis. Apocynin treatment of LDLR-null mice preserved ($P < 0.05$) maximal intracavernosal pressure, and reversed ($P < 0.05$) the abnormalities in protein expressions of $gp67^{phox}$ and $gp47^{phox}$, 4-HNE, P-VASP-Ser-239, and eNOS uncoupling in the penis. Apocynin treatment of WT mice did not affect any of these parameters. Protein expressions of P-eNOS-Ser-1177 and total eNOS were unaffected by hypercholesterolemia.

Conclusion.—Activated NAD(P)H oxidase in the penis is an initial source of oxidative stress resulting in eNOS uncoupling, thus providing a mechanism of eNOS uncoupling and endothelial dysfunction in hypercholesterolemia-induced ED.

▶ The molecular mechanisms underlying hypercholesterolemia-induced erectile dysfunction (ED) are investigated in this mouse study. The authors determined that the nicotinamide adenine dinucleotide phosphate (NAD[P]H) oxidase is activated in low-density lipoprotein receptor—deficient mice (a model system for familial hypercholesterolemia) fed a high-fat diet to induce hyperlipidemia. This activation was associated with declines in average intracavernosal pressure (ICP) response to cavernous nerve electrostimulation and decreased activity of endothelial nitric oxide synthase. The decline in maximal ICP was prevented by treatment with the NAD[P]H oxidase inhibitor apocynin, although the more precise metric of ICP area (the total area under the pressure transducer curve during cavernous nerve electrostimulation, a more accurate assessment of total erectile response) was not entirely normalized by treatment with apocynin. It is implied that numerous pathways are likely involved in the pathogenesis of hyperlipidemia-associated erectile impairment, and NAD[P]H oxidase is one of the more critical ones.

NAD[P]H oxidase is a potent mediator of oxidative stress, and hence these data highlight the importance of reactive oxygen species in the pathogenesis of hyperlipidemia-associated vascular disease. This study is of benefit in that it does help to elucidate mechanisms by which research on interventions for hyperlipidemia-induced ED may proceed; however, it is clear that a more direct (if more difficult) approach to manage this problem would be to take steps to prevent the development of hyperlipidemia in the first place.

A. Shindel, MD

Atorvastatin improves the response to sildenafil in hypercholesterolemic men with erectile dysfunction not initially responsive to sildenafil
Dadkhah F, Safarinejad MR, Asgari MA, et al (Shahid Beheshti Univ (MC), Tehran, Iran)
Int J Impot Res 22:51-60, 2010

Despite the initial enthusiasm, the significant number of patients in whom sildenafil is contraindicated or ineffective is a major challenge to all urologists. Our aim was to determine the safety and efficacy of adjunctive atorvastatin in restoring normal erectile function in hypercholesterolemic (low-density lipoprotein (LDL) cholesterol >120 mg per 100 ml) sildenafil nonresponders. The study comprised 131 men with ED not responding to sildenafil citrate. They were randomized either to 40 mg atorvastatin daily ($n = 66$, group 1) or matching placebo ($n = 65$, group 2) for 12 weeks while they were taking on-demand 100 mg sildenafil. Erectile function was subjectively assessed using the 5-item version of the International Index of Erectile Function (IIEF-5) questionnaire and response to the global efficacy question (GEQ). Serum biochemical and lipid profile (total cholesterol, triglycerides, LDL cholesterol and high-density lipoprotein cholesterol) analyses were performed at baseline and repeated at post-treatment weeks 6 and 12. Compared with the placebo group (59 patients, mean age ± s.d. 61.9 ± 6.1, mean years ED 3.9 ± 1.8), the atorvastatin group (59 patients, mean age ± s.d. 63.9 ± 6.9, mean years ED 3.7 ± 1.6) had significantly greater improvements in all IIEF-5 questions ($P = 0.01$) and GEQ ($P = 0.001$). Subgroup analyses did reveal trends in the atorvastatin group to indicate that a change in the IIEF-5 score is affected by age, severity of ED and baseline serum levels of LDL. Patients with moderate ($r = 0.28$, $P = 0.01$) and severe ($r = 0.20$, $P = 0.01$) ED had better positive response rates to adjunctive atorvastatin than patients with mild to moderate ED. None of the patients taking atorvastatin achieved a response of 5 to the IIEF-5 questions and none of the patients regained normal erectile function as defined by the IIEF-5 score >21. Subjects experienced a statistically significant but modest improvement in erectile function. Further investigation is needed to test the usefulness of long-term atorvastatin administration to restore erectile function in sildenafil nonresponders.

▶ A growing body of evidence supports the use of adjunctive measures for men initially refractory to phosphodiesterase type 5 inhibitors. Testosterone supplementation, exercise, weight loss, and dose escalation have all been advanced as means to enhance responsiveness to treatment in this population of men. In this double-blind, placebo-controlled, randomized study, adjunctive treatment with atorvastatin 40 mg or placebo for 12 weeks was instituted in 118 men with erectile dysfunction (ED) not responsive to sildenafil, who were not hypercholesterolemic (ie, total cholesterol level less than 200 mg per 100 mL and low-density lipoprotein level less than 160 mg per 100 mL). Men continued with on-demand sildenafil during this treatment period. It was found that there was a significant but modest improvement in the mean International Index of Erectile Function 5 scores, a difference that was more pronounced in patients with moderate or severe ED at baseline. Thirty-seven percent of the patients given atorvastatin reported statistically significant improvement in response to sildenafil relative to 12% of the patients in the placebo group ($P < .01$). No patients, however, normalized their erectile function scores, implying that this treatment is not a complete amelioration of the condition.

It is possible that some of these nonresponder patients improved with re-education on proper use of the medication, although the subjects in this study had apparently failed even after a previous attempt at re-education, so this seems somewhat less likely. It is logical to speculate that the positive endothelial effects of statin medications may improve penile hemodynamics; this slight benefit must be weighed against the similarly slight but finite risk of hepatotoxicity or other complications from this medical therapy.

A. Shindel, MD

Is Testosterone a Friend or a Foe of the Prostate?

Jannini EA, Gravina GL, Mortengaler A, et al (Univ of L'Aquila, Italy; Harvard Med School, Boston, MA; et al)
J Sex Med 8:946-955, 2011

Introduction.—Is there any unequivocal evidence that testosterone (T) can stimulate growth and aggravate symptoms in men with locally advanced and metastatic prostate cancer (PCa)? This is not a controversial point: the answer is yes. However, this evidence does not imply that PCa is a result of T or therapy with T (TTh) of hypogonadal men. Furthermore, currently adequately powered and optimally designed long-term prostate disease data are not available to determine if there is an additional risk from normal T values in cured patients for PCa.

Methods.—This Controversy is introduced by an endocrinologist, the section editor (E.A.J.) with G.L.G., a fellow urologist and radiotherapist expert in basic research on PCa. Two outstanding urologists, A.M and W.J.G.H., debate clinical data and clinical guidelines, respectively. Finally, other controversial issues are discussed by another leader in the field (A.M.) and a radiation oncologist and sexologist who is actually president of the International Society for Sexuality and Cancer (L.I.).

Main Outcome Measure.—Expert opinion supported by the critical review of the currently available literature.

Result.—The answer to the main question "is the prostate a really T-dependent tissue?" is definitively yes, but T stimulates the prostatic tissue in a dose—dependent fashion only to a saturation point, achieved at low T concentrations. At these low T concentrations, stimulation is near maximal, and T supplementation above this level would not lead to significantly greater stimulation. Furthermore, there is no conclusive evidence that TTh increases the risk of PCa or even prostatic hyperplasia. There is also no evidence that TTh will convert subclinical PCa to clinically detectable PCa. However, there is a limited clinical experience of TTh after successful treatment of PCa. So far, just 48 patients have been studied in the three published articles.

Conclusions.—It is evident that the issue is still controversial and much more research is needed. However, the available data suggest to the expert in sexual medicine that TTh can be cautiously considered in selected hypogonadal men previously treated for curative intent of low-risk PCa and without evidence of active disease.

▶ For decades, it was the prevailing opinion of the medical community that testosterone therapy increased the odds of prostate cancer and that hypogonadism should never be treated with testosterone in men who carried the diagnosis of prostate or breast cancer. This conventional wisdom has been challenged in the past several decades, and a bevy of publications, many by the authors of this review article, have reported on the use of testosterone in men with prostate cancer and the relationship between testosterone and prostate tissue.

The principle proponents of testosterone therapy hypothesize that while testosterone exerts a trophic effect on prostate cancer, this effect occurs at relatively low levels of serum testosterone; supplementation above that level does not appreciably enhance the risks of stimulating prostate cancer development or growth. This saturation hypothesis is interesting and has some support based on studies (cited in this review) in which androgen supplementation to even supraphysiological levels did not induce changes in the prostate. However, controversy about this hypothesis exists, and further work needs to be done to validate or reject it. Many (but not all) of the authors of this article suggest judicious and cautious use of testosterone in men with prostate cancer, and all advocate for more research on the use of testosterone therapy in these men. Particular caution is indicated in cases of high-risk prostate cancer; studies on men with low- or intermediate-risk prostate cancer should precede investigation of the role of testosterone therapy in men with aggressive disease.

A. Shindel, MD

Physical Activity and PDE5 Inhibitors in the Treatment of Erectile Dysfunction: Results of a Randomized Controlled Study
Maio G, Saraeb S, Marchiori A (Policlinico Abano Terme, Padova, Italy; S. Antonio Hosp, Padova, Italy)
J Sex Med 7:2201-2208, 2010

Introduction.—Physical activity (PhA) has proven to be a protective factor for normal erectile function in numerous epidemiological studies.

Aim.—The aim of this study was to establish if PhA could have a therapeutic role in the treatment of erectile dysfunction (ED).

Methods.—This was a randomized, open-label study. A total of 60 patients complaining of ED were studied. Patients were assessed at baseline and after 3 months of study treatment. At baseline, patients were randomized to receive phosphodiesterase type 5 inhibitor (PDE5i) alone (group A) or PDE5i plus regular ($\geq$3 hours/week), aerobic, non-agonistic PhA (group B).

Main Outcome Measures.—All subjects completed the International Index of Erectile Function (IIEF-15) questionnaire and performed total testosterone (TT).

Results.—Mean PhA was 3.4 hours/week in group B vs. 0.43 in group A; mean energy expenditure in group B was 1,868 kcal/week or 22.8 metabolic equivalent (MET)/week. IIEF restoration of ED occurred in 77.8% (intervention group) vs. 39.3% (control) ($P < 0.004$). The IIEF-15 score resulted in statistical improvement in intervention group in all the domains but one (orgasm): erectile function 24.7 vs. 26.8 ($P = 0.003$); confidence (Q15) 3.53 vs. 4.07 ($P = 0.006$); sexual desire 6.46 vs. 7.18 ($P = 0.028$); intercourse satisfaction 9.85 vs. 11.25 ($P = 0.001$); total satisfaction 7.17 vs. 8.07 ($P = 0.009$); total score 56.2 vs. 61.07 ($P = 0.007$). TT was statistically similar in the two groups; separate analysis in each group showed statistical increase in group B 4.24 vs. 4.55 ($P = 0.012$). At multivariate logistic regression analysis, PhA was the only independent variable for normal erection ($P = 0.010$) (95% confidence interval [CI] 0.036–0.643), higher sexual satisfaction ($P = 0.022$) (95% CI 0.084–0.821) and normal total IIEF-15 score ($P = 0.023$) (95% CI 0.85–0.83).

Conclusion.—In this randomized controlled pilot study, PDE5i plus PhA was more effective than PDE5i alone in the treatment of ED.

► Exercise interventions are particularly challenging to investigate, given the impossibility of blinding. Nevertheless, it is widely accepted that exercise may have important health and sexual benefits. In this randomized open-label study, 55 men with erectile dysfunction (ED) and less than 2 hours per week of exercise activity at baseline were treated with either phosphodiesterase type 5 inhibitors (PDE5I) alone and general advice about the importance of physical activity or PDE5I with a regimented program of moderate physical activity (55%-64% of maximum heart rate) 3 to 5 days a week for a weekly total of at least 3 hours for a period of 3 months. Men in the physical activity arm had the option of participating in whatever form of exercise was most appealing to them. Men in this group engaged in a mean of 3.4 hours of aerobic activity per week compared with less than half an hour of such activity in the PDE5I-alone group. Seventy-eight percent of men in the physical activity group experienced restoration of erectile function compared with 39% of the control group. Men in the exercise group also experienced significantly greater mean improvement in the International Index of Erectile Function domain scores for desire, sexual satisfaction, overall satisfaction, and confidence with erections. After multivariable adjustment, physical activity remained independently associated with enhanced sexual function.

It is abundantly clear that physical activity is protective against erectile function. These data go further to suggest that exercise may either reverse pathological processes and/or enhance response to ED therapies. It behooves practitioners to encourage their patients to make healthy lifestyle choices as part of their overall sexual dysfunction treatment regimen; this will likely improve treatment efficacy and general markers of health.

A. Shindel, MD

Adverse Events Associated with Testosterone Administration

Basaria S, Coviello AD, Travison TG, et al (Boston Univ School of Medicine and Boston Med Ctr, MA; et al)
N Engl J Med 363:109-122, 2010

Background.—Testosterone supplementation has been shown to increase muscle mass and strength in healthy older men. The safety and efficacy of testosterone treatment in older men who have limitations in mobility have not been studied.

Methods.—Community-dwelling men, 65 years of age or older, with limitations in mobility and a total serum testosterone level of 100 to 350 ng per deciliter (3.5 to 12.1 nmol per liter) or a free serum testosterone level of less than 50 pg per milliliter (173 pmol per liter) were randomly assigned to receive placebo gel or testosterone gel, to be applied daily for 6 months. Adverse events were categorized with the use of the Medical Dictionary for Regulatory Activities classification. The data and safety monitoring board recommended that the trial be discontinued early because there was a significantly higher rate of adverse cardiovascular events in the testosterone group than in the placebo group.

Results.—A total of 209 men (mean age, 74 years) were enrolled at the time the trial was terminated. At baseline, there was a high prevalence of hypertension, diabetes, hyperlipidemia, and obesity among the participants. During the course of the study, the testosterone group had higher rates of cardiac, respiratory, and dermatologic events than did the placebo group. A total of 23 subjects in the testosterone group, as compared with 5 in the placebo group, had cardiovascular-related adverse events. The relative risk of a cardiovascular-related adverse event remained constant throughout the 6-month treatment period. As compared with the placebo group, the testosterone group had significantly greater improvements in leg-press and chest-press strength and in stair climbing while carrying a load.

Conclusions.—In this population of older men with limitations in mobility and a high prevalence of chronic disease, the application of a testosterone gel was associated with an increased risk of cardiovascular adverse events. The small size of the trial and the unique population prevent broader inferences from being made about the safety of testosterone therapy. (ClinicalTrials.gov number, NCT00240981.)

▶ In this important double-blind, placebo-controlled, randomized study, 209 elderly hypogonadal (total serum testosterone 100-350 ng/dL or free testosterone 50 pg/mL) men with limitations in their mobility received treatment with testosterone gel versus placebo. Men in the treatment group received testosterone dose titration such that their serum levels were between 500 and 1000 ng/dL. The study was terminated prematurely secondary to a significantly elevated rate of cardiac events in men in the testosterone arm versus placebo-treated men; after adjustment, testosterone-treated men had an odds ratio of 5.8 for cardiovascular-related events (defined in this study as vascular stenting and bypass procedures, peripheral edema, elevated blood pressure, arrhythmias, electrocardiographic changes, stroke, and syncope) based on 23 events in men in the treatment group and 5 in men in the placebo group. Atherosclerosis-related events (defined as myocardial infarction, sudden death, angioplasty, coronary-artery bypass surgery, and stroke) occurred in 7 men in the treatment group and 1 in the placebo group. The number of adverse events deemed life threatening was higher in the testosterone treatment group, although the difference did not attain statistical significance. Of minor note, testosterone-treated men did experience significantly greater improvement in chest and leg strength as well as ability to climb stairs while carrying weight.

Interestingly, there was a slight but significant difference in the racial makeup of the 2 groups; African American men accounted for 4% of the placebo group and 14% of the treatment group. Furthermore, the mean free testosterone was higher in the treatment group at baseline, and more men in the treatment group were on antihypertensive and/or statin therapy and carried the diagnosis of hyperlipidemia. However, after multivariate analysis these baseline statistics did not account for the difference in rate of adverse events.

The authors enumerate a number of limitations of this study; it was not designed to detect differences in cardiac morbidity, it enrolled elderly men with numerous chronic comorbid conditions (differing from many other studies of testosterone therapy), and there was no one type of cardiovascular event that drove the significant differences, making a parsimonious physiological explanation difficult to conjure, although prior studies indicate a number of possible explanations. Furthermore, early termination of the study might have compromised the true predictive capacity of the overall trial. Be that as it may, the decision to terminate this particular study was certainly reasonable and prudent.

These data are important for physicians providing testosterone supplementation to men. Men who derive benefit from testosterone therapy should not be instantaneously taken off of such therapy or denied access to it, but a frank and honest discussion of these new findings should become part of the conversation men have with their doctors about the risks and potential benefits of testosterone therapy.

A. Shindel, MD

Adipose Tissue-Derived Stem Cells Secrete CXCL5 Cytokine with Neurotrophic Effects on Cavernous Nerve Regeneration

Zhang H, Yang R, Wang Z, et al (Univ of California, San Francisco; Ninth People's Hosp Affiliated to Med College of Shanghai Jiao-Tong Univ, China)
J Sex Med 8:437-446, 2011

Introduction.—Previously we reported that paracrine actions likely mediated the therapeutic effects of adipose tissue-derived stem cells (ADSCs) on a rat model of cavernous nerve (CN) injury.

Aim.—To identify potential neurotrophic factors in ADSC's secretion, test the most promising one, and identify the molecular mechanism of its neurotrophic action.

Methods.—Rat major pelvic ganglia (MPG) were cultured in conditioned media of ADSC and penile smooth muscle cells (PSMCs). Cytokine expression in these two media was probed with a cytokine antibody array. CXCL5 cytokine was quantified in these two media by enzyme-linked immunosorbent assay (ELISA). Activation of Janus Kinase/Signal Transducer and Activator of Transcription (JAK/STAT) by CXCL5 was tested in neuroblastoma cell lines BE(2)C and SH-SY5Y as well as in Schwann cell line RT4-D6P2T by Western blot. Involvement of CXCL5 and JAK/STAT in ADSC-conditioned medium's neurotrophic effects was confirmed with anti-CXCL5 antibody and JAK inhibitor AG490, respectively.

Main Outcome Measures.—Neurotrophic effects of ADSC and PSMC-conditioned media were quantified by measuring neurite length in MPG cultures. Secretion of CXCL5 in these two media was quantified by ELISA. Activation of JAK/STAT by CXCL5 was quantified by densitometry on Western blots for STAT1 and STAT3 phosphorylation.

Results.—MPG neurite length was significantly longer in ADSC than in PSMC-conditioned medium. CXCL5 was secreted eight times higher in ADSC than in PSMC-conditioned medium. Anti-CXCL5 antibody blocked the neurotrophic effects of ADSC-conditioned medium. CXCL5 activated JAK/STAT concentration-dependently from 0 to 50 ng/mL in RT4-D6P2T Schwann cells. At 50 ng/mL, CXCL5 activated JAK/STAT time-dependently, peaking at 45 minutes. AG490 blocked these activities as well as the neurotrophic effects of ADSC-conditioned medium.

Conclusions.—CXCL5 was secreted by ADSC at a high level, promoted MPG neurite growth, and activated JAK/STAT in Schwann cells. CXCL5 may contribute to ADSC's therapeutic efficacy on CN injury-induced ED.

▶ Stem cell therapy has shown promising results in the therapy of erectile dysfunction (ED) from a variety of sources. A persistent problem has been elucidation of the molecular mechanisms underlying these effects. A previous report from this laboratory indicated that a lysate of adipose-derived stem cells (ADSCs) was efficacious in reversing cavernous nerve injury–associated erectile impairment in a rat model.[1] This follow-up study suggests that the ADSC-derived cytokine CXCL5 may play an important role in this process.

Cultured fragments of the rat major pelvic ganglion (MPG) were shown to grow longer neurites when cultured with medium primed by ADSC, an affect that was attenuated when anti-CXCL5 antibody or an inhibitor of the Janus Kinase/Signal Transducer Activator of Transcription (JAK/STAT) was incubated with the specimens. While a direct upregulation of JAK/STAT by CXCL5 was not assessed in MPG fragments, a separate series of experiments indicated that this cytokine does upregulate JAK/STAT in cultured Schwann cells.

JAK/STAT is known to be involved in neurotrophic pathways, and hence, it seems likely that this effect may be responsible for the improvements in nerve function reported in prior studies of stem cell therapy for ED. Mechanistic studies such as these are paving the way for further progress in human application of stem cells for this troubling condition.

A. Shindel, MD

Reference

1. Albersen M, Fandel TM, Lin G, et al. Injections of adipose tissue-derived stem cells and stem cell lysate improve recovery of erectile function in a rat model of cavernous nerve injury. *J Sex Med.* 2010;7:3331-3340.

Testosterone Levels and Quality of Life in Diverse Male Patients With Cancers Unrelated to Androgens

Fleishman SB, Khan H, Homel P, et al (Beth Israel Med Ctr and St Luke's-Roosevelt Hosp, NY; Helen F. Graham Cancer Ctr, Newark, DE)

J Clin Oncol 28:5054-5060, 2010

Purpose.—Symptoms secondary to hormonal changes significantly impact quality of life (QoL) in patients with cancer. This cross-sectional study examines prevalence of hypogonadism and its correlation with QoL and sexual dysfunction.

Patients and Methods.—We collected blood and medical histories from 428 male patients with non—testosterone-related cancer at three cancer centers. Serum was analyzed for total testosterone (TT), free testosterone (FT), bioavailable testosterone (BAT), and sex hormone binding globulin (SHBG). The Functional Assessment of Cancer Therapy-Prostate (FACT-P) QoL questionnaire measured physical, social, emotional, and functional domains as well as sexual function. Exclusion criteria were prostate, testicular, or male breast cancer; known hypogonadism; and HIV.

Results.—Mean and median TTs were 337.46 and 310 ng/dL, respectively. The mean age of patients was 62.05 years. The crude prevalence of hypogonadism (ie, TT < 300 ng/dL) was 48%, and mean TT in hypogonadal patients was 176 ng/dL. The prevalences that were based on FT (ie, hypogonadal < 52 pg/dL) and BAT (ie, hypogonadal < 95 ng/dL) were 78% and 66%, respectively. The mean FT and BAT values in hypogonadal patients were 25 pg/dL and 45 ng/dL, respectively. Hypogonadal patients had decreased total QoL scores on FACT-P ($P = .01$) and decreased three-item sexual function subset ($P = .003$).

Conclusion.—The prevalence of hypogonadism was unexpectedly high. Measurement of FT or BAT detected a higher prevalence than TT alone, which confirmed previous studies. Correlation of T with FACT-P showed significant reduction of both overall QoL and sexual function for hypogonadal men. BAT and FT levels showed a stronger correlation than TT with overall FACT-P and subscales. The prevalence of symptomatic hypogonadism in male patients with cancer exceeds that found in comparable studies in noncancer populations.

▶ Androgens have been a topic of great interest in the study of prostate cancer and to a lesser extent in testicular and male breast cancer. The relationship between androgens and cancers with no known hormonal sensitivity is less well understood. In this prospective cohort of study of male patients with nonhormone-sensitive malignancies, it was determined that the prevalence of low testosterone (defined here as total testosterone < 300 ng/dL) was relatively high at 48%, with the rate even higher when stratified by free and bioavailable testosterone levels. Hypogonadism was present in 58% of men with respiratory cancers but in just 43% of men with gastrointestinal cancers; however, this difference was not statistically significant, and no specific type of cancer was associated with greater odds of hypogonadism.

Obesity, opioid use, white ethnicity, and poorer sexual function were all independently associated with greater odds of hypogonadism on logistic regression. Low testosterone state was associated with greater odds of sexual problems and lower overall quality of life.

The use of testosterone therapy in malignant disease is a topic in need of more thorough research. The potential benefits with respect to quality of life and vitality and weight maintenance might be considerable.

A. Shindel, MD

Can Low-Intensity Extracorporeal Shockwave Therapy Improve Erectile Function? A 6-Month Follow-up Pilot Study in Patients with Organic Erectile Dysfunction

Vardi Y, Appel B, Jacob G, et al (Rambam Healthcare Campus and the Technion, Haifa, Israel)

Eur Urol 58:243-248, 2010

Background.—Low-intensity extracorporeal shockwave therapy (LI-ESWT) is currently under investigation regarding its ability to promote neovascularization in different organs.

Objective.—To evaluate the effect of LI-ESWT on men with erectile dysfunction (ED) who have previously responded to oral phosphodiesterase type 5 inhibitors (PDE5-I).

Design, Setting, and Participants.—We screened 20 men with vasculogenic ED who had International Index of Erectile Function ED (IIEF-ED) domain scores between 5−19 (average: 13.5) and abnormal nocturnal penile tumescence (NPT) parameters. Shockwave therapy comprised two treatment sessions per week for 3 wk, which were repeated after a 3-wk no-treatment interval.

Intervention.—LI-ESWT was applied to the penile shaft and crura at five different sites.

Measurements.—Assessment of erectile function was performed at screening and at 1 mo after the end of the two treatment sessions using validated sexual function questionnaires, NPT parameters, and penile and systemic endothelial function testing. The IIEF-ED questionnaire was answered at the 3- and 6-mo follow-up examinations.

Results and Limitations.—We treated 20 middle-aged men (average age: 56.1 yr) with vasculogenic ED (mean duration: 34.7 mo). Eighteen had cardiovascular risk factors. At 1 mo follow-up, significant increases in IIEF-ED domain scores were recorded in all men (20.9 ± 5.8 vs

13.5 ± 4.1, $p < 0.001$); these remained unchanged at 6 mo. Moreover, significant increases in the duration of erection and penile rigidity, and significant improvement in penile endothelial function were demonstrated. Ten men did not require any PDE5-I therapy after 6-mo follow-up. No pain was reported from the treatment and no adverse events were noted during follow-up.

Conclusions.—This is the first study that assessed the efficacy of LI-ESWT for ED. This approach was tolerable and effective, suggesting a physiologic impact on cavernosal hemodynamics. Its main advantages are the potential to improve erectile function and to contribute to penile rehabilitation without pharmacotherapy. The short-term results are promising, yet demand further evaluation with larger sham-control cohorts and longer follow-up.

▶ Extracorporeal Shockwave Lithotripsy (ESWL) has been investigated for the treatment of Peyronie disease (PD) with marginal and conflicting results. Most sexual medicine experts no longer use this modality for treatment of PD. However, there has been new interest in low-intensity ESWL as a treatment for erectile dysfunction (ED); this approach has some preliminary evidence supporting its use in other vasculopathic conditions. In this pilot study, 20 men with mild/moderate to severe ED (International Index of Erectile Function [IIEF]-ED domain score 5-19) responsive to medical management with phosphodiesterase type 5 inhibitors (PDE5Is) were treated with ESWL for a total of 12 sessions over a 9-week period. Follow-up was carried out with assessment of penile endothelial function by measurement of flow-mediated dilation after penile vascular occlusion 1 month posttreatment and repeat survey with the IIEF-ED at 3 and 6 months posttreatment. A variety of other measures of sexual function were also obtained, including the Self-Esteem and Relationship Quality survey and nocturnal penile tumescence testing.

There were no adverse events in any patients. Endothelial function improved, and 14 of the men experienced at least a 5-point (clinically significant) improvement in IIEF-ED score. More importantly, half of the men reported that they no longer required PDE5I for sexual intercourse.

These results are compelling and suggest a new and potentially completely novel approach to the management of vasculogenic ED. Controlled studies of longer than 6 months duration are necessary to verify these results and to rule out placebo effect. It will also be of interest to elucidate the mechanisms underlying any putative benefit that is obtained with this approach and whether or not this approach would have any efficacy in patients who are not responsive to PDE5I.

A. Shindel, MD

A Cross-Sectional Study for the Analysis of Clinical, Sexual and Laboratory Conditions Associated to Peyronie's Disease

Rhoden EL, Riedner CE, Fuchs S, et al (Universidade Federal do Rio Grande do Sul (UFRGS)—Postgraduate Course in Med Sciences, Porto Alegre, RS, Brazil; Hospital Militar de Porto Alegre—Serviço de Urologia, Porto Alegre, Brazil; et al)
J Sex Med 7:1529-1537, 2010

Introduction.—Although Peyronie's Disease (PD) was first described over 250 years ago, its precise etiology remains obscure.

Aim.—Analyze a variety of potential associated factors with PD, including erectile dysfunction.

Materials and Methods.—This cross-sectional study included 83 consecutive men with PD and 252 age-matched controls. All men completed the International Index of Erectile Function (IIEF) and were evaluated regarding their clinical and demographic characteristics, comorbidities, and used medications. Anthropometric measures included body mass index and waist circumference (WC). Fasting blood glucose, lipid profile, total testosterone, and dehydroepiandrosterone-sulfate were determined.

Main Outcome Measures.—Clinical and laboratory characteristics associated to PD.

Results.—The mean age was 59.2 ± 10 years in the cases and 59.7 ± 12 years in the controls. Marital status, current smoking, and excessive consumption of alcoholic beverages were similar between groups ($P > 0.05$). PD was more common among white skin color males ($P = 0.001$). The mean score for each IIEF domain and the androgen levels were similar in the two groups. Thiazides were the only medication associated to PD ($P = 0.03$). Dupuytren's disease was more frequent among individuals with PD ($P = 0.001$). The distribution of all other comorbidities investigated was similar between groups ($P > 0.05$). The characteristics WC > 102 cm and levels of low-density lipoprotein (LDL) > 130 mg/dL were more prevalent in the controls ($P < 0.05$). After multivariate analysis, white skin color (OR: 8.47, 95%CI: 1.98—36.24) and thiazide use (OR: 2.29, 95%CI: 1.07—4.90) were associated to PD, and LDL > 130 mg/dL (OR: 0.55, 95%CI: 0.32—0.92) and WC > 102 cm (OR: 0.53, 95%CI: 0.29—0.96) were inversely associated to PD.

Conclusions.—In this study, PD was more common among white skin colored males. An inverse relationship with the presence of elevated serum levels of LDL and WC was observed. We found no association with medications other than thiazides and comorbidities other than Dupuytren's disease. Androgen serum levels and sexual dysfunction had also no association to PD.

▶ This review article investigates comorbidities and associations of Peyronie disease (PD). A study cohort of 83 men with PD was compared with an age-matched group of men (n = 252) without PD; all subjects were assessed using demographic characteristics, anthropomorphic measures, the International

Index of Erectile Function, and serum studies. On multivariate analysis, it was found that Caucasian men and those using thiazide diuretics were significantly more likely to have PD relative to controls, whereas hyperlipidemia (low-density lipoprotein > 130 mg/dL) and obesity (waist circumference greater than 102 cm) were associated with significantly lower odds of PD.

In this study, men were allocated to the PD arm based on physical examination findings rather than on clinical presentations, so the study cohort does not necessarily represent men who are primarily concerned with PD. Indeed, just 42% of the PD cohort was aware that they had a penile lesion. This recruitment method is the most likely reason why sexual dysfunction was not higher in men with PD, as many of these men likely had very mild disease with no deformity. Caucasian men represented a very large proportion of the total cohort (87.5%), so the higher prevalence of PD in this population will require more thorough investigation to verify this finding.

Of greater potential concern and interest is the association between thiazides and PD. Thiazides are associated with erectile dysfunction; it is unclear how these antihypertensive agents may be related to PD, and further studies are required to determine if, in fact, this relationship is consistent or causal. The relationship between PD and lipid parameters/waist circumference is puzzling. It is unlikely that these factors are intrinsically protective against PD, although it is conceivable that behavioral changes in men with vascular comorbidity may influence the risk factors for PD.

A. Shindel, MD

Role for Tyrosine Kinases in Contraction of Rat Penile Small Arteries
Villalba N, Kun A, Stankevicius E, et al (Univ of Aarhus, Denmark)
J Sex Med 7:2086-2095, 2010

Introduction.—The devasting effect of cancer and treatment thereof contribute to sexual dysfunction. Recently, a series of tyrosine kinase inhibitors have been approved either as add-on or for targeted treatment of cancer. However, tyrosine kinases are not only important for cell growth and proliferation, but also in regulation of vascular tone.

Aim.—The present study investigated whether tyrosine kinases contribute to contractility in rat penile arteries, and addressed whether they are involved in calcium entry and/or related to the RhoA/Rho-kinase pathway.

Methods.—Segments of the rat dorsal penile artery were mounted in microvascular myographs for simultaneous measurements of intracellular calcium concentration ($[Ca^{2+}]_i$) and tension, and tyrosine kinase activity, and phosphorylation of 20-kDa myosin light chain (MLC_{20}) was measured in dorsal penile artery homogenates.

Main Outcome Measures.—In vitro evidence for contractility and changes in intracellular Ca^{2+} in small penile arteries.

Results.—Sodium vanadate (Na_3VO_4, 1 mM), a tyrosine phosphatase inhibitor, increased $[Ca^{2+}]_i$ and tension. A L-type calcium channel blocker, nifedipine (1 μM), markedly reduced Na_3VO_4-evoked increases in $[Ca^{2+}]_i$ and tension. A thromboxane analog, U46619, increased TK activity. In contrast to the inactive analogue, genistein, a general TK inhibitor, concentration-dependently reduced both U46619-evoked contraction, and $[Ca^{2+}]_i$. U46619-induced contraction was markedly inhibited by tyrphostin A23 and bis-tyrphostin, whereas there was no effect of the tyrosine kinase c-Src inhibitor, herbimycin A. Tyrphostin A23 suppressed U46619-mediated phosphorylation of MLC_{20}.

Conclusions.—This study suggests that activation of tyrosine kinases is involved in contraction of rat penile smooth muscle probably by regulation of calcium entry through L-type calcium channels. These findings may have implications for the selections of novel add on anticancer treatments, e.g., inhibitors of tyrosine kinases, and for novel approaches to treat erectile dysfunction.

▶ Tyrosine kinase inhibitors (TKIs) are a relatively new class of chemotherapeutic agents that act by inhibiting TKs, a class of enzyme with a variety of functions, including cell proliferation. Interestingly, TK enzymes also appear to play a contributing role in vascular contraction of small arteries.

In this experiment, rat penile small arteries were harvested and subjected to organ bath experiments to elucidate the actions of TK and TKI in this model system. Through a series of inhibitor experiments, it was elucidated that TK enzymes are involved in smooth muscle contraction by modulating the phosphorylation status of the myosin light chain and the patency of membrane-bound calcium channels. The TKI, genistein blocked calcium influx and muscle tension in response to the thromboxane analog U46619 and phenylephrine. Additional experiments suggested that both nonselective and receptor-selective TKI were effective at attenuating U46619-mediated muscle contraction.

These data are clearly very preliminary. However, TK enzymes are an intriguing target for additional research on novel means to treat erectile dysfunction. It will also be of interest to gather additional data on the sexual side-effect profile of TKI as long-term data become available. While it may be too much to hope that this chemotherapeutic agent will have a beneficial effect on erectile function, these data are quite intriguing.

A. Shindel, MD

Amyloid β Precursor Protein Regulates Male Sexual Behavior

Park JH, Bonthius PJ, Tsai H-W, et al (Univ of Virginia School of Medicine, Charlottesville)
J Neurosci 30:9967-9972, 2010

Sexual behavior is variable between individuals, ranging from celibacy to sexual addictions. Within normal populations of individual men, ranging from young to middle aged, testosterone levels do not correlate with libido. To study the genetic mechanisms that contribute to individual differences in male sexual behavior, we used hybrid B6D2F1 male mice, which are a cross between two common inbred strains (C57BL/6J and DBA/2J). Unlike most laboratory rodent species in which male sexual behavior is highly dependent upon gonadal steroids, sexual behavior in a large proportion of these hybrid male mice after castration is independent of gonadal steroid hormones and their receptors; thus, we have the ability to discover novel genes involved in this behavior. Gene expression arrays, validation of gene candidates, and transgenic mice that overexpress one of the genes of interest were used to reveal genes involved in maintenance of male sexual behavior. Several genes related to neuroprotection and neurodegeneration were differentially expressed in the hypothalamus of males that continued to mate after castration. Male mice overexpressing the human form of one of these candidate genes, amyloid β precursor protein (*APP*), displayed enhanced sexual behavior before castration and maintained sexual activity for a longer duration after castration compared with controls. Our results reveal a novel and unexpected relationship between APP and male sexual behavior. We speculate that declining APP during normal aging in males may contribute to the loss of sexual function.

▶ In this study, the role of amyloid precursor protein (APP) in modulation of male sexual motivation was investigated in a strain of hybrid mice that exhibit patterns of sexual activity that appear to be independent of testosterone. The authors investigated sexual behaviors in these mice after castration and assessed differential gene expression in the medical preoptic nucleus and bed nucleus of the stria terminalis of mice that remained sexually active versus those that did not. Over 500 genes were noted to be differentially expressed, with 7 genes involved in neurophysiology and 6 involved in neurodegeneration, the most significant difference between groups. It was determined that higher expression of APP was associated with greater sexual activity before castration and longer mean maintenance of sexual activity after castration. Follow-up studies using transgenic mice with a gene designed to overexpress APP confirmed that upregulation of APP plays a direct stimulatory role in sexual behavior before and after castration in rats. Transgene studies were not performed in all 12 of the upregulated genes, but gene array data suggest that pathways involved in cell survival and neural degeneration are also involved in the modulation of sexual behavior in this model system.

APP is related to neuronal survival; the precise mechanism of APP in preserving and modulating sexual function is unclear at this time, but this will be a topic for further research. The ramifications of these data are at this stage unclear but suggest possible future directions for research into sexual motivation and, further down the road, potential treatments for distressing declines in sexual desire.

A. Shindel, MD

Predicting Erectile Function Recovery after Bilateral Nerve Sparing Radical Prostatectomy: A Proposal of a Novel Preoperative Risk Stratification

Briganti A, Gallina A, Suardi N, et al (Vita-Salute Univ San Raffaele, Milan, Italy)

J Sex Med 7:2521-2531, 2010

Introduction.—No multivariable model is currently available for the prediction of erectile function (EF) recovery after bilateral nerve sparing radical prostatectomy (BNSRP).

Aim.—The aim of this study was to develop a novel preoperative risk stratification aimed at assessing the probability of EF recovery after BNSRP.

Main Outcome Measure.—The International Index of Erectile Function (IIEF) was used to evaluate EF after BNSRP.

Methods.—This study included 435 patients treated with retropubic BNSRP between 2004 and 2008 at a single Institution. Preoperative data, including age, IIEF, Charlson comorbidity index (CCI), and body mass index (BMI) were available for all patients. Moreover, all patients were assessed postoperatively every 3 months and were asked to complete the IIEF during each visit. Cox regression models tested the association between preoperative predictors (age at surgery, preoperative IIEF-EF domain score, CCI, BMI) and EF recovery. Independent predictors of EF recovery were then used to stratify patients into three groups according to the risk of erectile dysfunction (ED) after surgery: low (age ≤ 65 years, IIEF-EF ≥ 26, CCI ≤ 1; n = 184), intermediate (age 66–69 years or IIEF-EF 11-25,CCI ≤ 1; n = 115), and high (age ≥ 70 years or IIEF-EF ≤ 10 or CCI ≥ 2; n = 136). Kaplan-Meier curves assessed the time to EF recovery (defined as IIEF-EF score ≥ 22). Predictive accuracy of our proposed classification was quantified using the AUC method.

Results.—Of 435 patients, 242 (55.6%) received phosphodiesterase type 5 inhibitors (PDE5-I) either on demand or every day for a period of 3–6 months. Overall, EF recovery rate was 58% at 3-year follow-up. Patients treated with PDE5-I had significantly higher 3-year EF recovery rate as compared with patients left untreated after surgery (73 vs. 37%; $P < 0.001$). Except for BMI ($P = 0.7$), all preoperative covariates showed a significant association with EF recovery (all $P \leq 0.04$). The 3-year EF recovery rate significantly differed between the three groups, being 85, 59, and 37% in patients with low, intermediate, and high risk of postoperative ED, respectively ($P < 0.001$). Multivariable Cox regression analysis confirmed a highly significant association between the risk classification and EF recovery ($P < 0.001$). The proposed patient stratification tool showed a 69.1% accuracy. Similar results were achieved when patients were stratified according to the use of ED treatment after surgery (all $P < 0.001$).

Conclusions.—We report the first preoperative risk stratification tool aimed at assessing the probability of EF recovery after BNSRP. It is based on routinely available baseline data such as patient age, preoperative erectile function, and comorbidity profile.

▶ It is clear and undeniable that the vast majority of men experience a worsening of sexual function after radical pelvic surgery even in cases where nerve sparing is accomplished. Some degree of recovery can be expected in those men who had erectile capacity prior to surgery, but the time course and odds for this are not entirely clear. In this study derived from a large cohort of men treated with nerve sparing radical prostatectomy for prostate cancer between 2004 and 2008, baseline and follow-up data were used to categorize men into low-, medium-, and high-risk groups for persistent erectile dysfunction (ED) based on known independent predictors of this outcome (age, baseline erectile function [EF] as assessed by the International Index of Erectile Function [IIEF], and number of comorbid conditions).[1] Interestingly, body mass index and prostate cancer characteristics (Gleason score, pathological stage, and margin status) were not associated with differences in odds of recovery.

Slightly over half of the men had recovered EF by 3 years postsurgery with the odds of recovery progressively lower in men with increasing risk factors for ED. Specifically, 85% of men who were younger than 65 years had normal EF at baseline (IIEF-EF domain score of 26 or greater), and a Charlson Comorbidity Index score of 1 or less recovered EF at 3 years. It is important to note that the criterion for recovery of EF at follow-up was an IIEF-EF domain score of 22 or greater, which, based on validated scoring for the 6-item IIEF-EF domain, corresponds to either mild or no ED.

Although the follow-up metric used to assess EF may not be quite the definition patients think when they hear the term EF recovery, this report is of value in that it provides a means to provide a rough estimate of the time course and odds of EF improvement using easily accessible clinical data points. The accuracy of 70% is not robust, but the ease of use may make this sort of classification system of interest to clinicians who wish to discuss postprostatectomy ED with their patients.

A. Shindel, MD

Reference

1. Cappelleri JC, Rosen RC, Smith MD, Mishra A, Osterloh IH. Diagnostic evaluation of the erectile function domain of the International Index of Erectile Function. *Urology.* 1999;54:346-351.

Investigation of the Neural Target Level of Hyperthyroidism in Premature Ejaculation in a Rat Model of Pharmacologically Induced Ejaculation
Cahangirov A, Cihan A, Murat N, et al (Dokuz Eylul Univ, Izmir, Turkey)
J Sex Med 8:90-96, 2011

Introduction.—Association between hyperthyroidism and premature ejaculation was demonstrated in clinical studies.

Aim.—The aim of this study is to determine the target level of changes on ejaculatory physiology under hyperthyroid states.

Methods.—p-Chloroamphetamine (PCA)-induced pharmacologic ejaculation model with 24 male Wistar rats was used in the study. Subcutaneous injection of L-thyroxine for 14 days was performed to induce hyperthyroidism. At the end of the injection period, thyroid hormone status was evaluated by serum thyroid-stimulating hormone measurements in all rats. At the beginning of the operations, complete spinal transections (tx) at the T8-T9 level were performed to half of the L-thyroxine-injected and control group rats. Thus, experimental groups were constructed as follows: Group 1—control-spinal intact (n = 6), group 2—control-spinal tx (n = 6), group 3—hyperthyroid-spinal intact (n = 6), and group 4—hyperthyroid-spinal tx (n = 6). Ejaculatory responses were recorded before and 30 minutes after intraperitoneal administration of 5 mg/kg PCA.

Main Outcome Measures.—During the operations, seminal vesicle (SV) catheterization and bulbospongiosus (BS) muscle dissections were performed in all rats to demonstrate SV pressure (SVP) BS electromyographic (EMG) activity changes.

Results.—Following PCA administration SVP tonic amplitude, SV phasic contraction (SVPC) frequency, SVPC maximal amplitude, and BS EMG area under curve values were higher in hyperthyroid intact rats than in control intact rats. The time interval between PCA administration and first ejaculation of hyperthyroid intact rats were significantly shorter than control intact rats (261 ± 7.30 seconds vs. 426 ± 49.6 seconds, $P = 0.008$). All of the changes in the ejaculatory parameters that were induced by hyperthyroidism were completely resolved after spinal transections at the T8-T9 level in group 4.

Conclusion.—In this study, we confirmed the recent data that hyperthyroidism affects both the emission and expulsion phases of ejaculation. The changes that were induced by hyperthyroidism on ejaculatory physiology probably take place in the supraspinal centers above T8 level.

▶ This interesting article investigates the physiological mechanisms underlying the association between premature ejaculation (PE) and hyperthyroidism. Hyperthyroidism has been associated with PE, but it is identified in a relatively small proportion of PE cases. Be that as it may, improvements in understanding of how hyperthyroidism may be related to PE may enhance research into other causes and treatment options for this common and clinically vexing condition.

These authors demonstrate convincingly that experimentally induced hyperthyroidism is associated with a decline in ejaculatory latency in rats. Spinal cord transection at T8-T9 had a number of effects on ejaculation latency as well as seminal vesicle contractility. Importantly, the impact of hyperthyroidism on these ejaculation parameters was not statistically significantly different between the spinal cord—injured and intact animals, suggesting that the actions of hyperthyroidism on ejaculation occur via a process occurring cephalad to the T7 spinal cord.

These data are far from clinical application but represent an important step forward in localization of targets for future therapy of ejaculation disorders.

A. Shindel, MD

Potential Mechanism of Action of Human Growth Hormone on Isolated Human Penile Erectile Tissue
Ückert S, Scheller F, Stief CG, et al (Hannover Med School, Germany; Ludwig-Maximilians-Univ, Munich, Germany; St Markus Academic Hosp, Frankfurt am Main, Germany)
Urology 75:968-973, 2010

Objectives.—To evaluate the mechanisms of growth hormone (GH) action on isolated human penile erectile tissue. Human GH (hGH) has been suggested to play a role in male reproductive function, including penile erection. Nevertheless, it still remains unclear which intracellular pathways mediate the physiological effects of GH on the human corpus cavernosum (HCC).

Methods.—Using the organ bath technique, the effects of GH were investigated on electrical field stimulation (EFS)-induced relaxation of isolated HCC in the absence and presence of the guanylyl cyclase inhibitor 1H-[1,2,4]oxadiazolo[4,3-a]quinoxalin-1-one (ODQ) and nitric oxide synthase (NOS) inhibitor N^G-nitro-L-arginine (L-NOARG, 10 μm). Effects of GH on the production of tissue cyclic guanosine monophosphate (cGMP) in the absence and presence of ODQ and L-NOARG were also elucidated using radioimmunoassay.

Results.—ODQ and L-NOARG abolished the relaxation of the tissue induced by EFS, whereas amplitudes were increased by physiological concentrations of GH (1-100 nm). The attenuation of EFS-induced amplitudes by L-NOARG but not ODQ was, in part, reversed by GH. The production of cGMP (pmol cGMP/mg protein) induced by 10 nm GH was abolished in the presence of 10 μm ODQ. In contrast, the combination of GH (10 nm) and L-NOARG (10 μm) maintained cGMP production significantly greater than baseline (0.68 ± 0.36 vs 1.07 ± 0.48 pmol cGMP/mg protein).

Conclusions.—Our data provide evidence that GH may act on human HCC by an NO-independent effect on guanylyl cyclase activity and may thus explain how growth factors, such as hGH, regulate male erectile function.

▶ The influence of hormonal factors on the processes of penile erection is an area of growing importance and interest. Human Growth Hormone (hGH) has a number of biological effects relating to the hypothalamic-pituitary-gonadal axis and tissue senescence. In this study, the direct effects of hGH on corporeal tissue (obtained from patients undergoing male-to-female gender reassignment surgery) were assessed in an organ bath. It was determined that hGH exerted an enhancing effect on the amplitude of strip relaxation that was similar to that seen with a phosphodiesterase type 5 inhibitor; tissue levels of cyclic guanosine monophosphate were also enhanced by hGH, suggesting a generally proerectile effect of this treatment. These effects were attenuated to a greater extent by inhibitors of guanylate cyclase than by inhibitors of nitric oxide synthase, suggesting that the effects of this hormone are greatest downstream of the nitric oxide release.

It must be considered that these subjects had received between 8 and 15 months of therapy with antiandrogens and estrogens prior to tissue procurement; this may have had important effects on the tissue, and caution must be therefore exercised in extrapolating these results to the general male population. Nevertheless, it provides some preliminary insight into how hGH may affect the male erectile system.

A. Shindel, MD

T-786C Polymorphism in Promoter of eNOS Gene as Genetic Risk Factor in Patients With Erectile Dysfunction in Turkish Population

Sinici İ, Güven EO, Şerefoğlu E, et al (Hacettepe Univ Faculty of Medicine, Ankara, Turkey; Mustafa Kemal Univ Faculty of Medicine, Antakya, Turkey; Atatürk Hosp, Ankara, Turkey)
Urology 75:955-960, 2010

Objectives.—To investigate the effect of 2 endothelial nitric oxide synthase gene polymorphisms, namely, variable number of 27-bp tandem repeats in intron 4 and T-786C in the promoter region, on the susceptibility to erectile dysfunction (ED) in Turkish population.

Methods.—A total of 72 patients with ED (mean age 54.3 ± 9.2 years) diagnosed by Doppler ultrasonography and 71 healthy controls (mean age 55.4 ± 8.2 years) were analyzed. Genotypes were determined through polymerase chain reaction with or without restriction endonuclease digestions.

Results.—Genotype distribution for CC genotype of T-786C polymorphism in promoter was significantly different between patients with ED and controls, the genotype frequency being 31.9% and 12.7%, respectively ($P = .019$). The univariate odds ratio (OR) associated with CC alleles revealed 3 times increased risk for ED (OR = 3.2; 95% confidence interval [CI], 1.4-7.6; $P = .006$). The risk also holds when excluding patients with hypertension and diabetes mellitus ($P = .012$, OR = 3.1; 95% CI, 1.2-7.7) as well as obesity ($P = .05$, OR = 4; 95% CI, 1.05-15.3). Patients with CC genotype of promoter present earlier symptoms of ED (51.7%) compared with controls (10.7%) ($P < .001$). No significant correlation was observed with variable number of tandem repeats in intron 4 and with the type of vascular insufficiency.

Conclusions.—The CC genotype of T-786C polymorphism in the promoter of eNOS gene is associated with increased risk of ED in Turkish population. Earlier onset of ED with CC genotype suggests that CC allele is an independent risk factor for endothelial dysfunction in the absence of other risk factors (hypertension, diabetes mellitus, obesity). An impaired NO production because of CC alleles may account for pathophysiology of ED.

▶ It is becoming increasingly clear that genetic influences play a role in the susceptibility to many disease states, including sexual dysfunctions. In this report, 72 Turkish men with erectile dysfunction (ED) were compared with age-matched controls without ED. Genotype was determined by application of polymerase chain reaction to peripheral blood samples. Men with ED were significantly more likely than men without ED (32% vs 13%, respectively) to be homozygous for the T-786C polymorphism in the endothelial nitric oxide synthase (eNOS) promoter region; this allele has been shown in previous studies to result in a decline in the activity of the eNOS gene promoter. Men with this polymorphism had earlier onset of ED and increased risk of ED even after adjustment for vascular comorbidities. Interestingly, an area of variable tandem repeats in intron 4 of the eNOS gene (shown to be associated with better response to sildenafil in 1 study) was also assayed and found not to differ in prevalence between men with and without ED.

While genotype information is of great interest, it will be necessary to more clearly identify differences in protein expression between these groups; although genes may dictate to some extent which proteins are expressed, a variety of post-transcriptional modifications to messenger RNA may substantially alter the final product of a given genome.

A. Shindel, MD

Erectile Dysfunction Drug Receipt, Risky Sexual Behavior and Sexually Transmitted Diseases in HIV-infected and HIV-uninfected Men
Cook RL, McGinnis KA, Samet JH, et al (Univ of Florida, Gainesville; Pittsburgh VA Healthcare System, PA; Boston Univ, MA; et al)
J Gen Intern Med 25:115-121, 2010

Background.—Health care providers may be concerned that prescribing erectile dysfunction drugs (EDD) will contribute to risky sexual behavior.

Objectives.—To identify characteristics of men who received EDD prescriptions, determine whether EDD receipt is associated with risky sexual behavior and sexually transmitted diseases (STDs), and determine whether these relationships vary for certain sub-groups.

Design.—Cross-sectional study.

Participants.—Two thousand seven hundred and eighty-seven sexually-active, HIV-infected and HIV-uninfected men recruited from eight Veterans Health Affairs outpatient clinics. Data were obtained from participant surveys, electronic medical records, and administrative pharmacy data.

Measures.—EDD receipt was defined as two or more prescriptions for an EDD, risky sex as having unprotected sex with a partner of serodiscordant or unknown HIV status, and STDs, according to self-report.

Results.—Overall, 28% of men received EDD in the previous year. Eleven percent of men reported unprotected sex with a serodiscordant/ unknown partner in the past year (HIV-infected 15%, HIV-uninfected 6%, P<0.001). Compared to men who did not receive EDD, men who received EDD were equally likely to report risky sexual behavior (11% vs. 10%, p=0.9) and STDs (7% vs 7%, p=0.7). In multivariate analyses, EDD receipt was not significantly associated with risky sexual behavior or STDs in the entire sample or in subgroups of substance users or men who had sex with men.

Conclusion.—EDD receipt was common but not associated with risky sexual behavior or STDs in this sample of HIV-infected and uninfected men. However, risky sexual behaviors persist in a minority of HIV-infected men, indicating ongoing need for prevention interventions.

▶ Physicians are rightfully concerned about potential abuses of medications they might prescribe. In some cases the consequences of medication misuse may be minor, in others potentially criminal, and in some potentially life threatening. A particularly ethically challenging example of this is provision of erectile dysfunction (ED) treatments to men infected with human immunodeficiency virus (HIV). While these medications are generally safe in this population, some physicians have feared that providing treatments for ED in HIV+ men may lead to spread of the virus that would not occur in the absence of effective erectogenic agents. While there is little legal precedent for criminal charges against a prescribing doctor in those circumstances, public health and ethical concerns about this practice are legitimate.

In this study, 2787 men (1469 of whom were HIV+) were recruited from the VA health system. The authors determined that 28% of the patients had received a medical treatment for ED. Unprotected sex with a partner of serodiscordant or unknown HIV status occurred in 15% of the HIV+ men and in 6% of the HIV− men (*P* for difference <.001). However, having received a medical treatment for ED was not associated with a greater likelihood of risky sexual behavior or acquisition of sexually transmitted disease.

It is obvious and critical that education on safer sex practices be a part of our practice for patients who receive treatment for ED. Data such as these suggest that prescription of such treatments does not predispose patients to greater risk taking; this stands in contrast to some previous reports that have associated phosphodiesterase type 5 inhibitor use with high-risk sexual behavior in men who have sex with men. While there is little doubt that these drugs can be abused, it seems parsimonious to speculate that some individuals with no or mild ED may choose to enhance their erectile performance with medications at the time of engaging in high-risk sexual activity; the drug itself is not the determining factor in electing to engage in high-risk activity. More studies are needed.

A. Shindel, MD

Upregulation of gp91^{phox} Subunit of NAD(P)H Oxidase Contributes to Erectile Dysfunction Caused by Long-term Nitric Oxide Inhibition in Rats: Reversion by Regular Physical Training

Claudino MA, Franco-Penteado CF, Priviero FBM, et al (Univ of Campinas (UNICAMP), São Paulo, Brazil; State Univ of São Paulo (UNESP), Rio Claro, Brazil; Univ of São Paulo, (USP), Brazil)

Urology 75:961-967, 2010

Objectives.—To test the hypothesis that glyco protein 91phox (gp91^{phox}) subunit of nicotinamide adenine dinucleotide phosphate [NAD(P)H] oxidase is a fundamental target for physical activity to ameliorate erectile dysfunction (ED). Vascular risk factors are reported to contribute to ED. Regular physical exercise prevents cardiovascular diseases by increasing nitric oxide (NO) production and/or decreasing NO inactivation.

Methods.—Male Wistar rats received the NO synthesis inhibitor N^{ω}-nitro-L-arginine methyl ester (L-NAME) for 4 weeks, after which animals were submitted to a run training program for another 4 weeks. Erectile functions were evaluated by in vitro cavernosal relaxations and intracavernous pressure measurements. Expressions of gp91^{phox} subunit and neuronal nitric oxidase synthase in erectile tissue, as well as superoxide dismutase activity and nitrite/nitrate (NO$_x$) levels were determined.

Results.—The in vitro acetylcholine- and electrical field stimulation-induced cavernosal relaxations, as well as the increases in intracavernous pressure were markedly reduced in sedentary rats treated with L-NAME. Run training significantly restored the impaired cavernosal relaxations. No alterations in the neuronal nitric oxidase synthase protein expression (and its variant penile neuronal nitric oxidase synthase) were detected. A reduction of NO$_x$ levels and superoxide dismutase activity was observed in L-NAME-treated animals, which was significantly reversed by physical training. Gene expression of subunit gp91^{phox} was enhanced by approximately 2-fold in erectile tissue of L-NAME-treated rats, and that was restored to basal levels by run training.

Conclusions.—Our study shows that ED seen after long-term L-NAME treatment is associated with gp91^{phox} subunit upregulation and decreased NO bioavailability. Exercise training reverses the increased oxidative stress in NO-deficient rats, ameliorating the ED.

▶ In this study, sedentary rats treated with the nitric oxide synthase (NOS) inhibitor N^{ω}-nitro-L-arginine methyl ester for 4 weeks had a decline in their expression of nitric oxide and the antioxidant superoxide dismutase in the penile tissues, a blunting of their erectile response to acetylcholine and electrical field stimulation, and an increase in expression of messenger RNA for the glycoprotein 91phox subunit of nicotinamide adenine dinucleotide phosphate. Completion of a program of 4-week run training (1.2 km per hour for 60 minutes per day, 5 days a week) appeared to ameliorate these changes and at least partially restore functional erectile capacity. Interestingly, there was no change after exercise training in protein expression of neuronal NOS, suggesting that it is not a directly neuronally mediated process that underlies the restoration of erectile capacity in these animals.

Clinical data abounds on the importance of physical exercise for maintenance and even restoration of erectile function. With data such as these, the physiological rationale for these observations comes into clearer focus.

A. Shindel, MD

The Effects of Beta-blockers on Endothelial Nitric Oxide Synthase Immunoreactivity in the Rat Corpus Cavernosum

Dogru MT, Aydos TR, Aktuna Z, et al (Univ of Kirikkale, Turkey; Hacettepe Univ, Ankara, Turkey)

Urology 75:589-597, 2010

Objectives.—To explain the mechanism of the effects of β-blockers on endothelial dysfunction and release of nitric oxide from the endothelium.

Methods.—A total of 72 Sprague-Dawley rats were divided into 9 different groups as follows: group 1: control (n = 10), group 2: metoprolol (Beloc) 100 mg/kg/d (n = 7), group 3: carvedilol (Dilatrend) 50 mg/kg/d (n = 7), group 4: nebivolol (Vasoxen) 10 mg/kg/d (n = 6), group 5: estrogen receptor (ER) antagonist ICI 182.780 (Fluvestrant) 50 μg/g (n = 10), group 6: nebivolol + ER antagonist (n = 8), group 7: androgen receptor (AR) antagonist (flutamide) 20 mg/kg (n = 7), group 8: nebivolol + AR antagonist (n = 7), and group 9: DMSO (solvent for ER antagonist) (n = 10). All β-blockers were applied with gastric gavage after dilution with 5 mL of serum physiological; ER and AR were both applied intraperitoneally (i.p.) for 14 days. In the isolated rat cavernous tissues, endothelial nitric oxide synthase (eNOS) and ER and AR immunoreactivity were analyzed quantitatively. One-way analysis of variance and Tukey test were used for statistical analysis.

Results.—Although increased eNOS immunoreactivity was observed with nebivolol and nebivolol-flutamide in endothelial cells laying cavernous tissue, a lower score was observed after ICI-182.780 application, when compared with control cases. AR immunoreactivity in cavernosal endothelium was clearly higher with nebivolol. Higher H score and ER immunoreactivity were observed in the cavernous endothelium and smooth muscles in the nebivolol, carvedilol, and metoprolol groups when compared with control cases.

Conclusions.—We showed that eNOS activity was increased in the nebivolol and nebivolol-flutamide groups, whereas it was decreased in the ICI 182.780 group. We believe that an ER-dependent mechanism triggered by nebivolol played a role in nitric oxide formation.

▶ β-blockers are one of the most commonly prescribed treatments for hypertension and hence have an important role to play in the prevention of vascular (including penile vascular) morbidity. Unfortunately, β-blockers themselves have been linked to erectile dysfunction in numerous studies, and sexual dysfunction is one of the most common reasons for the lack of medication adherence. The development of new and less side effect-prone β-blockers might play a very important role in improving patient compliance and quality of life.

In this study, healthy rats were treated with metoprolol, carvedilol, or the endothelial nitric oxide synthase (eNOS)-potentiating β-blocker, nebivolol. Also included in this study was a cohort of rats treated with nebivolol with or without either an estrogen receptor antagonist *or* an androgen receptor antagonist. All subject rats received treatment for 14 days and then underwent tissue harvest for histological studies. Animals that had received treatment with nebivolol alone or with nebivolol plus the androgen receptor antagonist manifested greater eNOS and smooth muscle positivity relative to animals that did not receive nebivolol; animals that received nebivolol also tended to manifest greater immunoreactivity for the androgen and estrogen receptors in corporeal tissue. The authors postulate that an estrogen receptor-dependent mechanism may be responsible for the endothelial effects of the drug.

This study is limited in that healthy rats were used and no functional testing was performed. Additional work will be required to more clearly elucidate the mechanisms of action by which nebivolol exerts its effects. Be that as it may, this β-blocker may prove to be a preferred treatment for hypertension or other cardiac indications in men concerned with their erectile function.

A. Shindel, MD

Characterization of the Effects of Various Drugs Likely to Affect Smooth Muscle Tension on Isolated Human Seminal Vesicle Tissue

Birowo P, Ückert S, Kedia GT, et al (Univ of Indonesia School of Medicine, Jakarta; Hannover Med School, Germany; Inst for Biochemical Res and Analysis, Hannover, Germany; et al)
Urology 75:974-978, 2010

Objectives.—To investigate the effects of different classes of drugs on the isometric tension of isolated human seminal vesicle (SV) tissue. The contractility of human SV contributes to the process of seminal emission during ejaculation. Different endogenous compounds, such as serotonin (5-HT), adenosine triphosphate (ATP), and nitric oxide, have been suggested to be involved in the control of contraction and relaxation of human SV smooth muscle. However, only limited data are available regarding the effects of compounds known to affect smooth musculature on SV contractile activity.

Methods.—Using the organ bath technique, the effects of increasing concentrations (10 nM-1 μM/10 μM) of norepinephrine (NE), phenylephrine, endothelin 1, ATP, and 5-HT on human SV tissue at basal tension were studied. In another set-up, SV strip preparations were preincubated with prazosin (α-adrenergic blocker), nifedipine and verapamil (Ca^{2+}-channel blockers), 2-aminoethoxydiphenyl borate [inositol 1,4,5-trisphosphate (IP_3) antagonist], cromakalim (K^+-channel opener), or Y-27632

(ROK inhibitor) (1 μM each, for 10 minutes), followed by the application of NE (0.1 μM, 1 μM, and 10 μM).

Results.—SV smooth muscle was most effectively contracted by NE (mean = 75% of calibrated scale), phenylephrine (mean = 82% of calibrated scale), and endothelin 1 (mean = 70% calibrated scale), whereas only minor responses to ATP (mean = 10.65% calibrated scale) and 5-HT (mean = 6.3% calibrated scale) were observed. The contraction induced by NE was significantly inhibited after pre-exposure of the tissue to prazosin (−92.4%), cromakalim (−83.7%), 2-aminoethoxydiphenyl borate (−43.1%), Y-27632 (−42.8%), and nifedipine (−32.7%).

Conclusions.—α-adrenoceptor antagonism, activation of potassium channels, and inhibition of Rho-kinase decrease the sympathetic contraction of SV smooth muscle. This might be of significance with regard to the identification of new pharmacologic avenues to affect the male ejaculatory system.

▶ There are currently no drugs approved for the treatment of ejaculatory dysfunction (either premature or delayed) in the United States. A short acting selective serotonin reuptake inhibitor (SSRI) medication has been approved for the treatment of premature ejaculation (PE) in Europe, and topical anesthetics and off-label SSRI are currently used with some efficacy in the United States. Nevertheless, there is obviously an unmet need for better solutions to the problem of ejaculatory dysfunction.

While existing therapies rely on modulation of peripheral nerves or serotonin in the central nervous system, different therapeutic targets may produce more desirable effects. This study is a hypothesis generating study on different mechanisms to influence smooth muscle contraction in the seminal vesicles (SVs). Seminal vesicle tissue was obtained from 32 men undergoing ablative surgery for lower urinary tract malignancy and subjected to organ bath testing. A variety of agents with known vasoconstrictive or vasodilatory activity were applied to tissue strips followed by treatment with norepinephrine to simulate the sympathetic activation of the SV during seminal emission. It was determined that the alpha-receptor blocker prazosin, the potassium channel opening drug cromakalim, and the Rho-kinase inhibitor Y-27632 significantly diminished the contractile-inducing capacity of norepinephrine. Interestingly, serotonin had little impact on the contractile activity in these tissues.

Targeting of these molecular pathways may lead to novel drug development for the management of PE. These preliminary findings are intriguing and suggest the possibility that new medical therapies may be brought to bear in the problem of PE or even delayed ejaculation. Much research will be required, however, to determine which agents have acceptable side-effect profiles and produce SV tissue levels that are capable of inducing desired results (either pro- or anti-ejaculatory).

A. Shindel, MD

A Multicenter, Double-blind, Placebo-controlled Trial to Assess The Efficacy of Sildenafil Citrate in Men With Unrecognized Erectile Dysfunction

Shabsigh R, Kaufman J, Magee M, et al (Maimonides Med Ctr, Brooklyn, NY; Columbia Univ, NY; Urology Res Options, Aurora, CO; et al)
Urology 76:373-379, 2010

Objective.—Erectile dysfunction (ED) may be present but unrecognized in men with other comorbidities, such as cardiovascular disease (CVD), diabetes, or lower urinary tract symptoms (LUTS). The efficacy of sildenafil citrate treatment for ED in men who did not self-identify with or were unsure about whether they had ED, but had ED based on International Index of Erectile Function Erectile Function domain (IIEF-EF) scores, was evaluated.

Methods.—Men with an ED associated comorbidity were asked, "Do you have ED?" Those who answered "no" or "unsure" and were diagnosed with ED (score of ≤25 IIEF-EF) were invited to participate in a parallel-group, multicenter, flexible-dose, double-blind, randomized, placebo-controlled trial, followed by an open-label extension. Erectile function and emotional/ psychosocial benefits of sildenafil treatment were assessed.

Results.—Men with ED at baseline were randomized to sildenafil (n = 150) or placebo (n = 155). The mean ± SD number of ED risk factors in the sildenafil and placebo groups was 3.5 ± 1.8 and 3.3 ± 1.7, respectively. Hypertension, hypercholesterolemia, smoking, obesity (body mass index ≥30 kg/m^2), and waist circumference ≥40 inches were the most frequently reported risk factors. Sildenafil-treated men had improved scores on both functional and psychosocial measures. Most adverse events were mild to moderate.

Conclusions.—Many men do not recognize that they have ED; sildenafil treatment improved sexual function and satisfaction in these men. Because ED affects quality of life, it should be suspected and assessed in men with risk factors for ED.

▶ This rather interesting randomized blinded study investigates a population of men who either denied or weren't sure that they had erectile dysfunction (ED) based on response to a single-item question but had International Index of Erectile Function-erectile function (IIEF-EF) domain scores that suggested clinically significant erectile impairment. Over two-thirds of subjects who denied ED had evidence of the diagnosis based on IIEF-EF score. Three hundred and five subjects who elected to participate in the trial received either placebo or sildenafil 50 mg with the option of dose titration over the course of an 8-week study. Substantial improvements in erectile function were noted in the treatment group, which is not surprising. Interestingly, substantial improvements in Self-Esteem and Relationship score and sexual encounter profile affirmative responses were also detected in the treatment group, implying improvement in the broader sexual relationship.

It may be speculated that some of these men viewed ED as just part of getting older or had some other sort of stoic sense of acceptance regarding the situation. Clearly, even these men experienced a number of benefits from ED therapy. The question then becomes how vigorous providers should be about encouraging treatment for male patients who deny a problem with sexual function but have evidence of erectile impairment. This is an ethical/philosophical question that cannot be answered by data of this sort. Nevertheless, this does provide evidence that men who are on the fence about treatment should seriously consider the manifold benefits of taking steps to improve their sexual lives, be it with pharmacotherapy or other intervention.

A. Shindel, MD

Molecular Mechanisms of Vacuum Therapy in Penile Rehabilitation: A Novel Animal Study

Yuan J, Lin H, Li P, et al (Sichuan Univ, Chengdu, China; Nanjing Univ School of Medicine, China; Univ of Texas M.D. Anderson Cancer Ctr, Houston; et al)
Eur Urol 58:773-780, 2010

Background.—Penile rehabilitation (PR) is widely applied after radical prostatectomy. Vacuum erectile device (VED) therapy is the one of three PR methods used in the clinical setting that improve erectile function (EF) and is the only PR method which may preserve penile length. However, its unknown mechanism hampered doctors' recommendations and patients' compliance.

Objectives.—To assess the effects of VED therapy on erectile dysfunction (ED) in a rat model of bilateral cavernous nerve crush (BCNC) and to investigate the molecular mechanism of VED in postprostatectomy ED.

Design, Setting, and Participants.—This was an experimental study using Sprague-Dawley rats in three groups: sham, BCNC, and BCNC plus VED.

Intervention.—Intervention included BCNC, electrical stimulation of the cavernous nerve (CNS), and VED therapy.

Measurements.—At the end of a 4-wk period, CNS was used to assess EF by maximum intracavernosal pressure (ICP)/mean arterial pressure (MAP) ratio and duration (area under the curve [AUC]). For the structural analyses, whole rat penis was harvested. Terminal deoxynucleotidyl transferase biotin-dUTP nick end labeling assay was used for the assessment of apoptotic indices (AI). Immunohistochemistry was performed for endothelial nitric oxide synthase (eNOS), α-smooth muscle actin (ASMA), transforming growth factor beta 1 (TGF-β1), and hypoxia inducible factor-1α (HIF-1α). Staining for Masson's trichrome was utilized to calculate the smooth muscle/collagen ratios.

Results and Limitations.—EF was improved with VED therapy measured by ICP/MAP ratios and AUC. VED therapy reduced HIF-1α expression and AI significantly compared with control. Animals exposed to VED therapy had decreased TGF-β1 expression, increased smooth muscle/collagen ratios, and preserved ASMA and eNOS expression.

Conclusions.—To our knowledge, this is the first scientific study to suggest that VED therapy in the BCNC rat model preserves EF through antihypoxic, antiapoptotic, and antifibrotic mechanisms.

▶ This rather interesting study (sponsored by 2 manufacturers of vacuum tumescence devices [VTDs]) investigates histological and molecular changes in the rat penis after cavernous nerve injury with or without application of a VTD for 4 weeks postinjury. Fifteen rats comprised the study group and were divided into a sham surgery group, a cavernous nerve injury without VTD application group, and a group that had cavernous nerve injury with subsequent VTD application twice daily for a 5-minute period starting 2 weeks after injury. Rats that were treated with a protocol of VTD application manifested superior penile hemodynamics during cavernous nerve electrostimulation. At the tissue level, VTD treated animals had less apoptosis, better preservation of smooth muscle to collagen ratio, less evidence for hypoxia, and preservation of endothelial nitric oxide synthase expression.

Application of the VTD after radical prostatectomy is a viable option as part of penile rehabilitation and offers the benefit of relatively lower cost over the long-term when compared with oral therapy with phosphodiesterase type 5 inhibitors. Problems remain, however, with patient compliance. Data such as these should hopefully provide impetus for further studies, which, if positive, will give providers caring for sexual health in the postprostatectomy patient more talking points to convince men to adhere to this type of therapy for recovery of erectile function. However, the question remains whether or not this therapy will produce clinically beneficial results in men after radical pelvic surgery.

A. Shindel, MD

Activated RhoA/Rho Kinase Impairs Erectile Function After Cavernous Nerve Injury in Rats

Gratzke C, Strong TD, Gebska MA, et al (Ludwig-Maximilians-Univ Munich, Germany; Johns Hopkins Med Insts, Baltimore, MD; Univ of Iowa Hosps and Clinics, Iowa City; et al)
J Urol 184:2197-2204, 2010

Purpose.—RhoA and rho kinase serve as key regulators of penile vascular homeostasis. The role of RhoA/rho kinase signaling in the penis after cavernous nerve injury has not been fully investigated. We characterized the molecular expression profiles of RhoA/rho kinase signaling that occur in the penis after cavernous nerve injury. We hypothesized that erectile dysfunction after bilateral cavernous nerve injury is accompanied by up-regulation of RhoA/rho kinase activity in the rat penis.

Material and Methods.—We used 2 groups, including sham operation and bilateral cavernous nerve injury. At 14 days after nerve injury each group underwent cavernous nerve stimulation to determine erectile function at baseline and after intracavernous injection of the rho kinase inhibitor Y-27632 (Tocris Bioscience, Ellisville, Missouri). Penes were assessed at baseline for protein expression of neuronal nitric oxide synthase, RhoA, and rho kinase 1 and 2 by Western blot, immunoreactivity of neuronal nitric oxide synthase, rho kinase 1 and 2, RhoA-guanosine triphosphatase and rho kinase activity.

Results.—Erectile function was decreased in nerve injured rats. Neuronal nitric oxide synthase protein was significantly decreased while RhoA and rho kinase 2 protein levels were significantly increased in rat penes with nerve injury. Rho kinase 1 protein expression was equivalent. Rho kinase immunoreactivity was qualitatively increased in the corporeal smooth muscle of nerve injured rats. RhoA-guanosine triphosphatase and rho kinase activity was significantly increased in injured rat penes compared to that in sham operated penes. Intracavernous injection of Y-27632 caused a significantly greater increase in intracavernous pressure in nerve injured rats compared to that in sham operated rats, suggesting increased rho kinase activity.

Conclusions.—Data suggest that RhoA/rho kinase up-regulation in response to cavernous nerve injury contributes to penile vasculature dysfunction after cavernous nerve injury. Thus, the RhoA/rho kinase pathway may be a suitable target for treating post-radical prostatectomy erectile dysfunction.

▶ In this study, it was demonstrated that cavernous nerve injury induces upregulation of the RhoA/rho-kinase pathway in the penes of rats. Blockade of rho-kinase activity increased intracavernous erectile response to cavernous nerve electrostimulation 14 days postinjury, suggesting that up-regulation of this pathway is at least partly culpable for postnerve injury erectile impairment in this model system.

The activity of RhoA/rho-kinase in vivo in erectile function is somewhat complex. Rho-kinase inhibits the activity of myosin light chain phosphatase and increases calcium sensitivity; the end result of this activity in vascular smooth muscle is increased myosin/actin cross-bridge activity with resultant higher muscle tone and vasoconstriction. A great deal of evidence has suggested that Rho-kinase activity is positively associated with risk of erectile impairment; data such as these suggest that this pathway may be a suitable target for future novel pharmacotherapies. This is of particular interest in the radical prostatectomy population, but it is entirely possible that development of drugs that influence calcium sensitivity in the penile vascular system will be of benefit to men with erectile dysfunction or other etiologies as well.

A. Shindel, MD

Genome-wide association study to identify single nucleotide polymorphisms (SNPS) associated with the development of erectile dysfunction in African-American men after radiotherapy for prostate cancer
Kerns SL, Ostrer H, Stock R, et al (New York Univ School of Medicine; Mount Sinai School of Medicine, NY; et al)
Int J Radiat Oncol Biol Phys 78:1292-1300, 2010

Purpose.—To identify single nucleotide polymorphisms (SNPs) associated with erectile dysfunction (ED) among African-American prostate cancer patients treated with external beam radiation therapy.

Methods and Materials.—A cohort of African-American prostate cancer patients treated with external beam radiation therapy was observed for the development of ED by use of the five-item Sexual Health Inventory for Men (SHIM) questionnaire. Final analysis included 27 cases (post-treatment SHIM score ≤ 7) and 52 control subjects (post-treatment SHIM score ≥ 16). A genome-wide association study was performed using approximately 909,000 SNPs genotyped on Affymetrix 6.0 arrays (Affymetrix, Santa Clara, CA).

Results.—We identified SNP rs2268363, located in the follicle-stimulating hormone receptor (FSHR) gene, as significantly associated with ED after correcting for multiple comparisons (unadjusted $p = 5.46 \times 10^{-8}$, Bonferroni $p = 0.028$). We identified four additional SNPs that tended toward a significant association with an unadjusted p value $< 10^{-6}$. Inference of population substructure showed that cases had a higher proportion of African ancestry than control subjects (77% vs. 60%, $p = 0.005$). A multivariate logistic regression model that incorporated estimated ancestry and four of the top-ranked SNPs was a more accurate classifier of ED than a model that included only clinical variables.

Conclusions.—To our knowledge, this is the first genome-wide association study to identify SNPs associated with adverse effects resulting from radiotherapy. It is important to note that the SNP that proved to be significantly associated with ED is located within a gene whose encoded product plays a role in male gonad development and function. Another key finding of this project is that the four SNPs most strongly associated with ED were specific to persons of African ancestry and would therefore not have been identified had a cohort of European ancestry been screened. This study demonstrates the feasibility of a genome-wide approach to investigate genetic predisposition to radiation injury.

▶ The era of genomic medicine is upon us! Standard clinical predictor variables for risk of long-term erectile dysfunction (ED) after prostate cancer therapy are well established. However, contemporary genomic testing offers the potential for therapies and prognostication that are based on an individual patient's unique genetic makeup. While we are early in the development of tools for such an individualized and in-depth assessment, it appears inevitable that better understanding of genetic variables will help us to plan for our patients' well-being in the future.

In this study of 79 African American men treated for prostate cancer with brachytherapy, it was determined that a single nucleotide polymorphism (SNP) of a gene for a follicle-stimulating hormone receptor was significantly more common in men who developed severe ED (Sexual Health Inventory for Men [SHIM] < 7) relative to men who had mild or no ED (SHIM > 16) at least 1 year after brachytherapy for prostate cancer. A similar relationship was identified for SNPs relating to a prostaglandin negative receptor regulator, although this relationship did not remain significant after adjustment for multiple comparisons. Also of interest, subjects with a genetic admixture that suggested a more predominantly African ancestry were also more likely to be in the severe ED group.

There were some (statistically insignificant) differences in hormone therapy and prostate cancer stage between the 2 groups. In the end, further research will be required to determine whether these findings are in fact germane or even accurate. But as a novel and important approach to this clinical problem, this article merits citation.

A. Shindel, MD

Exposure of Human Seminal Vesicle Tissue to Phosphodiesterase (PDE) Inhibitors Antagonizes the Contraction Induced by Norepinephrine and Increases Production of Cyclic Nucleotides

Birowo P, Ückert S, Kedia GT, et al (Univ of Indonesia School of Medicine, Jakarta; Hannover Med School, Germany; Inst for Biochemical Res and Analysis, Hannover, Germany; et al)
Urology 76:1518.e1-1518.e6, 2010

Objectives.—To investigate further the role of phosphodiesterase (PDE) isoenzymes in the control of human seminal vesicle (SV) smooth muscle contractility, we examined the functional responses of isolated SV tissue to various PDE inhibitors. It has been suggested that the application of inhibitors of the PDE type 5 may facilitate SV smooth muscle relaxation and, subsequently, retard ejaculatory response.

Methods.—Using the organ bath technique, strip preparations of human SV were exposed for 5 minutes to 1 μM of the PDE inhibitors milrinone (PDE3 inhibitor), rolipram, Ro 20-1724 (PDE4 inhibitors), and sildenafil (PDE5 inhibitor). Norepinephrine (NE, alpha agonist) was then added (0,1 μM, 1 μM, and 10 μM) and isometric responses were recorded. A contraction-response curve to NE in the absence of PDE inhibitors was also generated. Drug effects on the production of cyclic adenosine monophosphate (AMP) and cyclic guanosine monophosphate (GMP) were measured by means of radioimmunometric assays.

Results.—The contraction induced by NE was effectively antagonized by 1 μM of rolipram (83.3% inhibition), Ro 20-1724 (72.3% inhibition), sildenafil (41.6% inhibition), and milrinone (37.5% inhibition). The inhibition of force generation was paralleled by a 1.6-fold to 2.8-fold increase in tissue cyclic AMP (induced by milrinone, rolipram, Ro 20-1724), and a 12-fold rise in cyclic GMP (induced by sildenafil).

Conclusion.—The findings demonstrate that PDE inhibitors can counteract the contraction of human SV mediated by alpha-adrenergic receptors and enhance levels of cyclic nucleotides. This might be of importance with regard to the identification of new options for the pharmacological treatment of premature ejaculation.

▶ Phosphodiesterase type 5 (PDE5) inhibitors have been used in the management of premature ejaculation (PE) with some mixed results and will likely continue to be used in the future. To evaluate the physiological effects of these drugs on the organs of ejaculation, this article evaluates selective inhibitors of PDE isozymes 3, 4, and 5 in the inhibition of norepinephrine-induced contractions of isolated seminal vesicle (SV) strips in organ bath. The PDE4 inhibitor rolipram exerted a stronger inhibitory effect on SV contraction than either PDE3 or PDE5 inhibitors, although all of the compounds did indeed significantly impair contraction.

The clinical implications are not entirely clear, although it is speculated that delay/inhibition of SV contraction may be a novel means for treating PE. Further development and refinement of drug therapy options is necessary before a human clinical trial can be contemplated, but given the dearth of US Food and Drug Administration—approved drugs for the management of the troubling and prevalent problem of PE, additional avenues for research are certainly welcome.

A. Shindel, MD

Pentoxifylline Promotes Recovery of Erectile Function in a Rat Model of Postprostatectomy Erectile Dysfunction

Albersen M, Fandel TM, Zhang H, et al (Univ of California, San Francisco; et al)
Eur Urol 59:286-296, 2011

Background.—Cavernous nerve (CN) injury during radical prostatectomy (RP) causes CN degeneration and secondary penile fibrosis and smooth muscle cell (SMC) apoptosis. Pentoxifylline (PTX) is a phosphodiesterase inhibitor that further inhibits multiple cytokine pathways involved in nerve degeneration, apoptosis, and fibrosis.

Objectives.—To evaluate whether PTX enhances erectile function in a rat model of CN injury.

Design, Setting and Interventions.—Forty male Sprague-Dawley rats underwent CN crush injury and were randomized to oral gavage feeding of phosphate-buffered saline (vehicle) or PTX 25, PTX 50, or PTX 100 mg/kg per day. Ten animals underwent sham surgery and received vehicle treatment. Treatment continued for 28 d, followed by a washout period of 72 h. An additional eight rats underwent resection of the major pelvic ganglion (MPG) for tissue culture and examination of direct effects of PTX on neurite sprouting.

Measurements.—Intracavernous pressure recording on CN electrostimulation, immunohistologic examination of the penis and the CN distal to the injury site, and length of neurite sprouts in MPG culture.

Results.—Daily oral gavage feeding of PTX resulted in significant improvement of erectile function compared to vehicle treatment in all treated groups. After treatment with PTX 50 and PTX 100 mg/kg per day, the expression of neuronal nitric oxide synthase in the dorsal penile nerve was significantly higher than in vehicle-treated rats. Furthermore, PTX treatment prevented collagen deposition and SMC loss in the corpus cavernosum. In the CN, signs of Wallerian degeneration were ameliorated by PTX treatment. MPG culture in medium containing PTX resulted in a significant increase of neurite length.

Conclusions.—PTX treatment following CN injury in rats improved erectile recovery, enhanced nerve regeneration, and preserved the corpus cavernosum microarchitecture. The clinical availability of this compound merits application in penile rehabilitation studies following RP in the near future.

▶ In this study, pentoxifylline exerted a dose-dependent salubrious effect on the recovery of erectile function in an animal model of radical pelvic surgery with nerve injury. This improvement was associated with greater integrity of neurons (as assessed by neuronal nitric oxide synthase content and qualitative histological analysis) and smooth muscle and decreased accumulation of collagen (a marker for fibrosis). Interestingly, pentoxifylline appeared to exert a dose-dependent effect on the sprouting of neurites from cultured fragments of the major pelvic ganglion. Whether or not this sprouting effect is representative of a neurotrophic property is unclear, but the finding is of some interest.

Pentoxifylline has antifibrotic and phosphodiesterase inhibitory effects. It also downregulates transforming growth factor β, a cytokine shown to play an important role in the pathogenesis of Peyronie disease and other fibrotic conditions of the penis. Importantly, this medication is relatively inexpensive and fairly well tolerated; this makes it an appealing alternative to current medical treatments administered for penile rehabilitation after radical prostatectomy. While further research is warranted, this study does not constitute sufficient evidence to merit changes in practice pattern at this time.

A. Shindel, MD

Long-Term Infection Outcomes After Original Antibiotic Impregnated Inflatable Penile Prosthesis Implants: Up to 7.7 Years of Followup
Carson CC III, Mulcahy JJ, Harsch MR (Univ of North Carolina at Chapel Hill; Univ of Arizona, Tuscon; American Med Systems, Minnetonka, MN)
J Urol 185:614-618, 2011

Purpose.—Although some studies suggest that most infections associated with inflatable penile prosthesis implantation develop within year 1 after surgery, device related infections have been reported 5 years after implantation or later and the infection risk with time is not well characterized. We previously reported a statistically significantly lower infection rate for original inflatable penile prostheses impregnated with antibiotic treatment with minocycline and rifampin vs nonimpregnated inflatable penile prostheses at 1-year followup. Long-term data are now available on infection revision after initial implantation of antibiotic impregnated vs nonimpregnated prostheses.

Materials and Methods.—We retrospectively reviewed patient information forms voluntarily filed with the manufacturer after the initial implantation of more than 39,000 inflatable penile prostheses to compare the revision rate due to infection for antibiotic impregnated vs nonimpregnated implants between May 1, 2001 and December 31, 2008. Life table analysis was used to evaluate device survival from revision surgery.

Results.—On life table survival analysis initial revision events due to infection were significantly less common in the impregnated vs the nonimpregnated group (log rank p <0.0001). At up to 7.7 years of followup 1.1% of 35,737 vs 2.5% of 3,268 men with impregnated vs nonimpregnated implants underwent initial revision due to infection.

Conclusions.—To our knowledge this long-term outcome analysis provides the first substantial clinical evidence of a decrease in costly infection related revision using an antibiotic impregnated inflatable penile prosthesis.

▶ This report (derived from a company database of reported complications) highlights over 7 years of experience using antibiotic-impregnated penile implants for the management of refractory erectile dysfunction. The rate of infection was markedly decreased in men who received the antibiotic-impregnated device compared with those who received a nonimpregnated device. Interestingly, the antibiotic-impregnated devices were much more commonly used than the nonimpregnated implants, in a ratio of 10:1. Furthermore, the mean duration of follow-up was 40 months in the impregnated group compared with 77 months in the nonimpregnated group.

It is unclear if and how these differences may have influenced the outcomes of this study. The potential for late infection is small but not nil, so the rate of infections in this antibiotic-impregnated cohort might theoretically rise with longer follow-up. Furthermore, the nonimpregnated implants might have been more commonly used by lower volume implanters in locations remote from major centers; the potential influence of surgeon experience cannot be controlled for in a study such as this.

Regardless, there appears to be little or no reason not to adopt the use of antibiotic-impregnated implants for penile prosthetic surgery, assuming that patients are not allergic to the antibiotics in question. These devices should be seen as the modern standard of care.

A. Shindel, MD

Relationship of Asymmetric Dimethylarginine With Penile Doppler Ultrasound Parameters in Men with Vasculogenic Erectile Dysfunction

Ioakeimidis N, Vlachopoulos C, Rokkas K, et al (Hippokration Hosp, Athens, Greece)
Eur Urol 59:948-955, 2011

Background.—Asymmetric dimethylarginine (ADMA), a selective endogenous nitric oxide synthase inhibitor, is elevated in many conditions associated with erectile dysfunction (ED), such as hypertension, diabetes, hyperlipidemia, and renal failure; it is also increased in men with coronary artery disease and ED. The dynamic penile colour Doppler ultrasound is considered the gold standard for the evaluation of penile vascular damage.

Objective.—We investigated whether the extent of ultrasonographically documented penile vascular disease is associated with higher ADMA levels.

Design, Setting, and Participants.—One hundred four consecutive ED patients (mean age: 56 ± 9 yr) without manifest cardiovascular/atherosclerotic disease and 31 subjects with normal erectile function matched for age and traditional risk factors were studied.

Measurements.—We evaluated penile dynamic colour Doppler parameters of arterial insufficiency (peak systolic velocity) and veno-occlusive dysfunction (end diastolic velocity) and measured systemic inflammatory markers/mediators.

Results and Limitations.—Compared to men without ED, ED patients had significantly higher ADMA levels ($p < 0.001$). ADMA was significantly increased in patients with severe arterial insufficiency (PSV <25 cm/s) compared to subjects with borderline insufficiency and men with normal penile arterial function ($p < 0.001$, by analysis of variance). Multivariable analysis adjusting for age, mean pressure, other risk factors, high-sensitivity C-reactive protein, testosterone, and treatment showed independent inverse association between ADMA level and peak systolic velocity ($p < 0.01$). The combination of higher ADMA level with arterial insufficiency showed greater impact on 10-yr risk of a cardiovascular event compared to either parameter alone.

Conclusions.—ADMA level is independently associated with ultrasonographically documented poor penile arterial inflow. This finding underlines the important role of ADMA as a marker of penile arterial damage and implies a contribution of this compound to the pathophysiology of generalised vascular disease associated with ED.

▶ Asymmetric dimethylarginine (ADMA) is a competitive inhibitor of endothelial nitric oxide synthase (eNOS). eNOS is known to be important in generation of NO and subsequent vasodilation during penile erection, and it is therefore logical to speculate that ADMA may be an antagonist of erectile function in men. In this study, serum ADMA levels were shown to be markedly increased in men with impaired vascular response to injection of erectogenic agents; higher levels of ADMA were more common in men with the most severe degree of penile vascular dysfunction. These relationships were maintained even after multivariate adjustment.

The strength of these data is the acquisition of objective measurements of penile vascular function using Doppler ultrasound. Questionnaire-based data are of value but are subject to numerous potentially confounding factors. However, control subjects in this study did not undergo penile Doppler ultrasound, so the relationship between ADMA and cavernosal artery peak systolic velocity is unclear in men without clinical erectile dysfunction (Sexual Health Inventory for Men score > 22 in this study).

A. Shindel, MD

Regular Nonsteroidal Anti-Inflammatory Drug Use and Erectile Dysfunction
Gleason JM, Slezak JM, Jung H, et al (Kaiser Permanente Los Angeles Med Ctr, CA; Kaiser Permanente Southern California, San Diego, CA; et al)
J Urol 185:1388-1393, 2011

Purpose.—Previous data suggest a potential relationship between inflammation and erectile dysfunction. If it is causal, nonsteroidal anti-inflammatory drug use should be inversely associated with erectile dysfunction. To this end we examined the association between nonsteroidal anti-inflammatory drug use and erectile dysfunction in a large, ethnically diverse cohort of men enrolled in the California Men's Health Study.

Materials and Methods.—This prospective cohort study enrolled male members of the Kaiser Permanente managed care plans who were 45 to 69 years old beginning in 2002. Erectile dysfunction was assessed by questionnaire. Nonsteroidal anti-inflammatory drug exposure was determined by automated pharmacy data and self-reported use.

Results.—Of the 80,966 men in this study 47.4% were considered nonsteroidal anti-inflammatory drug users based on the definitions used and 29.3% reported moderate or severe erectile dysfunction. Nonsteroidal anti-inflammatory drug use and erectile dysfunction strongly correlated with age with regular drug use increasing from 34.5% in men at ages 45 to 49 years to 54.7% in men 60 to 69 years old with erectile dysfunction increasing from 13% to 42%. The unadjusted OR for the association of nonsteroidal anti-inflammatory drugs and erectile dysfunction was 2.40 (95% CI 2.27, 2.53). With adjustment for age, race/ethnicity, smoking status, diabetes mellitus, hypertension, hyperlipidemia, peripheral vascular disease, coronary artery disease and body mass index, a positive association persisted (adjusted OR 1.38). The association persisted when using a stricter definition of nonsteroidal anti-inflammatory drug exposure.

Conclusions.—These data suggest that regular nonsteroidal anti-inflammatory drug use is associated with erectile dysfunction beyond what would be expected due to age and comorbidity.

▶ This interesting study investigates the association between the use of nonsteroidal antiinflammatory drugs (NSAIDs) and erectile dysfunction in a large cohort of men aged 45 to 69 years who were enrolled in managed care health system in California. In the unadjusted analysis, the NSAID use (self-report of NSAID use > 5 days per week, dispensing of a 3-times daily NSAID, or dispensing of a 100-day supply of NSAID) was associated with erectile dysfunction (defined as a response of "never" or "sometimes" to a 4-response option question about ability to attain and maintain an erection for sexual intercourse in a dichotomous analysis). This relationship persisted after adjustment for comorbid vascular diseases known to be associated with erection dysfunction (ED). Similar results were obtained when the analysis was repeated, stratifying ED into severity categories based on the same question on penile erection (a response of "never" equating to severe ED, a response of "sometimes" or "usually" equating to moderate ED, and a response of "always" equating to no ED).

It must be borne in mind that correlation does not imply causality; men with pain issues related to NSAIDs may find sexual activity more difficult, which is secondary to functional issues relating to the body mechanics of sexual activity. Be that as it may, the possibility that NSAIDs exert a physiological influence on erectile hemodynamics is a worthy topic for further investigation.

A. Shindel, MD

Effect of Intensive Glycemic Therapy on Erectile Function in Men With Type 1 Diabetes

Wessells H, Diabetes Control and Complications Trial/Epidemiology of Diabetes Interventions and Complications Research Group (Univ of Washington School of Medicine, Seattle; et al)
J Urol 185:1828-1834, 2011

Purpose.—We determined whether intensive glycemic therapy reduces the risk of erectile dysfunction in men with type 1 diabetes enrolled in the Diabetes Control and Complications Trial.

Materials and Methods.—The Diabetes Control and Complications Trial randomized 761 men with type 1 diabetes to intensive or conventional glycemic therapy at 28 sites between 1983 and 1989, of whom 366 had diabetes for 1 to 5 years and no microvascular complications (primary prevention cohort), and 395 had diabetes for 1 to 15 years with nonproliferative retinopathy or microalbuminuria (secondary intervention cohort). Subjects were treated until 1993, and followed in the Epidemiology of Diabetes Interventions and Complications study. In 2003 we conducted an ancillary study using a validated assessment of erectile dysfunction in 571 men (80% participation rate), 291 in the primary cohort and 280 in the secondary cohort.

Results.—Of the participants 23% reported erectile dysfunction. The prevalence was significantly lower in the intensive vs conventional treatment group in the secondary cohort (12.8% vs 30.8%, p = 0.001) but not in the primary cohort (17% vs 20.3%, p = 0.49). The risk of erectile dysfunction in primary and secondary cohorts was directly associated with mean HbA1c during the Diabetes Control and Complications Trial, and Epidemiology of Diabetes Interventions and Complications combined. Age, peripheral neuropathy and lower urinary tract symptoms were other risk factors.

Conclusions.—A period of intensive therapy significantly reduced the prevalence of erectile dysfunction 10 years later among those men in the secondary intervention cohort but not in the primary prevention cohort. Higher HbA1c was significantly associated with risk in both cohorts. These findings provide further support for early implementation of intensive insulin therapy in young men with type 1 diabetes.

▶ This is a long-term follow-up study of erectile function outcomes in a cohort of men with diabetes mellitus type 1 (DM1) treated with intensive insulin therapy (multiple daily insulin injections and/or the use of a subcutaneous insulin pump with close monitoring of serum glucose) compared with standard insulin therapy (insulin treatment once or twice daily) between 1983 and 1993 as part of the Diabetes Control and Complications Trial (DCCT). Men were divided into an early DM1 arm (DM1 of 1-5 years duration with no complications) for primary prevention and a late DM1 arm (DM1 of 1-15 years with retinopathy or microalbuminuria) for secondary prevention. After conclusion of the trial in 1993, all subjects were instructed to initiate intensive insulin therapy. Interestingly, 10 years after cessation of the formal study in 1993, it was found that men in the secondary prevention group who had been treated with intensive insulin therapy had a lower odds of erectile dysfunction (defined as low or very low confidence in the ability to get and keep an erection) compared with men treated with standard therapy. No such difference was detected between treatment arms in the primary prevention arm.

It is very interesting that, based on prior reports cited in the "Methods" section of this article, more than 90% of men in both the intensive and conventional arms of the DCCT were using intensive therapy at 10-year follow-up and hemoglobin A1c levels had equalized between these 2 arms. It is implied from this that the early initiation of intensive insulin therapy is responsible for the erectile function benefit. This finding should hopefully provide motivation for men with diabetes to take prompt control of their disease state.

A. Shindel, MD

The Management of Peyronie's Disease: Evidence-based 2010 Guidelines

Ralph D, Gonzalez-Cadavid N, Mirone V, et al (Inst of Urology, London UK; UCLA; Univ of Naples "Federico II", Italy; et al)
J Sex Med 7:2359-2374, 2010

Introduction.—The field of Peyronie's disease is evolving and there is need for a state-of-the-art information in this area.

Aim.—To develop an evidence-based state-of-the-art consensus report on the management of Peyronie's disease.

Methods.—To provide state-of-the-art knowledge regarding the prevalence, etiology, medical and surgical management of Peyronie's Disease, representing the opinion of leading experts developed in a consensus process over a 2-year period.

Main Outcome Measures.—Expert opinion was based on grading of evidence-based medical literature, widespread internal committee discussion, public presentation, and debate.

Conclusions.—The real etiology of Peyronie's disease and the mechanisms of formation of the plaque still remain obscure. Although conservative management is obtaining a progressively larger consensus among the experts, surgical correction still remains the mainstay treatment for this condition.

▶ This article is a consensus statement from a number of experts on the management of Peyronie disease. While it represents the state of the art, it remains a great disappointment that there is so little understanding about what causes Peyronie disease and how it should be managed. It is concluded that the disorder is not rare (grade B evidence) and that the spontaneous resolution rate is quite low (grade C evidence). The evidence supporting what penile morphometric criteria should be assessed at baseline is weak (grade D) as is evidence on the role of common comorbid conditions (grade D). The authors conclude that nonsurgical therapy with intralesional injections is an option for men with disease that has been present less than 12 months (grade C for verapamil and grade B for interferon), but that there is no clear evidence for efficacy from oral therapy or shock wave lithotripsy at this time (grade B). It is agreed that surgical therapy is the most definitive management for Peyronie disease, but there is no clear evidence that 1 surgical approach is superior to others (grade C for both).

It is clear from the relatively low grading of evidence for this condition that more research is required for this common condition.

A. Shindel, MD

Effects of Testosterone Undecanoate on Cardiovascular Risk Factors and Atherosclerosis in Middle-Aged Men with Late-Onset Hypogonadism and Metabolic Syndrome: Results from a 24-month, Randomized, Double-Blind, Placebo-Controlled Study

Aversa A, Bruzziches R, Francomano D, et al (Sapienza Univ of Rome, Italy; et al)

J Sex Med 2010 [Epub ahead of print]

Introduction.—Longitudinal studies have demonstrated that male hypogonadism could be considered a surrogate marker of incident cardiovascular disease.

Aim.—To evaluate the effects of parenteral testosterone undecanoate (TU) in outclinic patients with metabolic syndrome (MS) and late-onset hypogonadism (total testosterone (T) at or below 11 nmol/L or free T at or below 250 pmol/L).

Methods.—This is a randomized, double-blind, double-dummy, placebo-controlled, parallel group, single-center study. Fifty patients (mean age 57 ± 8) were randomized (4:1) to receive TU 1,000 mg (every 12 weeks) or placebo (PLB) gel (3–6 g/daily) for 24 months.

Main Outcome Measures.—Homeostasis model assessment index of insulin resistance (HOMA-IR), carotid intima media thickness (CIMT), and high-sensitivity C-reactive protein (hsCRP).

Results.—At baseline, all patients fulfilled the National Cholesterol Education Program-Third Adult Treatment Panel (NCEP-ATPIII) and International Diabetes Federation (IDF) criteria for the definition of MS. An interim analysis conducted at 12 months showed that TU markedly improved HOMA-IR ($P < 0.001$), CIMT ($P < 0.0001$), and hsCRP ($P < 0.001$) compared with PLB; thus, all patients were shifted to TU treatment. After 24 months, 35% ($P < 0.0001$) and 58% ($P < 0.001$) of patients still presented MS as defined by NCEP-ATPIII and IDF criteria, respectively. Main determinants of changes were reduction in waist circumference ($P < 0.0001$), visceral fat mass ($P < 0.0001$), and improvement in HOMA-IR without changes in body mass index (BMI).

Conclusions.—TU reduced fasting glucose, waist circumference, and improved surrogate markers of atherosclerosis in hypogonadal men with MS. Resumption and maintenance of T levels in the normal range of young adults determines a remarkable reduction in cardiovascular risk factors clustered in MS without significant hematological and prostate adverse events.

▶ Testosterone is widely known as a hormone intimately involved in sexual desire and function; the other health benefits of testosterone supplementation have become topics of greater interest in recent years. This is all the more important given data suggesting that lower testosterone is associated with serious cardiovascular disease and that hypogonadal states may be predictors of serious morbidity.

In this study, symptomatic hypogonadal men (total testosterone < 300 ng/dL or free testosterone < 250 pmol/L) with the metabolic syndrome were randomized to treatment with depot testosterone undecanoate versus placebo gel for a 2-year period. At 1-year follow-up, men who had been treated with testosterone had significant declines in insulin resistance, inflammatory C-reactive protein, and carotid intimal thickness and hence all men were treated with testosterone for the second year of the study. At 2-year follow-up, improvements in waist circumference, visceral adiposity, and insulin sensitivity led to a number of men no longer meeting criteria for metabolic syndrome. There were no clinically significant adverse events ascribable to testosterone during the trial aside from mild erythrocytosis in 3 patients who were advised to discontinue the trial.

The authors used a double-dummy trial design so that all subjects received both an injection and a gel on the same dosing schedule. The longitudinal nature of the study makes it interesting, although the patient population is rather small. It is suggested that testosterone may be a useful treatment for general cardiovascular health in men with the metabolic syndrome, although larger prospective studies are indicated to verify that these biochemical changes are associated with testosterone use in other centers. It will also be of interest to determine whether or not these biochemical changes are associated with differences in undesirable outcomes such as myocardial infarction or cardiac death.

A. Shindel, MD

Adherence to Mediterranean Diet and Erectile Dysfunction in Men with Type 2 Diabetes

Giugliano F, Maiorino MI, Bellastella G, et al (Second Univ of Naples, Italy)
J Sex Med 7:1911-1917, 2010

Introduction.—There are no reported studies assessing the relation between diet and erectile dysfunction (ED) in men with diabetes.

Aim.—In the present study, we explored the relation between consumption of a Mediterranean-type diet and ED in a population of type 2 diabetic men.

Methods.—Patients with type 2 diabetes were enrolled if they had a diagnosis of type 2 diabetes for at least six months but less than 10 years, age 35–70 years, body mass index (BMI) of 24 or higher, HbA1c of 6.5% or higher, treatment with diet or oral drugs. All diabetic patients were invited to complete a food-frequency questionnaire and self-report measures of sexual function. A total of 555 (90.8%) of the 611 diabetic men completed both questionnaires and were analyzed in the present study.

Main Outcome Measures.—Adherence to a Mediterranean diet was assessed by a 9-point scale that incorporated the salient characteristics of this diet (range of scores, 0–9, with higher scores indicating greater adherence). ED was assessed with the International Index of Erectile Function-5.

Results.—Diabetic men with the highest scores (6–9) had lower BMI, waist circumference, and waist-to-hip ratio, a lower prevalence of obesity and metabolic syndrome, a higher level of physical activity, and better glucose and lipid profiles than the diabetic men who scored <3 points on the scale. The proportion of sexually active men showed a significant increase across tertiles of adherence to Mediterranean diet (from 65.1% to 74.4%, $P = 0.01$). Moreover, men with the highest score of adherence were more likely to have a lower prevalence of global ED (51.9% vs. 62%, $P = 0.01$) and severe ED (16.5% vs. 26.4%, $P = 0.01$) as compared with low adherers.

Conclusions.—In men with type 2 diabetes, greater adherence to Mediterranean diet is associated with a lower prevalence of ED.

▶ In this study, 555 men with type 2 diabetes were queried on their dietary habits to determine how closely their dietary intake reflects the Mediterranean diet, consisting primarily of fruits, vegetables, nuts, legumes, olive oil, fish, and moderate amounts of ethanol with a low intake of saturated fats and processed or red meat. Men who adhered to a Mediterranean style diet over the year before the study tended to have lower body mass index, better lipid and glucose profiles, less depressive symptoms, and lower incidence of vascular comorbidities. After multivariable adjustment, men who ate a Mediterranean diet were also statistically more likely to be sexually active and be free from both erectile dysfunction (ED) and severe ED.

Dietary change is very difficult to effect, and it is likely that many patients with sexual dysfunction would be resistant to radical changes in their diet. However, data such as these suggest that encouraging our diabetic patients to make prudent dietary choices is likely to yield benefits in sexual functioning in addition to other health benefits. Additional studies should be undertaken to investigate other healthy diets as means to ameliorate the effects of sexual dysfunction.

A. Shindel, MD

Association of Episodic Physical and Sexual Activity With Triggering of Acute Cardiac Events: Systematic Review and Meta-analysis
Dahabreh IJ, Paulus JK (Tufts Med Ctr, Boston, MA; Tufts Univ, Medford, MA)
JAMA 305:1225-1233, 2010

Context.—Evidence has suggested that physical and sexual activity might be triggers of acute cardiac events.

Objective.—To assess the effect of episodic physical and sexual activity on acute cardiac events using data from case-crossover studies.

Data Sources.—MEDLINE and EMBASE (through February 2, 2011) and Web of Science (through October 6, 2010).

Study Selection.—Case-crossover studies investigating the association between episodic physical or sexual activity and myocardial infarction (MI) or sudden cardiac death (SCD).

Data Extraction.—Two reviewers extracted descriptive and quantitative information from each study. We calculated summary relative risks (RRs) using random-effects metaanalysis and absolute event rates based on US data for the incidence of MI and SCD. We used the Fisher *P* value synthesis method to test whether habitual physical activity levels modify the triggering effect and meta-regression to quantify the interaction between habitual levels of physical activity and the triggering effect.

Results.—We identified 10 studies investigating episodic physical activity, 3 studies investigating sexual activity, and 1 study investigating both exposures. The outcomes of interest were MI (10 studies), acute coronary syndrome (1 study), and SCD (3 studies). Episodic physical and sexual activity were associated with an increase in the risk of MI (RR=3.45; 95% confidence interval [CI], 2.33-5.13, and RR=2.70; 95% CI, 1.48-4.91, respectively). Episodic physical activity was associated with SCD (RR=4.98; 95% CI, 1.47-16.91). The effect of triggers on the absolute rate of events was limited because exposure to physical and sexual activity is infrequent and their effect is transient; the absolute risk increase associated with 1 hour of additional physical or sexual activity per week was estimated as 2 to 3 per 10 000 person-years for MI and 1 per 10 000 person-years for SCD. Habitual activity levels significantly affected the association of episodic physical activity and MI ($P<.001$), episodic physical activity and SCD ($P<.001$), and sexual activity and MI ($P=.04$); in all cases, individuals with lower habitual activity levels had an increased RR for the triggering effect. For every additional time per week an individual was habitually exposed to physical activity, the RR for MI decreased by approximately 45%, and the RR for SCD decreased by 30%.

Conclusion.—Acute cardiac events were significantly associated with episodic physical and sexual activity; this association was attenuated among persons with high levels of habitual physical activity.

▶ This important meta-analysis investigates the effects of intermittent physical exertion and sexual activity as risk factors for acute myocardial infarction (MI) and sudden cardiac death (SCD). The authors reviewed published case-crossover studies in Pubmed. Three studies specifically investigated sexual activity. It was determined that for each hour of additional sexual activity per week there is approximately a 2 to 3 per 10 000 person-year increase in MI, and a 1 per 10 000 person-year increase in SCD; these effects were attenuated in part because exposure to these physical activities was relatively rare. Most importantly, regular physical activity (ie, exercise) was protective against both MI and SCD; for each hour routinely spent in physical activity, there was a 45% and 30% decline in relative risk for MI and SCD during intermittent physical/sexual activity, respectively.

Exercise is known to be protective against development of erectile dysfunction (ED). This study makes it clear that exercise is also important for minimizing the slight but potentially devastating risk of serious cardiac events during sexual activity. Physicians prescribing erectogenic therapy for men with ED would be well advised to keep this in mind when counseling their patients about sexual activity.

A. Shindel, MD

Five-Year Follow-Up of Peyronie's Graft Surgery: Outcomes and Patient Satisfaction
Chung E, Clendinning E, Lessard L, et al (St Joseph Health Care—Urology, London, Ontario, Canada; Univ of Western Ontario, London, Ontario, Canada)
J Sex Med 8:594-600, 2011

Introduction.—Graft surgery for Peyronie's disease (PD) is associated with significant long-term risks.

Aim.—To evaluate the clinical and functional outcomes of graft repairs with a minimum of 5-year follow-up.

Methods.—A retrospective review of database and third party telephone survey was undertaken in all men who underwent reconstructive graft procedures for PD between May 1999 and May 2005.

Main Outcome Measures.—Patient demographics, International Index of Erectile Function (IIEF-5) scores, and penile Doppler ultrasonography were performed preoperative. Follow-up assessments included surgical outcomes and overall patient satisfactions.

Results.—A total of 86 patients with an average age of 54.6 (34 to 73) years underwent Peyronie's graft repair. The average follow-up was 98 (61 to 120) months. Twenty patients received dermal graft whereas 33 patients underwent Tutoplast graft and 33 patients had Stratasis small intestinal submucosa graft. Penile curvature greater than 60 degrees was more common in the Tutoplast and Stratasis groups. Twelve patients used phosphodiesterase type 5 inhibitors or intracavenous agents preoperatively. At the time of review, only 46 (53%) patients were able to be contacted and consented for telephone interview. Although 6 months of postoperative follow-up showed excellent resolution, or significantly less, penile curvature, this figures decreased to 50% in dermal, 87% in Tutoplast, and 76% in Stratasis patients. Further penile length shortening was also reported on patient self-assessment at the recent follow-up. Worsening of IIEF-5 scores were noted with the development of erectile dysfunction was more pronounced in the diabetic cohort ($P < 0.01$). The overall satisfaction on a 5-point scale was 2.6 with more than 65% of patients dissatisfied with the outcomes of the Peyronie's graft surgery.

Conclusions.—The recurrence of penile curvature, penile length loss, and the new-onset of ED are not uncommon sequelae and are associated with a significant patient dissatisfaction rate when a 5-year follow-up is achieved.

▶ This report is limited, as all retrospective cohort studies must be, by patient attrition. However, among the slightly over half of eligible patients who were able to be contacted at follow-up (mean 98 months postoperatively), dissatisfaction with penile patch grafting for repair of pronounced penile deformity from Peyronie disease (PD) was quite high. The 5-year minimum follow-up provides a better sense of long-term durability of this type of repair. The durability of the repair at time of follow-up was slightly less at final follow-up compared with 6 months, and a greater number of patients were reliant on erectogenic therapies at follow-up. Tellingly, almost two-thirds of subjects were dissatisfied with the surgery.

This study was derived from a patient population seen at a center of excellence in management of PD, so it may be reasonably concluded that these are near optimal outcomes for the clinical scenarios and types of graft material used. Furthermore, 90% of these men had adequate arterial inflow, and 100% had no evidence of venous leak as determined by Doppler ultrasound of the penis at baseline.

A legitimate critique is that natural progression of either PD or vascular disease may be to blame for the greater incidence of penile foreshortening and erectile dysfunction (ED) at the time of follow-up. Be that as it may, an increase in ED incidence after patch graft surgery has been previously reported, and this most recent study only adds to the evidence that ED is a potentially serious outcome of this approach.

Regardless of etiology, it is clear from these data that current outcomes for men with PD who undergo grafting surgery are far from optimal. More research is required, and men contemplating this repair need to have a well-informed discussion with their provider about expectations.

A. Shindel, MD

The Effect of Intracavernous Injection of Adipose Tissue-Derived Stem Cells on Hyperlipidemia-Associated Erectile Dysfunction in a Rat Model
Huang Y-C, Ning H, Shindel AW, et al (Univ of California, San Francisco)
J Sex Med 7:1391-1400, 2010

Introduction.—Hyperlipidemia has been associated with erectile dysfunction (ED) via damage to the cavernous endothelium and nerves. Adipose tissue-derived stem cells (ADSC) have been shown to differentiate into endothelial cells and secrete vasculotrophic and neurotrophic factors.

Aim.—To assess whether ADSC have therapeutic effects on hyperlipidemia-associated ED.

Methods.—Twenty-eight male rats were induced to develop hyperlipidemia with a high-fat diet (hyperlipidemic rats, HR). Ten additional male rats were fed a normal diet to serve as controls (normal rats, NR). Five months later, all rats were subjected to ADSC isolation from paragonadal fat. The cells were cultured for 1 week, labeled with 5-ethynyl-2'-deoxyuridine (EdU), and then injected autologously into the corpus cavernosum of 18 HR. The remaining 10 HR rats were injected with phosphate buffered saline (PBS). At 2 and 14 days post-transplantation, four rats in the HR + ADSC group were sacrificed for tracking of the transplanted cells. At 28 days post-transplantation, all remaining rats were analyzed for serum biochemistry, erectile function, and penile histology.

Main Outcome Measures.—Erectile function was assessed by intracavernous pressure (ICP) measurement during electrostimulation of the cavernous nerve. Cavernous nerves, endothelium, and smooth muscle were assessed by immunohistochemistry.

Results.—Serum total cholesterol and low-density lipoprotein levels were significantly higher in HR than in NR. High-density lipoprotein level was significantly lower in HR than in NR. Mean ICP/mean arterial pressure ratio was significantly lower in HR + PBS than in NR + PBS or HR + ADSC. Neuronal nitric oxide synthase (nNOS)-positive nerve fibers and endothelial cells were fewer in HR + PBS than in HR + ADSC. Smooth muscle content was significantly higher in both HR groups than in NR.

Conclusions.—Hyperlipidemia is associated with abnormalities in both the nerves and endothelium. Treatment with ADSC ameliorates these adverse effects and holds promise as a potential new therapy for ED.

▶ In this study, cultured vascular stem cells derived from autologous adipose tissue were injected into the cavernous tissues of rats with diet-induced hyperlipidemia. Rats were sacrificed for cell localization at 2, 14, and 28 days after injection, and functional studies were performed 28 days after injection. Rats that were treated with the stem cell preparation had significantly better intracavernous pressure response during cavernous nerve electrostimulation; tissue studies confirmed that treated rats had higher content of neuronal nitric oxide synthase, endothelial cells, and smooth muscle. Interestingly, labeled stem cells were scant at the 28-day time point.

These data suggest that stem cells may be used to reverse the penile tissue effects of hyperlipidemia. Indeed, the improvements that were noted involved virtually every penile tissue type thought to be important in penile erection. Questions remain, however, with respect to the mechanism of action. Do cells transform into tissues of interest? The relative scarcity of stem cells at the 28-day time point suggests that the cells do not persist in the corporeal tissues or at the very least that they divide and dilute the intensity of the label staining such that they are no longer visualized. An alternate explanation for the efficacy of this treatment could be prompting survival/regeneration of native tissues by release of trophic factors. Further research on the basic mechanisms is certainly warranted before clinical trials are initiated.

A. Shindel, MD

Genetic and Environmental Influences on Self-Reported G-Spots in Women: A Twin Study
Burri AV, Cherkas L, Spector TD (King's College London, UK)
J Sex Med 7:1842-1852, 2010

Introduction.—There is an ongoing debate around the existence of the G-spot—an allegedly highly sensitive area on the anterior wall of the human vagina. The existence of the G-spot seems to be widely accepted among women, despite the failure of numerous behavioral, anatomical, and biochemical studies to prove its existence. Heritability has been demonstrated in all other genuine anatomical traits studied so far.

Aim.—To investigate whether the self-reported G-spot has an underlying genetic basis.

Methods.—1804 unselected female twins aged 22—83 completed a questionnaire that included questions about female sexuality and asked about the presence or absence of a G-spot. The relative contribution of genetic and environmental factors to variation in the reported existence of a G-spot was assessed using a variance components model fitting approach.

Main Outcome Measures.—Genetic variance component analysis of self-reported G-spot.

Results.—We found 56% of women reported having a G-spot. The prevalence decreased with age. Variance component analyses revealed that variation in G-spot reported frequency is almost entirely a result of individual experiences and random measurement error (>89%) with no detectable genetic influence. Correlations with associated general sexual behavior, relationship satisfaction, and attitudes toward sexuality suggest that the self-reported G-spot is to be a secondary pseudo-phenomenon.

Conclusions.—To our knowledge, this is the largest study investigating the prevalence of the G-spot and the first one to explore an underlying genetic basis. A possible explanation for the lack of heritability may be that women differ in their ability to detect their own (true) G-spots. However, we postulate that the reason for the lack of genetic variation—in contrast to other anatomical and physiological traits studied—is that there is no physiological or physical basis for the G-spot.

▶ An enormous self-help industry has been built around the concept of the G-spot, an anatomical area within the anterior vaginal wall, which is purportedly a potential source of intense sexual pleasure for women. However, it has proved exceedingly difficult to prove the existence of such an anatomical structure using imaging or tissue studies. Some authors have even argued that the G-spot is a quasi-Freudian concept designed to encourage women to focus on penetrative sexual acts at the possible expense of attention to the generally more orgasmically reliable and sensitive clitoris. The controversy surrounding the G-spot has not, however, dampened enthusiasm about this alleged magic button for female sexual pleasure.

In this study, 1840 heterosexual female twins (average age 55 years) completed a series of questions relating to their sexuality and perception of the G-spot. Over half of the subjects reported that they had a G-spot, with younger women reporting a G-spot more frequently than older women. It was found that the variance in self-report of having a G-spot was not likely because of genetic factors but rather environmental cues and random error. In this population, orgasm was most reliably obtained by clitoral stimulation even in women who reported having a G-spot; indeed, among women who had a G-spot, a significantly greater proportion preferred clitoral versus vaginal orgasm (42% vs 27%, respectively).

Fundamentally, whether the G-spot exists as a discrete structure, a nexus of nervous tissue, or a collective delusion is of little import. Some women may find stimulation of the anterior vaginal wall pleasurable and conducive to orgasm, whereas others may not. It would seem that our patients' interests will be best served by providers who neither herald nor deny the G-spot but rather encourage their female patients to experiment and explore which types of sensations feel good to them sexually. There is no reason for women not to engage in directed stimulation of the anterior vaginal wall during masturbation or partnered intercourse. Those women who enjoy that type of stimulation should use that as a part of their sexual repertoire; by the same token, those women (and their partners) who do not find it particularly pleasurable and/or conducive to orgasm should not be made to feel defective or deficient.

A. Shindel, MD

Radiofrequency Treatment of Vaginal Laxity after Vaginal Delivery: Nonsurgical Vaginal Tightening

Millheiser LS, Pauls RN, Herbst SJ, et al (Stanford Univ School of Medicine, CA; Good Samaritan Hosp, Cincinnati, OH; Inst for Women's Health, West Palm Beach, FL)
J Sex Med 2010 [Epub ahead of print]

Introduction.—All women who have given birth vaginally experience stretching of their vaginal tissue. Long-term physical and psychological consequences may occur, including loss of sensation and sexual dissatisfaction. One significant issue is the laxity of the vaginal introitus.

Aim.—To evaluate safety and tolerability of nonsurgical radiofrequency (RF) thermal therapy for treatment of laxity of the vaginal introitus after vaginal delivery. We also explored the utility of self-report questionnaires in assessing subjective effectiveness of this device.

Methods.—Pilot study to treat 24 women (25—44 years) once using reverse gradient RF energy (75—90 joules/cm^2), delivered through the vaginal mucosa. Post treatment assessments were at 10 days, 1, 3, and 6 months.

Main Outcome Measures.—Pelvic examinations and adverse event reports to assess safety. The author modified Female Sexual Function Index (mv-FSFI) and Female Sexual Distress Scale-Revised (FSDS-R), Vaginal Laxity and Sexual Satisfaction Questionnaires (designed for this study) to evaluate both safety and effectiveness, and the Global Response Assessment to assess treatment responses.

Results.—No adverse events were reported; no topical anesthetics were required. Self-reported vaginal tightness improved in 67% of subjects at one month post-treatment; in 87% at 6 months ($P < 0.001$). Mean sexual function scores improved: mv-FSFI total score before treatment was 27.6 ± 3.6, increasing to 32.0 ± 3.0 at 6 months ($P < 0.001$); FSDS-R score before treatment was 13.6 ± 8.7, declining to 4.3 ± 5.0 at month 6 post-treatment ($P < 0.001$). Twelve of 24 women who expressed diminished sexual satisfaction following their delivery; all reported sustained improvements on SSQ at 6 months after treatment ($P = 0.002$).

Conclusion.—The RF treatment was well tolerated and showed an excellent 6-month safety profile in this pilot study. Responses to the questionnaires suggest subjective improvement in self-reported vaginal tightness, sexual function and decreased sexual distress. These findings warrant further study.

▶ There is no shortage of tips, techniques, devices, maneuvers, exercises, and interventions that are promulgated by the mass media and purported experts with the intention of enhancing sexual satisfaction in men and women. Indubitably, much of this advice can be of value to the public, but it is essential that claims of efficacy be supported by objective independent data before they are widely embraced or even accepted, particularly by the medical community.

There has been a marked increase over the past several years in minor procedures designed to resolve perceived or real deficits in the female genitalia. The Internet is awash with practices offering office-based vulvovaginal procedures including laser therapy, minor surgery, and other interventions purported to enhance female sexual experience. While improvement in sexual satisfaction is a laudable goal, it is essential that such procedures undergo a thorough, unbiased, independent evaluation for safety and efficacy before they are widely disseminated as cures for sexual woes.

This research is an attempt to quantify the efficacy of a single episode of radiofrequency-based thermal therapy for vaginal laxity after parturition. Twenty-four heterosexual women in monogamous relationships with complaints of sexual dissatisfaction related to vaginal laxity after vaginal delivery were treated with radiofrequency therapy to the vaginal mucosa. There were no adverse events, and most patients reported subjective improvement in sexual function; there was also a significant improvement in validated measures used for the assessment of sexual function.

The data rely on subjective recollection of predelivery vaginal laxity as well as completely subjective assessment of change in laxity; no vaginal plethysmography or manometry was performed, so it is difficult to determine if there was any objective change in vaginal tightness. This lack of objectivity is a particular concern given the lack of a control group; a placebo effect cannot be ruled out. Assessment of the broader relationship and partner situation in women who receive this treatment will be of interest in future studies.

Further studies are necessary before this treatment can be considered an evidence-based management tactic for this sexual problem. Independent corroboration of results will also be essential as 3 of the 4 authors of this study have financial interests in the device manufacturer.

A. Shindel, MD

Effects of exposure to a mobile phone on sexual behavior in adult male rabbit: an observational study

Salama N, Kishimoto T, Kanayama H-o, et al (Tokushima School of Medicine, Japan)
Int J Impot Res 22:127-133, 2010

The accumulating effects of exposure to electromagnetic radiation emitted by a conventional mobile phone (MP) on male sexual behaviour have not yet been analyzed. Therefore, we studied these effects in 18 male rabbits that were randomly divided into phone and control groups. Six female teasers were taken successively to the male's cage and the copulatory behavior was recorded. Serum total testosterone, dopamine and cortisol were evaluated. The animals of the phone group were exposed to MPs (800 MHz) in a standby position for 8 h daily for 12 weeks. At the end of the study, the copulatory behavior and hormonal assays were re-evaluated. Mounts without ejaculation were the main mounts in the phone group and its duration and frequency increased significantly compared with the controls, whereas the reverse was observed in its mounts with ejaculation. Ejaculation frequency dropped significantly, biting/grasping against teasers increased notably and mounting latency in accumulated means from the first to the fourth teasers were noted in the phone group. The hormonal assays did not show any significant differences between the study groups. Therefore, the pulsed radiofrequency emitted by a conventional MP, which was kept on a standby position, could affect the sexual behavior in the rabbit.

▶ In this study, sexually experienced male rabbits were exposed to a mobile phone operating on an 800 Mhz frequency in the standby mode for 8 hours daily over a 12-week course. A control group was kept in a similar cage with the cell phone switched off, and a third group of rabbits had no exposure to the cage or the cell phone. Hormone assays were performed before and after the initiation of the study. The primary end point was mount and ejaculatory behavior after exposure to an estrous female rabbit over a 2-week period after the intervention. There was no difference in weight or in hormone profiles. During the mating period, animals that had been exposed to the cell phone in the standby position had a 56% rate of mounts without ejaculation compared with 26% to 27% in the other 2 groups. Mount duration without ejaculation was significantly higher in the phone-exposed group; conversely, mount duration with ejaculation was significantly lower in the phone-exposed group.

The methodology of this study is obviously difficult to extrapolate to human beings who have a much more complex set of rules and motivations for sexual activity. Nevertheless, the possibility that cell phone usage is exerting a subtle but potentially important effect on sexual function must be taken seriously, given the ubiquity of cellular phone use in the modern era. Additional human studies are needed, although it will be quite challenging to definitively ascribe findings to the cell phones themselves, as numerous potential confounders exist, and it may be highly impossible to recruit a group of noncell phone users these days.

A. Shindel, MD

A Protein Tyrosine Kinase Inhibitor, Imatinib Mesylate (Gleevec), Improves Erectile and Vascular Function Secondary to a Reduction of Hyperglycemia in Diabetic Rats
Gur S, Kadowitz PJ, Hellstrom WJG (Tulane Univ Health Sciences Ctr, New Orleans, LA)
J Sex Med 2010 [Epub ahead of print]

Introduction.—Erectile dysfunction (ED) afflicts 50% of diabetic men, many of whom experience poor results with phosphodiesterase type 5 inhibitors. The protein tyrosine kinase (PTK) inhibitor imatinib (Gleevec, Novartis Pharmaceuticals, Basel, Switzerland) has therapeutic potential in diabetic men by maintaining β-cell function.

Aim.—To determine if imatinib has a beneficial effect on erectile and vascular function in diabetic rats.

Methods.—Male Sprague-Dawley rats were divided into six groups: (i) control; (ii) imatinib (50 mg/kg, daily gavage)- treated control; (iii) diabetic; (iv) preventive imatinib (8 weeks); (v) reversal imatinib (4 weeks untreated diabetes and 4 weeks of treatment); and (vi) insulin (8 weeks)-treated diabetic rats.

Main Outcome Measures.—After 8 weeks, all groups underwent cavernosal nerve stimulation and measurements of intracavernosal pressure (ICP) and mean arterial pressure (MAP). Contractile and relaxation responses were evaluated using isolated strips of corpus cavernosum smooth muscle (CCSM) and aorta.

Results.—Diabetic rats exhibited a 32% decrease in weight and fivefold increase in blood glucose levels. Imatinibtreated diabetic rats gained weight and partially improved blood glucose levels. Diabetic rats displayed a decrease in ICP/MAP. While maximum electrical field stimulation- and acetylcholine (ACh)-induced relaxations in CCSM strips from the diabetics were reduced, preventive imatinib or insulin treatment normalized ICP/MAP ratios and improved relaxation responses. ACh responses in diabetic aortas were diminished by 50.1% and restored by imatinib. While contractile responses to phenylephrine in diabetic CCSM were not altered, there was a significant enhancement (59.4 %) in the aortic contractile response in diabetic rats, which was restored by imatinib and insulin treatment.

Conclusions.—In diabetic rats, prolonged therapy with imatinib improves diabetes-related ED and vascular function, which may involve normalization of high glucose levels and restoration of PTK activation.

Future studies are needed to elaborate on the actions of imatinib on diabetic vascular complications.

▶ Tyrosine kinases are a family of enzymes that facilitate phosphorylation of cellular proteins important for a variety of processes including cell growth, division, and death. The protein tyrosine kinase inhibitor imatinib (Gleevec) is commonly used for the treatment of chronic myeloid leukemia but has also been shown in animal models to help reduce insulin resistance in diabetes and prevent development of type I diabetes in a rat model system.

In this 8-week study, rats with streptozotocin-induced diabetes were treated with imatinib, insulin, or placebo. Rats that received imatinib treatment had significantly less blood glucose elevation relative to untreated diabetic rats, although imatinib was not as efficacious as insulin at maintaining normal blood glucose levels. Functional studies of erectile response using cavernous nerve electrostimulation in vivo and contractility studies of corpora strips ex vivo indicated better preservation of erectile capacity in diabetic rats treated with imatinib relative to those treated with placebo. The most pronounced effects were noted in rats that were treated with imatinib for the entire 8-week duration of the study rather than those that received just 4 weeks of treatment. In addition to the erectile tissue benefits, decreased adrenergic receptor mediated contractility of the aorta, suggesting a more widespread vascular benefit to this drug in these diabetic animals.

The mechanism(s) underlying these observed effects are not at this time clear; the authors speculate that preservation of nonadrenergic noncholinergic neurons and the corporal endothelium is the most likely explanation for these observations, but this is by no means certain. Clearly, further studies investigating the efficacy of this type of intervention in animals and humans with type II diabetes (rather than the diabetes mellitus type I model used in this study) are warranted.

A. Shindel, MD

Is Obesity a Further Cardiovascular Risk Factor in Patients with Erectile Dysfunction?
Corona G, Monami M, Boddi V, et al (Univ of Florence, Italy; et al)
J Sex Med 7:2538-2546, 2010

Introduction.—Erectile dysfunction (ED) and, in particular, arteriogenic ED have been proposed as new markers of risk for incident major adverse cardiovascular events (MACE). Reduced penile blood flow is more common in obese people than in leaner ED subjects.

Aim.—To explore the interaction of overweight/obesity and penile blood flow in the prediction of incident MACE.

Methods.—This is an observational prospective cohort study evaluating a consecutive series of 1,687 patients attending our andrological unit for

ED. Different clinical, biochemical, and instrumental (penile flow at color Doppler ultrasound: PCDU) parameters were evaluated.

Main Outcomes Measures.—According to body mass index (BMI), subjects were divided into three groups: normal weight (BMI = 18.5–24.9 kg/m^2), overweight (BMI = 25.0–29.9 kg/m^2), and obese (BMI ≥ 30.0 kg/m^2). Information on MACE was obtained through the City of Florence Registry Office.

Results.—Among patients studied, 39.8% were normal weight, while 44.1% and 16.1% showed BMI 25–29.9 and 30 kg/m^2 or higher, respectively. During a mean follow-up of 4.3 ± 2.6 years, 139 MACE, 15 of which were fatal, were observed. Cox regression model, after adjusting for age and Chronic Diseases Score, showed that obesity classes along with the presence of arteriogenic ED (peak systolic velocity at PCDU <25 cm/second) were significantly and independently associated with incident MACE (hazard ratio = 1.47 [1.1–1.95], $P < 0.05$ and 2.58 [1.28–5.09], $P < 0.001$, respectively). When a separate analysis was performed for classes of obesity, reduced peak systolic velocity at PCDU (<25 cm/second) was significantly associated with incident MACE in obese (BMI ≥ 30 kg/m^2), but not in leaner, subjects.

Conclusions.—In obese subjects, more than in leaner ED subjects, impaired penile blood flow is associated with an increased risk of incident cardiovascular disease. The interaction with concomitant risk factors, such as obesity, should be taken into account when assessing the predictive value of penile blood flow for cardiovascular diseases.

▶ Numerous studies in recent years have made clear the association between self-reported erectile dysfunction (ED) and incident adverse cardiovascular events including death. This large prospective cohort study of 1687 men (957 of whom underwent color duplex ultrasound of the penis for evaluation of vascular ED) seen in an andrology clinic investigates which factors are independent predictors of major adverse cardiovascular events (MACE) over a greater than 4-year follow-up period. MACE were observed in 8% of the study population during this time period; it was determined that arterial peak systolic velocity less than 25 cm/s during duplex scan was an independent predictor of MACE, particularly in men with body mass indices greater than 30. Obesity was another particularly important predictor of MACE.

Data such as these do not dramatically change the already well-established connection between ED and incident cardiovascular events; however, the objective data linking lower peak systolic velocity to MACE verify that it is vascular ED that drives the greater mortality rate in men with ED.

A. Shindel, MD

Time Course of Recovery of Erectile Function After Radical Retropubic Prostatectomy: Does Anyone Recover After 2 Years?

Rabbani F, Schiff J, Piecuch M, et al (Montefiore Medical Center, Bronx, NY)
J Sex Med 2010 [Epub ahead of print]

Introduction.—Given the paucity of literature on the time course of recovery of erectile function (EF) after radical prostatectomy (RP), many publications have led patients and clinicians to believe that erections are unlikely to recover beyond 2 years after RP.

Aims.—We sought to determine the time course of recovery of EF beyond 2 years after bilateral nerve sparing (BNS) RP and to determine factors predictive of continued improved recovery beyond 2 years.

Methods.—EF was assessed prospectively on a 5-point scale: (i) full erections; (ii) diminished erections routinely sufficient for intercourse; (iii) partial erections occasionally satisfactory for intercourse; (iv) partial erections unsatisfactory for intercourse; and (v) no erections. From 01/1999 to 01/2007, 136 preoperatively potent (levels 1–2) men who underwent BNS RP without prior treatment and who had not recovered consistently functional erections (levels 1–2) at 24 months had further follow-up regarding EF. Median follow-up after the 2-year visit was 36.0 months.

Main Outcome Measures.—Recovery of improved erections at a later date: recovery of EF level 1–2 in those with level 3 EF at 2 years and recovery of EF level 1–3 in those with level 4–5 EF at 2 years.

Results.—The actuarial rates of further improved recovery of EF to level 1–2 in those with level 3 EF at 2 years and to level 1–3 in those with level 4–5 EF at 2 years were 8%, 20%, and 23% at 3, 4, and 5 years postoperatively, and 5%, 17%, and 21% at 3, 4, and 5 years postoperatively, respectively. Younger age was predictive of greater likelihood of recovery beyond 2 years.

Conclusion.—There is continued improvement in EF beyond 2 years after BNS RP. Discussion of this prolonged time course of recovery may allow patients to have a more realistic expectation.

▶ In this study, long-term recovery of erectile function was assessed in 136 men who were potent on at least most attempts at intercourse before radical prostatectomy but had not covered reliable erectile function 2 years after radical prostatectomy. The authors used a 5-point scale for erectile functionality and assessed for improvement to at least some capacity for erections in men who were unable to have intercourse at the 2-year point and improvement to reliable erections in men who were occasionally successful at the 2-year point. The actuarial estimate for functional improvement by these criteria in both categories was just shy of one-quarter of all subjects at 5 years after prostatectomy with about 30% of men who had occasionally usable erections at the 2-year point progressing to a better function at 6 years after prostatectomy; no further improvements were noted after this date in any group. Younger age was associated with greater odds of erectile recovery more than 2 years after radical prostatectomy; no other factors were found to be associated with odds of recovery.

Use of phosphodiesterase type 5 inhibitors was permitted, with erectile dysfunction diagnosed only in the cases where second- or third-line therapies were required to produce effects. Given the general benignity of these drugs, this is not necessarily of major clinical concern but may confound the results in that normal potency (defined by most patients as nonmedication-assisted erections) may not be what was occurring in these men greater than 2 years after radical prostatectomy. Further research on the relationship and psychological variables that may influence recovery more than 2 years after radical prostatectomy is necessary.

A. Shindel, MD

Adherence to Mediterranean Diet and Sexual Function in Women with Type 2 Diabetes

Giugliano F, Maiorino MI, Di Palo C, et al (Second Univ of Naples, Italy)
J Sex Med 7:1883-1890, 2010

Introduction.—There are no reported studies assessing the relation between diet and sexual function in women with diabetes.

Aim.—In the present study, we explored the relation between consumption of a Mediterranean-type diet and sexual function in a population of type 2 diabetic women.

Methods.—Patients with type 2 diabetes were enrolled if they had a diagnosis of type 2 diabetes for at least six months but less than 10 years, age 35–70 years, body mass index (BMI) of 24 or higher, HbA1c of 6.5% or higher, treatment with diet or oral drugs. All diabetic patients were invited to complete a food-frequency questionnaire and self-report measures of sexual function. A total of 595 (90.2%) of the 659 women completed both questionnaires and were analyzed in the present study.

Main Outcome Measures.—Adherence to a Mediterranean diet was assessed by a 9-point scale that incorporated the salient characteristics of this diet (range of scores, 0–9, with higher scores indicating greater adherence). The Female Sexual Function Index (FSFI) was used for assessing the key dimensions of female sexual function.

Results.—Diabetic women with the highest scores (6–9) had lower BMI, waist circumference, and waist-to-hip ratio, a lower prevalence of depression, obesity and metabolic syndrome, a higher level of physical activity, and better glucose and lipid profiles than the diabetic women who scored <3 points on the scale. The proportion of sexually active women showed a significant increase across tertiles of adherence to Mediterranean diet (from 54.2% to 65.1%, P = 0.01). Based on the FSFI cutoff score for female sexual dysfunction (FSD) of 23, women with the highest score of adherence had a lower prevalence of sexual dysfunction as compared with women of lower tertiles (47.6%, 53.9%, and 57.8%, higher, middle, and lower tertile, respectively, $P = 0.01$). These associations remained significant after adjustment for many potential confounders.

Conclusions.—In women with type 2 diabetes, greater adherence to Mediterranean diet is associated with a lower prevalence of FSD.

▶ The strong associations between vascular disease and sexual dysfunction that exist in men have not been quite as clearly determined in women. This likely stems from the relative dearth of research into women's sexuality, although it is also possible that the physiological processes of sexual function in women are of lesser import for their overall sexual satisfaction, and therefore, vascular disease is less prone to cause sexual dysfunction with distress. Be that as it may, there can be little doubt that healthy lifestyle factors, including a prudent diet and routine exercise are unlikely to have a negative impact on female sexual function and may substantially enhance sexual function for some women.

In this study, 595 women with type 2 diabetes were queried on their dietary habits to determine how closely their dietary intake reflects the Mediterranean diet, consisting primarily of fruits, vegetables, nuts, legumes, olive oil, fish, and moderate amounts of ethanol with a low intake of saturated fats and processed or red meat. Women who adhered to a Mediterranean style diet over the year before the study tended to have lower body mass index, better lipid and glucose profiles, less depressive symptoms, and lower incidence of vascular comorbidities. After multivariable adjustment, greater adherence to a Mediterranean diet was associated with greater likelihood of being sexually active and better scores on the Female Sexual Function Index (FSFI) total score, suggesting that better sexual function was associated with this diet. Interestingly, while all FSFI domain scores were higher in women with Mediterranean diets, only the sexual satisfaction domain score attained statistically significant mean difference, suggesting that this diet had a subtle but global positive impact on female sexual function.

Dietary change is very difficult to effect, and it is likely that many patients with sexual function would be resistant to radical changes in diet. However, data such as these suggest that encouraging our female patients to make prudent dietary choices is likely to yield benefits in sexual functioning. Additional studies should be undertaken to investigate other healthy diets as means to ameliorate the effects of sexual dysfunction.

A. Shindel, MD

Activation of NMDA Receptors in Lumbar Spinothalamic Cells is Required for Ejaculation

Staudt MD, de Oliveira CVR, Lehman MN, et al (The Univ of Western Ontario—Dept of Anatomy and Cell Biology, London, Canada; The Univ of Western Ontario—Dept of Physiology and Pharmacology, London, Canada; et al)
J Sex Med 8:1015-1026, 2011

Introduction.—The sexual reflex ejaculation is controlled by a spinal ejaculation generator located in the lumbosacral spinal cord. A population of spinothalamic (LSt) neurons forms a key component of this generator, as manipulations of LSt cells either block or trigger ejaculation. However, it is currently unknown which afferent signals contribute to the activation of LSt cells and ejaculation.

Aim.—The current study tested the hypothesis that glutamate, via activation of N-Methyl-D-aspartic acid (NMDA) receptors in LSt cells, is a key regulator of ejaculation.

Methods.—Expression of phosphorylated NMDA receptor subunit 1 (NR1) was investigated following mating, or following ejaculation induced by electrical stimulation of the dorsal penile nerve (DPN) in anesthetized, spinalized male rats. Next, the effects of intraspinal delivery of NMDA receptor antagonist AP-5 on DPN stimulation-induced ejaculation were examined. Moreover, the ability of intraspinal delivery of NMDA to trigger ejaculation was examined. Finally, the site of action of NMDA was determined by studying effects of NMDA in male rats with LSt cell-specific lesions.

Main Outcome Measures.—Expression of NR1 and phosphorylated NR1 in LSt cells was analyzed. Electromyographic recordings of the bulbocavernosus muscle (BCM) were recorded in anesthetized, spinalized rats following stimulation of the DPN and delivery of AP-5 or NMDA.

Results.—Results indicate that the NR1 receptors are activated in LSt cells following ejaculation in mating animals or induced by DPN stimulation in anesthetized, spinalized animals. Moreover, NR1 activation in LSt cells is an essential trigger for rhythmic BCM bursting, as DPN stimulation-induced reflexes were absent following administration of NMDA receptor antagonist in the L3-L4 spinal area, and were triggered by NMDA. NMDA effects were dependent on intact LSt cells and were absent in LSt-lesioned males.

Conclusion.—These results demonstrate that glutamate, via activation of NMDA receptors in LSt cells, is a key afferent signal for ejaculation.

▶ This study investigated the role of glutamatergic activation of *N*-methyl-D-aspartic acid (NMDA) receptors in the lumbar spinothalamic tracts of rats, as it pertains to ejaculation. It was demonstrated that activation of these receptors was associated with both ejaculation from copulation and experimentally induced ejaculation. Furthermore, abolition of NDMA signaling via the NMDA antagonist AP-5 inhibited experimentally induced ejaculation.

These results are not of any clear and immediate clinical relevance. However, it is apparent from these data that novel targets for the modulation of the ejaculatory reflex exist. This may have implications for patients taking agents that affect glutamate metabolism in the central nervous system. Furthermore, it may lead to the development of targeted therapies for disorders of ejaculation in men. In the United States, contemporary medical treatments for premature ejaculation are composed entirely of off-label use of selective serotonin reuptake inhibitors and topical anesthetics. There are very little data on the efficacy of treatments for delayed ejaculation. Research such as this will hopefully spearhead further improvements in our ability to address disorders of ejaculation and orgasm in our male patients.

A. Shindel, MD

Morphological and Functional Evidence for the Contribution of the Pudendal Artery in Aging-Induced Erectile Dysfunction
Hannan JL, Blaser MC, Oldfield L, et al (Queen's Univ, Kingston, Ontario, Canada)
J Sex Med 7:3373-3384, 2010

Introduction.—Aging increases the risk of both erectile dysfunction (ED) and cardiovascular disease. These conditions have similar etiologies and commonly coexist. One unifying concept is the role of arterial insufficiency which is a primary factor in the onset of age-related ED.

Aim.—Based on the novel finding that the pudendal arteries contribute 70% of the total penile vascular resistance, our objective was to morphometrically and functionally characterize this vessel in young and old normotensive rats.

Methods.—Erectile function was monitored in 15- and 77-week Sprague-Dawley rats using the apomorphine bioassay (80 mg/kg, s.c.). Anesthetized animals were perfusion-fixed, aortic, renal, and internal pudendal arteries were excised, embedded, sectioned, stained, and morphometrically assessed using light microscopy. Hearts were excised, separated, and weighed prior to perfusion. Contractile and relaxation responses to acetylcholine (ACh) and phenylephrine (PE) were assessed by wire myograph.

Main Outcome Measures.—Erectile function, morphological measurements, concentration response curves to ACh and PE.

Results.—With age, there were marked decreases in erectile responses compared to younger rats (2.8 ± 0.87 vs. 0.3 ± 0.58). The pudendal arteries had a relatively small lumen (303 ± 13.8 μm) and a thick medial layer (47 ± 2.2 μm). In aged pudendal arteries, the lumen diameter did not change, and yet the medial layer, cross sectional area, and extracellular matrix were markedly increased. In contrast, the lumen diameter and wall thickness of the aorta and renal arteries in aged rats increased proportionally. An increase in small, round, smooth muscle cells was seen in aged pudendal arteries. Functionally, there were no differences in contractile responses to PE; however, ACh-induced relaxation decreased with age.

Conclusions.—In aged rats, erectile function was severely diminished when pudendal arteries had undergone marked phenotypic changes. Specifically, there was endothelial dysfunction and pathological remodeling of this vessel with age, characterized by medial thickening, impaired vasodilation and significantly reduced capacity for penile blood flow.

▶ This study investigates histological and functional differences in pudendal artery specimens from young and aged rats. Diminished erectile response in the aged versus the young animals was verified by testing with apomorphine before euthanasia and tissue harvest. Interestingly, the relaxant response of the pudendal artery to acetylcholine was diminished (signifying impaired endothelium-dependent relaxation) in the aged animals compared with what was observed in the young animals. This was associated with the thickening of the medial wall in the aged animals but no significant differences in luminal diameter. No difference was detected in acetylcholine response of mesenteric arteries between young and aged rats, implying that the pudendal artery is more susceptible to age-related changes in functionality.

The relevance of this finding is underscored by a previous report from this group, indicating that most vascular resistance in the penile circulation is attributable to the pudendal artery.[1] It is interesting that the luminal diameter as assessed histologically did not differ significantly between young and old rats; it is implied that the defect is a functional rather than a structural one. While there may not be immediate implications for this study, it does imply that modulation of pudendal artery blood flow may have use in the future management of erectile dysfunction.

A. Shindel, MD

Reference

1. Manabe K, Heaton JP, Morales A, Kumon H, Adams MA. Pre-penile arteries are dominant in the regulation of penile vascular resistance in the rat. *Int J Impot Res.* 2000;12:183-189.

Improved Ejaculatory Latency, Control and Sexual Satisfaction When PSD502 is Applied Topically in Men with Premature Ejaculation: Results of a Phase III, Double-Blind, Placebo-Controlled Study
Carson C, Wyllie M (Univ of North Carolina, Chapel Hill; Plethora Solutions, Ltd High Holborn, London, UK)
J Sex Med 2010 [Epub ahead of print]

Introduction.—PSD502 is a novel aerosolized, lidocaine-prilocaine, spray being developed for the treatment of lifelong premature ejaculation. The clinical profile of PSD502 is described in one of two double-blind, placebo-controlled, phase III studies.

Aim.—To determine the effect of PSD502 on the Index of Premature Ejaculation (IPE) and intravaginal ejaculatory latency (IELT) of men with lifelong PE.

Methods.—Men with lifelong PE who documented an IELT ≤ 1 minute with two or more of the first three sexual encounters during a 4-week baseline period were randomized to receive double-blind treatment with PSD502 or placebo for 3 months. Patients completed IPE and Premature Ejaculation Profile questionnaires at entry and monthly visits, and recorded stop-watch timed IELT during each encounter. Safety was assessed by collecting adverse event data and standard safety measures.

Main Outcome Measures.—Stopwatch timed IELT recordings and a patient-reported outcome questionnaire the IPE were used in this study to determine the effect of PSD502 applied topically 5 minutes before intercourse.

Results.—Two hundred fifty-six men with PE were randomized from 38 centers in the U.S., Canada, and Poland. The geometric mean IELT over the 3-month treatment period increased from a baseline of 0.56 minute and 0.53 minute in the PSD502 and placebo group respectively to 2.60 and 0.80 minute. There were significantly greater increases in the scores for the IPE domains of ejaculatory control, sexual satisfaction and distress in the PSD502 group than in the placebo group, with a mean 5.0 point difference between treatments in change from baseline in the IPE domain for ejaculatory control, 4.6 point difference in change from baseline in the IPE domain for sexual satisfaction, and a 2.5 point difference in change from baseline in the IPE domain for distress. This was supported by improvements in all secondary endpoints.

Conclusion.—In this study, PSD502 applied topically to the glans penis 5 minutes before intercourse showed significantly improved ejaculatory latency, ejaculatory control, sexual satisfaction and distress and was shown to be well tolerated by patients and partners.

▶ This double-blinded, placebo-controlled, industry-sponsored 3-month trial investigates the use of a eutectic (ie, liquid at body temperature) topical mixture of prilocaine and lidocaine as a treatment for 256 men with lifelong premature ejaculation (PE) (defined as ejaculation within 1 minute of penetration on at least 2 of 3 attempts at intercourse during baseline evaluation). Patients were instructed to apply treatment 5 minutes before intercourse. Men in the treatment group experienced a 5-fold increase in ejaculatory latency as well as clinically and statistically significant improvements in their sense of control over ejaculation, sexual satisfaction, ejaculation-related distress, and assessment of their overall satisfaction with their sexual relationship. Side effects were generally mild and consisted of excessive penile numbness in the patients and vaginal irritation/burning in the sexual partner; these effects were noted in about 10% of the subjects and partners in the treatment arm and 1% to 3% of the subjects in the control arm.

A short-acting selective serotonin reuptake inhibitor (dapoxetine) has been approved for treatment of PE in Europe, but no US Food and Drug Administration (FDA)-approved treatment for PE currently exists. Data such as these may serve as a foundation for future approval of an on-demand fast-acting treatment for PE in the United States, with the added advantage that this topical mixture is unlikely to contribute to mood or psychiatric disturbances (which was a major contributor to FDA's rejection of dapoxetine for PE).

A. Shindel, MD

Intracavernous Delivery of Synthetic Angiopoietin-1 Protein as a Novel
Therapeutic Strategy for Erectile Dysfunction in the Type II Diabetic
db/db Mouse
Jin H-R, Kim WJ, Song JS, et al (Inha Univ School of Medicine, Incheon,
Korea; et al)
J Sex Med 7:3635-3646, 2010

Introduction.—Patients with erectile dysfunction (ED) associated with
type II diabetes often have impaired endothelial function and tend to
respond poorly to oral phosphodiesterase type 5 inhibitors. Therefore,
neovascularization is a promising strategy for curing diabetic ED.

Aim.—To determine the effectiveness of a soluble, stable, and potent
angiopoietin-1 (Ang1) variant, cartilage oligomeric matrix protein
(COMP)-Ang1, in promoting cavernous angiogenesis and erectile function
in a mouse model of type II diabetic ED.

Methods.—Sixteen-week-old male *db/db* mice (in which obesity and
type II diabetes are caused by a mutation in the leptin receptor) and control
C57BL/6J mice were used and divided into four groups (N = 14 per
group): agematched controls; *db/db* mice receiving two successive intracavernous injections of phosphate-buffered saline (PBS) (days −3 and 0;
20 μL); *db/db* mice receiving a single intracavernous injection of COMP-
Ang1 protein (day 0; 5.8 μg/20 μL); and *db/db* mice receiving two successive intracavernous injections of COMP-Ang1 protein (days −3 and 0;
5.8 μg/20 μL).

Main Outcome Measures.—Two weeks later, erectile function was
measured by electrical stimulation of the cavernous nerve. The penis was
then harvested and stained with antibodies to platelet/endothelial cell adhe-
sion molecule-1 (PECAM-1) (endothelial cell marker), phosphohistone H3
(PH3, a nuclear protein indicative of cell proliferation), phospho-endothelial
nitric oxide synthase (eNOS), and eNOS. Penis specimens from a separate
group of animals were used for cyclic guanosine monophosphate (cGMP)
and cyclic adenosine monophosphate (cAMP) quantification.

Results.—Local delivery of COMP-Ang1 protein significantly increased
eNOS phosphorylation and cGMP and cAMP expression compared with
that in the group treated with PBS. Repeated intracavernous injections
of COMP-Ang1 protein completely restored erectile function and
cavernous endothelial content through enhanced cavernous neoangiogen-
esis as evaluated by PECAM-1 and PH3 immunohistochemistry and
terminal deoxynucleotidyl transferase-mediated deoxyuridine triphosphate nick end labeling assay, whereas a single injection of COMPAng1
protein elicited partial improvement.

Conclusion.—Cavernous neovascularization using recombinant Ang1
protein is a novel therapeutic strategy for the treatment of ED resulting
from type II diabetes.

► In this study, application of a synthetic analog of the angiogenic cytokine
angiopoietin-1 was used as a therapy for mice with erectile impairment

associated with diabetes. At the tissue level, this treatment was associated with improved endothelial cell content, indications of endothelial cell proliferation, and lower levels of endothelial cell apoptosis, suggesting restoration and preservation of endothelial cells with this treatment. Levels of cyclic guanosine monophosphate and cyclic adenosine monophosphate were also increased in the treated *db/db* animals. Treated animals also manifested superior penile hemodynamic response to cavernous nerve electrostimulation.

This mouse model system (*db/db* mutant) is preferable to streptozotocin-treated rats in that diabetes in this model animal more closely reflects type 2 rather than type 1 diabetes. Whether or not this sort of focal cytokine therapy will be of use in the future for human patients remains an open question, but it is a topic worthy of further consideration, particularly in light of the increasing burden of diabetes and subsequent vascular disease in the American population.

A. Shindel, MD

The Role of PDE5 Inhibitors in Penile Septal Scar Remodeling: Assessment of Clinical and Radiological Outcomes
Chung E, DeYoung L, Brock GB (St Joseph Health Care, London, Ontario, Canada)
J Sex Med 2011 [Epub ahead of print]

Introduction.—Effective oral medication for use in men with Peyronie's disease (PD) has been an area of interest of the medical community and lay public for decades. Isolated septal scars (ISS) without evidence of penile deformity is a relatively new clinical entity, and at present, there is paucity in the published literature regarding its treatment. Current research into the use of phosphodiesterase type 5 (PDE5) inhibitors in regulating penile erectile response has revealed an alternative role for PDE5 inhibitors in decreasing oxidative stress-associated inflammatory change as seen in PD.

Aim.—To examine the presence of ISS and assess the efficacy of PDE5 inhibitor use in septal scar remodeling.

Methods.—Retrospective review of prospective database on all men who underwent penile Doppler ultrasound between December 2007 and December 2009.

Main Outcome Measures.—Of the 65 men with ultrasonographic-confirmed ISS, 35 men received tadalafil 2.5 mg daily over a 6-month period. The clinical outcomes between the two groups were compared using International Index of Erectile Function (IIEF)-5 score and 6 months penile Doppler ultrasound follow up.

Results.—The mean age for the tadalafil group was 43.2 (20—65) years, similar to the control group at 44.2 (34—72) years. The length of time from onset to presentation was 22 (6 to 40) months. The majority of ultrasonographic-proven ISS was not clinically palpable and complaint of decreased penile rigidity (66%) was the predominant feature. Treatment with low-dose daily tadalafil did not result in any significant side effects (such as headache and flushing) or discontinuation. The tadalafil group reported higher IIEF-5 score (pretreatment 11/25 to post-treatment 18/25) ($P < 0.01$) and resolution of septal scar were recorded in 24 patients (69%) compared to three patients (10%) in the control group.

Conclusion.—Low-dose daily tadalafil is a safe and effective treatment option in septal scar remodeling.

▶ Peyronie disease (PD) is currently a protean condition. While it seems likely that there may be a unifying pathway leading to the disease, it may also be that the conditions we currently diagnose as PD represent a collection of processes that differ in subtle but important ways. This article advances the concept of a PD variant known as septal scar or septal fibrosis. As opposed to the classic concept of PD as a condition associated with curvature, septal fibrosis curvature may be absent but narrowing, pain, and/or erectile dysfunction may occur. Ultrasonography is required for diagnosis of the sometimes nonpalpable lesion.

This report details outcomes in a cohort of men with septal fibrosis treated with low-dose tadalafil for 6 months; the treatment group was compared with a control group that did not receive treatment. A significant improvement was noted in the subjective erectile function of tadalafil-treated men; furthermore, many more men in the tadalafil group experienced a resolution of the septal fibrotic process.

Although baseline physiological and sexual function parameters were similar between the 2 groups, lack of randomization makes definitive conclusions on the efficacy of tadalafil based on these data impossible. Furthermore, in the absence of blinding, the conclusions about differences in the rate of fibrosis resolution must be interpreted cautiously. Further studies are warranted to determine if in fact phosphodiesterase type 5 inhibitors may be useful for the treatment of this condition.

A. Shindel, MD

Bioengineered corporal tissue for structural and functional restoration of the penis

Chen K-L, Eberli D, Yoo JJ, et al (Wake Forest Univ Health Sciences, Winston-Salem, NC)

Proc Natl Acad Sci U S A 107:3346-3350, 2010

Various reconstructive procedures have been attempted to restore a cosmetically acceptable phallus that would allow normal reproductive, sexual, and urinary function in patients requiring penile reconstruction. However, these procedures are limited by a shortage of native penile tissue. We previously demonstrated that a short segment of the penile corporal body can be replaced using naturally derived collagen matrices with autologous cells. In the current study, we examined the feasibility of engineering the entire pendular penile corporal bodies in a rabbit model. Neocorpora were engineered from cavernosal collagen matrices seeded with autologous cells using a multistep static/dynamic procedure, and these were implanted to replace the excised corpora. The bioengineered corpora demonstrated structural and functional parameters similar to native tissue and male rabbits receiving the bilateral implants were able to successfully impregnate females. This study demonstrates that neocorpora can be engineered for total pendular penile corporal body replacement. This technology has considerable potential for patients requiring penile reconstruction.

▶ Penile loss due to cancer or trauma is a rare but incredibly devastating occurrence for men. Aside from the obvious difficulties with urinary and sexual function in a man who loses his penis, the psychological toll of losing the part of his anatomy that is central to his identity as a man can be tremendous.

In this article, one of the foremost experts in tissue regenerative therapies for urology reports preliminary data on corporal replacement in a rabbit model system. Endothelial and smooth muscle cells were harvested and expanded in vitro. These expanded cells were then seeded onto a decellularized collagen matrix derived from donor corpora cavernosa with unseeded collagen matrices used as controls. Engineered corpora were then transplanted to recipient rabbits that had undergone corpora excision; functional and histological studies were performed at 1, 3, and 6 months. Rabbits that had received the seeded implants demonstrated intracavernous pressure and normalized mating behavior, including successful establishment of pregnancy in female rabbits. Organ bath studies confirmed that the seeded grafts were responsive to nitric oxide, phenylephrine, and electrical field stimulation.

This technology is very new, and numerous studies are required before human trials can be contemplated. However, this is a very exciting breakthrough that might lead (one day) to restoration of a functional penis in men who have lost some or all of their phallus. Conceivably it may also have a role to play in men with severe erectile dysfunction who desire tissue regeneration.

A. Shindel, MD

Erectile Dysfunction Predicts Cardiovascular Events in High-Risk Patients Receiving Telmisartan, Ramipril, or Both: The ONgoing Telmisartan Alone and in combination with Ramipril Global Endpoint Trial/Telmisartan Randomized AssessmeNt Study in ACE iNtolerant subjects with cardiovascular Disease (ONTARGET/TRANSCEND) Trials

Böhm M, for the ONTARGET/TRANSCEND Erectile Dysfunction Substudy Investigators (Univ of the Saarland, Saarbrücken, Germany; et al)
Circulation 121:1439-1446, 2010

Background.—Although erectile dysfunction (ED) is associated with cardiovascular risk factors and atherosclerosis, it is not known whether the presence of ED is predictive of future events in individuals with cardiovascular disease. We evaluated whether ED is predictive of mortality and cardiovascular outcomes, and because inhibition of the renin-angiotensin system in high-risk patients reduces cardiovascular events, we also tested the effects on ED of randomized treatments with telmisartan, ramipril, and the combination of the 2 drugs (ONTARGET), as well as with telmisartan or placebo in patients who were intolerant of angiotensin-converting enzyme inhibitors (TRANSCEND).

Methods and Results.—In a prespecified substudy, 1549 patients underwent double-blind randomization, with 400 participants assigned to receive ramipril, 395 telmisartan, and 381 the combination thereof (ONTARGET), as well as 171 participants assigned to receive telmisartan and 202 placebo (TRANSCEND). ED was evaluated at baseline, at 2-year follow-up, and at the penultimate visit before closeout. ED was predictive of all-cause death (hazard ratio [HR] 1.84, 95% confidence interval [CI] 1.21 to 2.81, $P=0.005$) and the composite primary outcome (HR 1.42, 95% CI 1.04 to 1.94, $P=0.029$), which consisted of cardiovascular death (HR 1.93, 95% CI 1.13 to 3.29, $P=0.016$), myocardial infarction (HR 2.02, 95% CI 1.13 to 3.58, $P=0.017$), hospitalization for heart failure (HR 1.2, 95% CI 0.64 to 2.26, $P=0.563$), and stroke (HR 1.1, 95% CI 0.64 to 1.9, $P=0.742$). The study medications did not influence the course or development of ED.

Conclusions.—ED is a potent predictor of all-cause death and the composite of cardiovascular death, myocardial infarction, stroke, and heart failure in men with cardiovascular disease. Trial treatment did not significantly improve or worsen ED.

Clinical Trial Registration.—URL: http://www.clinicaltrials.gov. Unique identifier: NCT 00153101.

▶ This large randomized controlled trial underscores yet again the sentinel nature of erectile dysfunction (ED) as a predictor of cardiovascular morbidity and mortality. Men were randomized to receive the angiotensin-converting enzyme inhibitor (ACEI), ramipril, the angiotensin receptor blocker (ARB), telmisartan, both, or a placebo. ED was assessed at baseline and at study follow-up. It was found that having ED as baseline significantly increased the hazard of all-cause death (hazard ratio [HR] 1.84) and the composite measure of cardiovascular morbidity, including cardiac death, myocardial infarction, hospitalization for heart failure, and stroke (HR 1.42). The study medications did not appear to have an influence or association with prevalent or incident ED.

This large and well-designed study provides compelling proof of the importance of ED as a sentinel event for serious vascular morbidity. It also lends credence to the growing body of data that ACEI and ARB are antihypertensive agents with generally favorable sexual side-effect profiles in men. This is particularly important news in light of the generally favorable effects of these drugs on reducing the hazard of serious cardiovascular events in high-risk patients.

A. Shindel, MD

Smoking-Cessation and Adherence Intervention Among Chinese Patients with Erectile Dysfunction
Chan SSC, Leung DYP, Abdullah ASM, et al (The Univ of Hong Kong; Boston Univ, School of Public Health, MA; et al)
Am J Prev Med 39:251-258, 2010

Background.—Whether the association between smoking and erectile dysfunction is causal is uncertain. No RCTs have been previously conducted on cessation counseling and additional nicotine replacement therapy (NRT) adherence counseling among smokers with erectile dysfunction.

Purpose.—The aim of the study was to determine if smoking-cessation counseling in conjunction with NRT increases quitting and NRT adherence compared to usual care, and if stopping smoking would improve erectile function among Chinese erectile dysfunction patients who smoke.

Design.—An RCT was conducted. Data were collected in 2004–2007 and analyzed in 2008.

Setting/Participants.—The sample included 719 Chinese adult erectile dysfunction patients who smoked at least 1 cigarette per day, intended to quit smoking within the next 7 days, and would use NRT.

Interventions.—Group A1 received 15-minute smoking-cessation and 3-minute NRT adherence counseling at baseline, 1 week, and 4 weeks with free NRT for 2 weeks. Group A2 received the same treatment, except for the adherence counseling. Group B received 10 minutes of quitting advice. All subjects received a self-help quitting booklet at first contact.

Main Outcome Measures.—Self-reported 7-day tobacco abstinence at 6 months, 4-week NRT adherence at 1 month, and improvement in erectile dysfunction condition at 6 months.

Results.—The intervention groups (A1 + A2) achieved higher rates of abstinence, both self-reported (23% vs 12.8%, RR = 1.79, 95% CI = 1.22, 2.62) and biochemically validated (11.4% vs 5.5%, RR = 2.07, 95% CI = 1.13, 3.77), than the control group. The NRT adherence rate did not differ between Groups A1 and A2 (13.7% vs 12.7%, RR = 1.08, 95% CI = 0.69, 1.69). An improvement in erectile dysfunction status from baseline to 6 months was associated with self-reported quitting at 6 months but not with intervention status.

Conclusions.—Although quitting smoking was associated with improvement in erectile dysfunction, this study found significant outcome differences among the means used to achieve smoking cessation.

Trial Registration.—ISRCTN13070778.

▶ Numerous previous reports have linked tobacco use to erectile dysfunction (ED) and other sexual problems, and data have suggested that tobacco cessation improves vascular parameters. In this prospective study in 719 Chinese men (523 of whom completed the study) who used tobacco, tobacco cessation by any means was associated with a statistically significant, approximately 2-fold increase in the likelihood of at least 1-stage improvement in erectile function (ie, change from severe to moderate ED or mild to no ED, as assessed by International Index of Erectile Function-erectile function [IIEF-EF] domain score) at 6-month follow-up. Ninety-five percent of these men had IIEF-EF domain scores consistent with at least mild ED at baseline.

Evidence about the importance of lifestyle factors in the pathogenesis and treatment of ED continues to accumulate. Prospective data such as these strengthen the evidence underscoring the potential utility of tobacco cessation in managing sexual concerns in men. Clearly, it is incumbent on the physician treating the tobacco-using patient with ED to make completely clear the relationship between tobacco use and ED and the potential benefits (sexual and otherwise) of quitting smoking.

A. Shindel, MD

Sexually Transmitted Diseases Among Users of Erectile Dysfunction Drugs: Analysis of Claims Data
Jena AB, Goldman DP, Kamdar A, et al (Harvard Med School, Boston, MA; Univ of Southern California, Los Angeles, CA; Univ of Chicago Booth Graduate School of Business, IL; et al)
Ann Intern Med 153:1-7, 2010

Background.—Pharmacologic treatments for erectile dysfunction (ED) have gained popularity among middle-aged and older men. Increased sexual activity among those who use these drugs raises concerns about sexually transmitted diseases (STDs).

Objective.—To examine the rates of STDs in men who use and do not use ED drugs.

Design.—Retrospective cohort study.

Setting.—Database of claims from 1997 to 2006 for 1 410 806 men older than age 40 years with private, employer-based insurance from 44 large companies.

Patients.—33 968 men with at least 1 filled prescription for an ED drug and 1 376 838 patients with no prescription.

Measurements.—STD prevalence among users and nonusers of ED drugs.

Results.—Users of ED drugs had higher rates of STDs than nonusers the year before initiating ED drug therapy (214 vs. 106 annually per 100 000 persons; $P = 0.003$) and the year after (105 vs. 65; $P = 0.004$). After adjustment for age and other comorbid conditions, users of ED drugs had an odds ratio (OR) for an STD of 2.80 (95% CI, 2.10 to 3.75) in the year before initiating drug therapy; the OR was 2.65 (CI, 1.84 to 3.81) in the year after. These differences were largely due to infections with HIV. The OR for HIV infection was 3.32 (CI, 2.38 to 4.36) in the year before and 3.19 (CI, 2.11 to 4.83) in the year after an ED drug prescription was filled. Significant changes in STD rates from the year before to the year after the first ED drug prescription was filled were not documented (adjusted OR for STD for users before vs. after the first ED drug prescription was filled, 0.96 [CI, 0.87 to 1.06]).

Limitation.—Selection bias precludes conclusions about whether use of ED treatments directly leads to increases in STDs.

Conclusion.—Men who use ED drugs have higher rates of STDs, particularly HIV infection, both in the year before and after use of these drugs. The observed association between ED drug use and STDs may have more to do with the types of patients using ED drugs rather than a direct effect of ED drug availability on STD rates. Counseling about safe sexual practices and screening for STDs should accompany the prescription of ED drugs.

▶ Safer sex-practice education has generally not targeted older Americans. This is of particular concern, as many older Americans became sexually active before human immunodeficiency virus (HIV) became an acknowledged and understood risk of sexual activity. Because these individuals are often not experienced with safer sex and are typically not concerned about unwanted pregnancy, they may be less likely to use condoms when resuming sexual activity with new partners after being widowed, divorced, or separated.

As demand for erectogenic drugs is higher in older individuals, it behooves practitioners to consider safer sex education when considering a patient for erectile dysfunction (ED) therapy. This investigation from a large claims database explores the relationship between receipt of an erectogenic drug and subsequent diagnosis of sexually transmitted infection (STI). The rate of STI in men who received an erectogenic medication was higher both before and after prescription of the drug; no significant change was detected in the rate of STI after prescription of an erectogenic drug.

This study appears to indicate that ED drugs in and of themselves do not change the rate of STI in men, but men who use ED drugs appear to be at greater risk. The reasons for the higher rate of STI at baseline cannot be gleaned from this study; however, one theory could be that men with marginal erectile function may be less inclined to use condoms as the interference from the barrier may further exacerbate trouble-maintaining erection.

Regardless of interpretation, 2 important points are apparent, (1) provision of ED medication should be accompanied by an assessment of safer sex practices and education of the patient as needed, and (2) there is no clear evidence that ED medication in and of itself predisposes individuals to unsafe sex practices. Therefore, practitioners have no clear rationale to deny patients with HIV infection treatment for ED unless there is a compelling reason to suspect the patient will be particularly careless with the health of their sexual partner(s).

A. Shindel, MD

The use of high-resolution magnetic resonance imaging in the management of patients presenting with priapism

Ralph DJ, Borley NC, Allen C, et al (Univ College London Hosps, UK)
BJU Int 106:1714-1718, 2010

Objective.—To investigate the use of magnetic resonance imaging (MRI) of the penis during an episode of priapism and assess the viability of the corpus cavernosum (CC) smooth muscle, as prolonged ischaemic priapism is associated with a high rate of long-term erectile dysfunction (ED), and the viability of CC smooth muscle influences the subsequent management in ischaemic priapism.

Patients and Methods.—The study was set in a single centre based in a large university teaching hospital. We investigated the correlation of T2-weighted gadolinium- enhanced MRI with the histology from CC biopsies in the same patients. In all, 38 patients (mean age 42 years) presenting with priapism over a 3-year period had MRI of the penis. The scans were reported by two dedicated uroradiologists who graded the MR images as showing viable or nonviable erectile tissue. One pathologist assessed the CC biopsies for necrosis. The findings were then correlated. Where no biopsies were taken a clinical follow-up was used to assess erectile function.

Results.—In 23 patients undergoing both a CC biopsy and MRI, the sensitivity of MRI in predicting nonviable smooth muscle was 100%. In a further 10 patients MRI showed nonviable CC smooth muscle, but no biopsy was taken in these patients; on clinical follow-up all of these patients subsequently developed ED. In a further five patients the imaging showed viable smooth muscle and these patients subsequently maintained erectile function on clinical follow up.

Conclusions.—Penile MRI provides an accurate imaging method to assess smooth muscle viability in patients presenting with priapism.

▶ In this study, the utility of gadolinium-enhanced MRI in the prediction of erectile function recovery after ischemic priapism was assessed. MRI had excellent (100%) predictive capacity for smooth muscle necrosis in the 23 men who had both MRI and corporal biopsy. Most men in this group underwent placement of a penile implant at the time of corporal biopsy although a few declined; all of the men who declined did develop erectile dysfunction (ED). In men who did not have tissue biopsy for confirmation of tissue MRI findings, clinical outcomes (ED vs no ED) were in-line with MRI findings (ie, men with evidence of viable corporal tissue recovered erectile function, whereas men without evidence of viable tissue did not).

The authors are relatively scant on detail regarding how erectile function versus dysfunction was classified at follow-up; it may be presumed that this was determined by patient report rather than a validated quantitative instrument such as the International Index of Erectile Function or Sexual Health Inventory for Men. For this reason, these data must be interpreted with caution. Nevertheless, this is an interesting report on a novel (albeit expensive) way to triage patients with ischemic priapism.

A. Shindel, MD

Oral L-Citrulline Supplementation Improves Erection Hardness in Men With Mild Erectile Dysfunction
Cormio L, De Siati M, Lorusso F, et al (Univ of Foggia, Italy)
Urology 77:119-122, 2011

Objectives.—To test the efficacy and safety of oral L-citrulline supplementation in improving erection hardness in patients with mild erectile dysfunction (ED). L-arginine supplementation improves nitric oxide-mediated vasodilation and endothelial function; however, oral administration has been hampered by extensive presystemic metabolism. In contrast, L-citrulline escapes presystemic metabolism and is converted to L-arginine, thus setting the rationale for oral L-citrulline supplementation as a donor for the L-arginine/nitric oxide pathway of penile erection.

Methods.—In the present single-blind study, men with mild ED (erection hardness score of 3) received a placebo for 1 month and L-citrulline, 1.5 g/d, for another month. The erection hardness score, number of intercourses per month, treatment satisfaction, and adverse events were recorded.

Results.—A total of 24 patients, mean age 56.5 ± 9.8 years, were entered and concluded the study without adverse events. The improvement in the erection hardness score from 3 (mild ED) to 4 (normal erectile function) occurred in 2 (8.3%) of the 24 men when taking placebo and 12 (50%) of the 24 men when taking L-citrulline ($P < .01$). The mean number of intercourses per month increased from 1.37 ± 0.93 at baseline to 1.53 ± 1.00 at the end of the placebo phase ($P = .57$) and 2.3 ± 1.37 at the end of the treatment phase ($P < .01$). All patients reporting an erection hardness score improvement from 3 to 4 reported being very satisfied.

Conclusions.—Although less effective than phosphodiesterase type-5 enzyme inhibitors, at least in the short term, L-citrulline supplementation has been proved to be safe and psychologically well accepted by patients. Its role as an alternative treatment for mild to moderate ED, particularly in patients with a psychological fear of phosphodiesterase type-5 enzyme inhibitors, deserves further research.

► Alternative medications and dietary supplements claiming to enhance sexual function are ubiquitous and probably have been since the dawn of human history. The rise of the Internet has enhanced the ability of individuals/groups marketing these treatments to advertise their wares and reach out to a huge population of men who may be too embarrassed to seek out formal medical evaluation. Indubitably, some individuals advocating for these treatments are genuinely interested in the good of their clients, and there is evidence that these treatments may be efficacious in some circumstances. This small crossover study (n = 24) suggests that oral administration of the arginine precursor citrulline may benefit men with mild erectile dysfunction; less than 10% of patients treated with placebo had improvement in their erectile function, whereas half of the men treated with citrulline noted improvement. While not dramatic, the tolerability and relatively sound physiological rationale for use of this medication makes it worthy of further study.

A. Shindel, MD

Impact of nasal polyposis on erectile dysfunction
Gunhan K, Zoron F, Uz U, et al (Celal Bayar Univ, Manisa, Turkey)
Am J Rhinol Allergy 25:112-115, 2011

Background.—Our male patients with chronic rhinosinusitis with nasal polyposis (NP) declare a better sexual function after functional endoscopic sinus surgery (FESS) with polypectomy. This study was planned to conduct the first prospective, controlled trial evaluating the possible relation between erectile dysfunction (ED) and NP by subjective and objective parameters.

Methods.—Thirty-three male patients with NP and thirty randomly selected male control subjects were evaluated. All subjects underwent assessments of nasal endoscopy, rhinomanometry, body mass index (BMI), Epworth Sleepiness Scale, full in-laboratory polysomnograpy and serum levels of glucose, thyroid hormones, lipid profile, and testosterone. ED was evaluated by the erectile function domain of the International Index of Erectile Function (IIEF-EF) subjectively and nocturnal penile tumescence (NPT) objectively. The NP group was reassessed 6 months after FESS.

Results.—The mean age, BMI, and laboratory tests of the patients and the control subjects had no significant difference. The well-recognized risk factors for ED were eliminated. Preoperative evaluation of the patients revealed that ED was present in 34 and 24% of the patients by IIEF-EF and NPT, respectively, which was significantly higher than the control group ($p = 0.009$ and $p = 0.018$, respectively). There was a significant improvement of ED in the assessment of IIEF-EF and NPT postoperatively ($p = 0.014$ and $p = 0.037$, respectively).

Conclusion.—ED was determined in a high percentage of patients with NP and significantly ameliorated after FESS. NP might present a risk factor in the development of ED.

▶ This rather interesting if modest study investigates penile erection in 33 men undergoing functional endoscopic sinus surgery (FESS) for treatment of nasal polyposis with chronic rhinosinusitis. Subjects completed the International Index of Erectile Function erectile function domain (IIEF-EF) and nocturnal penile tumescence testing at baseline and 6 months posttreatment. Importantly, 3 patients were excluded because of obstructive sleep apnea. At baseline, an age and body mass index—matched control group of healthy men had a 3.3%

prevalence of erectile dysfunction (ED) (defined here as IIEF-EF < 25) compared with a 34% prevalence in patients with nasal polyposis. The rate of ED declined to 10% 6 months postoperatively; mean IIEF-EF score for the treatment group improved from 22.1 at baseline to 26.5 at follow-up.

A direct pathophysiological relationship between nasal polyposis and ED is difficult to conceptualize, although disruption of sleep and/or oxygenation may be potential explanations for these observations. It is also possible that general improvements in health and sense of well-being account for better subjective sexual function posttreatment. While FESS cannot be advocated as a treatment for ED it is suggested from this study that treatment of seemingly unrelated health problems can have beneficial effects on sexual function. Urologists should be supportive and/or encouraging of their patients seeking appropriate treatment for conditions outside of standard urologic practice.

A. Shindel, MD

The effects of three phosphodiesterase type 5 inhibitors on ejaculation latency time in lifelong premature ejaculators: a double-blind laboratory setting study
Gökçe A, Halis F, Demirtas A, et al (Erciyes Univ Med Faculty, Kayseri, Turkey)
BJU Int 107:1274-1277, 2010

Objective.—• To evaluate the effects of three phosphodiesterase type 5 (PDE5) inhibitors on the ejaculation process in men with lifelong premature ejaculation using adouble-blind laboratory setting.

Patients and Methods.—• Eighty men with lifelong premature ejaculation, 20 in each group, received placebo, vardenafil (10 mg), sildenafil (50 mg) or tadalafil (20 mg) in a doubleblind study design. Placebo or PDE5 inhibitor was ingested after at least 2 h fasting and non-smoking. The subjects were placed in a silent room immediately and real-time penile rigidity and tumescence was monitored.

• Subjects read some magazines or newspapers without any sexually stimulating material for 1.5 h. At the end of this period audiovisual sexual stimulation began with a video film and after the 8th minute the subject began vibratory stimulation to the frenular area.

• At the beginning of ejaculation the patient stopped stimulation. When the patient began and stopped stimulation, the light near the observer turned on and off and the observer calculated the ejaculation period with a chronometer. The elapsed time was the ejaculation latency time (ELT) in seconds.

• There was no interaction between subjects and observer during the test. The ELT, and the qualities of base and tip rigidities during ELT and after ejaculation were calculated.

Results.—• Median age of patients was 29 (range 22—39) years and median duration of premature ejaculation was 60 (range 7—180) months and there was no significant difference between groups. Median duration of vibratory stimulation (ELT) of subjects who received placebo was

48.5 s: 53.5 s for sildenafil, 70.0 s for tadalafil and 82.5 s for vardenafil. Compared with the placebo group, ELT was significantly longer only in subjects receiving vardenafil ($P = 0.019$).

• In the post-ejaculatory refractory period, times to last recorded base rigidities were significantly longer than placebo in vardenafil and sildenafil groups with better erection quality ($P < 0.01$ for each).

Conclusions.—• The PDE5 inhibitors seem to prolong ELT and the quality of penile rigidity is better with PDE5 inhibitors in post-ejaculatory period.

• These findings suggest that PDE5 inhibitors might have some beneficial effects in men with lifelong premature ejaculation.

▶ In this rather interesting randomized study, men with lifelong premature ejaculation (PE) and no erectile dysfunction were treated with placebo, starting dose vardenafil or sildenafil (10 and 50 mg, respectively) or maximum dose tadalafil (20 mg), and then subjected to penile vibratory stimulation to induce ejaculation. Men treated with the vardenafil had a slight but statistically significant prolongation of ejaculatory latency relative to what was observed in placebo-treated men.

This study differs from many prior investigations of ejaculatory latency in that data were collected in a laboratory setting using vibratory stimulation of the frenulum rather than stopwatched intravaginal ejaculatory latency time (IELT). The laboratory setting, while clearly artificial, may have some unique strengths in that interpersonal variables may be theoretically less likely to interfere with acquisition of physiological data. However, the relatively modest (34 seconds) difference in mean ejaculatory latency between the placebo and vardenafil group does not explain the 3- to 7- fold increase in IELT from clinical trials of phosphodiesterase type 5 inhibitor (PDE5I) in PE. Although a physiological effect may be at work, it is likely that much of the clinical benefit of PDE5I in PE is derived from greater erectile rigidity and reliability and resultant increased sexual confidence. It would have also been of greater interest to gather data in a crossover fashion so that each man could serve as his own control after testing with the various PDE5I.

A. Shindel, MD

Characterizing Behavior of Corpus Cavernosum in Chloride-free Condition
Lau L-C, Adaikan PG, Armugam A, et al (Natl Univ of Singapore)
Urology 77:1265.e17-1265.e22, 2011

Objective.—To elucidate the role of chloride currents in erectile function through characterizing the behavior of corpus cavernosum (CC) in chloride-free (Cf) medium, which has not been evaluated before.

Methods.—Isolated rabbit CC strips were suspended in thermo-regulated organ baths containing oxygenated Tyrode for isometric tension recording. Cf Tyrode was prepared by substituting sodium chloride, calcium chloride, and potassium chloride (KCl) with equivalent molar concentrations of sodium acetate, calcium acetate, and potassium acetate salts. Resting cavernosal tone and contractions by noradrenaline, histamine, and KCl were assessed in Cf Tyrode with or without chloride channel blockers, niflumic acid (NFA), and anthracene-9-carboxylic acid (A9C).

Results.—Withdrawal of extracellular chloride caused myogenic contractions in the unstimulated CC strips (n = 18). In addition, peak contractions by noradrenaline (n = 14) and histamine (n = 13) were augmented in Cf buffer by 47.2 ± 5.9% and 85.4 ± 13.2%, respectively (*P* <.05), whereas KCl contractions were not significantly altered (17.6 ± 4.6%; n = 7). Interestingly, Cf buffer exerted opposing effects, potentiation and reduction, respectively, on the plateau phase of contractions mediated by noradrenaline and histamine. The stimulatory effect of Cf buffer on the intrinsic myogenic tone was diminished by NFA (30 μM), and A9C (300 μM−1 mM) NFA (30-100 μM), however, specifically reduced the plateau phase without significantly modifying the peak contraction of noradrenaline in Cf buffer.

Conclusions.—These results reiterate the importance of chloride currents as a mechanism underlying the maintenance of penile cavernosal tone. Thus, chloride channel could be an effective alternative target to regulate penile erection.

▶ This article examines chloride metabolism as a modulator of contractile state of cavernous smooth muscle cells. Smooth muscle contraction and resultant vasoconstriction is mediated in large part by membrane hyperpolarization, and chloride is the principle anion contributing to this differential. In this study, chloride-free medium was used to incubate segments of smooth muscle from the corpora cavernosa of rabbits. This unique medium induced unstimulated contraction of the smooth muscle segments as well as enhancing contractile response to adrenaline and histamine. These effects were attenuated by the addition of various chloride channel blockers, suggesting that efflux of chloride might play a role in penile erection and/or serve as a target for future pharmacotherapies.

Smooth muscle hyperpolarization has been investigated as a means to retard contraction and vasoconstriction in penile tissues by modulation of intracellular calcium levels.[1] Further progress in chloride channel modulation will require development of selective drugs that target the chloride channels present in cavernosal tissue specifically; this represents a new and potentially important therapeutic target.

A. Shindel, MD

Reference

1. Schiff JD, Melman A. Ion channel gene therapy for smooth muscle disorders: relaxing smooth muscles to treat erectile dysfunction. *Assay Drug Dev Technol.* 2006;4:89-95.

10 Urethral Reconstruction

Tissue-engineered autologous urethras for patients who need reconstruction: an observational study
Raya-Rivera A, Esquiliano DR, Yoo JJ, et al (Wake Forest Univ School of Medicine, Winston-Salem, NC; et al)
Lancet 377:1175-1182, 2011

Background.—Complex urethral problems can occur as a result of injury, disease, or congenital defects and treatment options are often limited. Urethras, similar to other long tubularised tissues, can stricture after reconstruction. We aimed to assess the effectiveness of tissue-engineered urethras using patients' own cells in patients who needed urethral reconstruction.

Methods.—Five boys who had urethral defects were included in the study. A tissue biopsy was taken from each patient, and the muscle and epithelial cells were expanded and seeded onto tubularised polyglycolic acid:poly(lactide-coglycolide acid) scaff olds. Patients then underwent urethral reconstruction with the tissue-engineered tubularised urethras. We took patient history, asked patients to complete questionnaires from the International Continence Society (ICS), and did urine analyses, cystourethroscopy, cystourethrography, and flow measurements at 3, 6, 12, 24, 36, 48, 60, and 72 months after surgery. We did serial endoscopic cup biopsies at 3, 12, and 36 months, each time in a different area of the engineered urethras.

Findings.—Patients had surgery between March 19, 2004, and July 20, 2007. Follow-up was completed by July 31, 2010. Median age was 11 years (range 10–14) at time of surgery and median follow-up was 71 months (range 36–76 months). AE1/AE3, α actin, desmin, and myosin antibodies confirmed the presence of cells of epithelial and muscle lineages on all cultures. The median end maximum urinary flow rate was $27 \cdot 1$ mL/s (range 16–28), and serial radiographic and endoscopic studies showed the maintenance of wide urethral calibres without strictures. Urethral biopsies showed that the engineered grafts had developed a normal appearing architecture by 3 months after implantation.

Interpretation.—Tubularised urethras can be engineered and remain functional in a clinical setting for up to 6 years. These engineered urethras can be used in patients who need complex urethral reconstruction.

▶ The authors report long-term follow-up on urethral placement using constructs created using bladder mucosal and smooth muscle cells. All 5 men had a history of traumatic posterior urethral injury. The urethral defects were between 4 and 6 cm, and the scaffolds were constructed to give a 16F diameter. Biopsy, cell culture, and construction of the neourethra took up to 7 weeks. This is not all that important because these urethral reconstructions are elective procedures. After excision of scar tissue (and, presumably, creation of a healthy bed for placement), a mucosal anastomosis was performed to the healthy native urethra. The postoperative imaging and flow rates show excellent results. While an onlay to a healthy residual plate or staged repair with grafting typically has good outcomes, tubularized grafts have very poor success rates. The bulbar/posterior urethra is typically a very vascular area that is more likely to support angiogenesis and neovascularization. This study shows that an engineered tubularized urethra can give good long-term outcomes. It is unknown if the same success can be achieved in the anterior urethra or if long-term outcomes will be equivalent or better than that achieved with a staged reconstruction using either a skin or buccal mucosal graft.

D. E. Coplen, MD

Developing biodegradable scaffolds for tissue engineering of the urethra
Selim M, Bullock AJ, Blackwood KA, et al (Menoufia Teaching Hosp, Egypt; Univ of Sheffield, South Yorkshire, UK; et al)
BJU Int 107:296-302, 2010

Objective.—To develop a synthetic biodegradable alternative to using human allodermis for the production of tissue-engineered buccal mucosa for substitution urethroplasty, looking specifically at issues of sterilization and cell-seeding protocols and, comparing the results to native buccal mucosa.

Material and Methods.—Three methods of sterilization, peracetic acid (PAA), γ-irradiation and ethanol, were evaluated for their effects on a biodegradable electrospun scaffold of polylactide-co-glycolide (PLGA, 85: 15), to identify a sterilization method with minimal adverse effects on the scaffolds. Two protocols for seeding oral cells on the scaffold were compared, co-culture of fibroblasts and keratinocytes on the scaffolds for 14 days, and seeding fibroblasts for 5 days then adding keratinocytes for a further 10 days. Cell viability and proliferation on the scaffolds, scaffold contraction and mechanical properties of the scaffolds with and without cells were examined.

Results.—γ-irradiation and PAA sterilized scaffolds remained sterile for >3 months when incubated in antibiotic-free culture medium, while ethanol sterilized and unsterilized samples became infected within 2–14 days. All scaffolds showed extensive contraction (up to 50% over 14 days) irrespective of the method of sterilization or the presence of cells. All methods of sterilization, particularly ethanol, reduced the tensile strength of the scaffolds. The addition of cells tended to further reduce mechanical properties but increased elasticity. The cell-seeding protocol of adding fibroblasts for 5 days followed by keratinocytes for 10 days was the most promising, achieving a mean (sem) ultimate tensile stress of 1.20 (0.24) $\times$ 10^5 N/m^2 compared to 3.77 (1.05) $\times$ 10^5 N/m^2 for native buccal mucosa, and a Young's modulus of 2.40 (0.25) MPa, compared to 0.73 (0.09) MPa for the native buccal mucosa.

Conclusion.—This study adds to our understanding of how sterilization and cell seeding affect the physical properties of scaffolds. Both PAA and γ-irradiation appear to be suitable methods for sterilizing PLGA scaffolds, although both reduce the tensile properties of the scaffolds. Cells grow well on the sterilized scaffolds, and with our current protocol produce constructs which have ≈30% of the mechanical strength and elasticity of the native buccal mucosa. We conclude that sterilized PLGA 85: 15 is a promising material for producing tissue-engineered buccal mucosa.

▶ Instead of developing a template for urethral tissue engineering using urothelial cells, the authors used oral mucosa. Presumably, buccal mucosa was used because of its known excellent compatibility in urethral replacement and the relative ease of oral biopsy compared with open bladder biopsy. The scaffold can be modified to achieve the desired tensile and mechanical properties. Because a tissue-engineered urethra can be grafted onto a recipient bed, this technology holds great promise. Clinical application and success will be achieved much earlier than, for example, the development of a tissue-engineered bladder.

D. E. Coplen, MD

11 Urinary Reconstruction

Long-Term Complications of Conduit Urinary Diversion

Shimko MS, Tollefson MK, Umbreit EC, et al (Mayo Med School and Mayo Clinic, Rochester, MN)
J Urol 185:562-567, 2011

Purpose.—We evaluated long-term surgical complications and clinical outcomes in a large group of patients treated with conduit urinary diversion.

Materials and Methods.—We identified 1,057 patients who underwent radical cystectomy with conduit urinary diversion using ileum or colon at our institution from 1980 to 1998 with complete followup information. Patients were followed for long-term clinical outcomes and analyzed for the incidence of diversion specific complications.

Results.—A total of 844 patients died at a median of 4.1 years (range 0.1 to 28.1) following cystectomy. Median followup of the surviving 213 patients was 15.5 years (range 0.3 to 29.1). There were 643 (60.8%) patients with 1,453 complications directly attributable to the urinary diversion performed with a mean of 2.3 complications per patient. Bowel complications were the most common, occurring in 215 patients (20.3%), followed by renal complications in 213 (20.2%), infectious complications in 174 (16.5%), stomal complications in 163 (15.4%) and urolithiasis in 162 (15.3%). The least common were metabolic abnormalities, which occurred in 135 patients (12.8%), and structural complications, which occurred in 122 (11.5%). Increasing age at cystectomy (HR 1.21, p <0.001), increasing Eastern Cooperative Oncology Group performance status (HR 1.23, p = 0.02) and recent era of surgery (HR 1.68, p <0.001) were significantly associated with a higher incidence of complications.

Conclusions.—Conduit urinary diversion is associated with a high overall complication rate but a low reoperation rate. Long-term followup of these patients is necessary to closely monitor for potential complications from the urinary diversion that can occur decades later.

▶ Conduit urinary diversion is infrequently used in children with benign lower urinary tract disease because with long-term follow-up, renal deterioration was identified in a significant portion of children. Continent orthotopic or cutaneous reconstruction has been used to possibly improve quality of life, but incontinent diversion remains the most common reconstruction after cystectomy. Long-term follow-up is somewhat difficult in the adult population because most patients succumb to malignancy within 10 years of cystectomy. In this series, a 15-year follow-up is available in 215 patients. Fig 2 in the original article shows that the incidence of complications continues to increase over time. Even though nearly 80% of the patients had at least 1 complication, only 6% of patients required reoperation. Bowel complications occur in 20% of the patients, and that incidence is likely independent of the type of diversion performed. New onset renal insufficiency developed in 20% of the patients. It is impossible to know whether this incidence is any different than in patients with a history of continent reconstruction. The data show the importance of long-term follow-up of patients after urinary diversion.

D. E. Coplen, MD

Intermediate Term Outcomes Associated With the Surveillance of Ureteropelvic Junction Obstruction in Adults

Gurbuz C, Best SL, Donnally C, et al (Univ of Texas Southwestern Med Ctr, Dallas)
J Urol 185:926-929, 2011

Purpose.—We determined the outcome of minimally symptomatic adult ureteropelvic junction obstruction in a group of patients treated conservatively with an active surveillance regimen.

Materials and Methods.—A total of 27 patients with asymptomatic or minimally symptomatic ureteropelvic junction obstruction were treated conservatively. All patients were evaluated with diuretic renograms. Ureteropelvic junction obstruction was defined by an obstructive pattern of the clearance curve and/or T1/2 greater than 20 minutes. Followup consisted of an office visit and renogram every 6 to 12 months. Cases of greater than 10% loss of relative renal function of the affected kidney, development of pyelonephritis and/or more than 1 episode of acute pain were considered active surveillance failures, and treatment was recommended.

Results.—Of the 27 patients 6 were lost to followup, leaving 21 (median age 47 years) with sufficient followup for analysis. In the 4 patients (19%) who initially presented with mild pain that led to the diagnosis of ureteropelvic junction obstruction, the pain completely resolved. Ipsilateral relative renal function decreased significantly in 2 patients (9.5%, mean reduction 14%). Pain worsened in 3 patients (14.3%) and de novo pain occurred in 1 (4.7%). Surgical intervention for ureteropelvic junction obstruction was required in 6 patients (29%) at an average of 34 months. In total 15 patients (71%) remained on surveillance with a mean followup of 48 months.

Conclusions.—Active surveillance seems to be a reasonable initial option for asymptomatic or mildly symptomatic adult patients with ureteropelvic junction obstruction because only approximately 30% have progression to surgical intervention within 4 years of diagnosis. This strategy offers the advantage of individualizing therapy according to symptoms and renographic findings.

▶ The authors evaluate observational management of 21 patients with incidentally identified or minimally symptomatic ureteropelvic junction (UPJ) obstruction. They define obstruction based on renal scan findings (curve pattern and drainage half-time), while better definitions of obstruction are loss of ipsilateral renal function over time or severe colic associated with intermittent renal obstruction. This is the same type of management plan that is routinely used in the pediatric patient with prenatally identified renal dilation, although I suspect that the degree of dilation that is followed in infants is significantly greater than the dilation in this adult population. In the pediatric population, children with normal split function and no drainage are often followed expectantly. Both patients with failure secondary to loss of function had only a 4.7% ipsilateral decrease that was less than the 10% threshold in the study protocol. While adult UPJ/hydronephrosis may have a different etiology than prenatally identified abnormalities, observation of the asymptomatic patient with good renal function is safe and advisable even when the drainage half-time is greater than the published normative limit of 20 minutes.

D. E. Coplen, MD

Irrigation of Continent Catheterizable Ileal Pouches: Tap Water Can Replace Sterile Solutions Because It Is Safe, Easy, and Economical
Birkhäuser FD, Zehnder P, Roth B, et al (Univ of Bern, Switzerland)
Eur Urol 59:518-523, 2011

Background.—Continent catheterizable ileal pouches require regular irrigations to reduce the risk of bacteriuria and urinary tract infections (UTIs).

Objective.—Our aim was to compare the UTI rate, patient friendliness, and costs of standard sterile irrigation versus irrigation with tap water.

Design, Setting, and Participants.—Twenty-three patients participated in a prospective randomized two-arm crossover single-center trial. Aseptic intermittent self-catheterization (ISC) combined with sterile sodium chloride (NaCl) 0.9% irrigation was compared with clean ISC and irrigation with tap water (H_2O) during two study periods of 90 d each.

Intervention.—Patients underwent daily pouch irrigations with NaCl 0.9% solution or tap water.

Measurements.—Urine nitrite dipstick tests were evaluated daily; urine culture (UC) and patient friendliness were evaluated monthly. Costs were documented.

Results and Limitations.—A total of 3916 study days with nitrite testing and irrigation were analyzed, 1876 (48%) in the NaCl arm and 2040 (52%) in the H_2O arm. In the NaCl arm, 418 study days (22%) with nitrite-positive dipsticks were recorded, 219 d (11%) in the H_2O arm, significantly fewer ($p = 0.01$). Of the 149 UCs, 96 (64%) were positive, 48 in each arm, revealing a total of 16 different germs. All patients preferred the H_2O method. Monthly costs were up to 20 times lower in the H_2O arm.

Conclusions.—Pouch irrigation with sterile NaCl 0.9% solution and tap water had comparable rates of positive UC. Irrigation with tap water significantly lowered the incidence of nitrite-positive study days and was substantially less costly and more patient friendly than NaCl irrigation. We therefore recommend the use of tap water (or bottled water) instead of sterile NaCl 0.9% solution for daily irrigation of continent catheterizable ileal pouches.

Trial registration.—Australian New Zealand Clinical Trials Registry, ACTRN12610000618055, http://www.ANZCTR.org.au/ACTRN1261 0000618055.aspx.

▶ The presence of mucus in continent urinary reservoirs or augmented bladders predisposes to bladder stone formation and likely facilitates bacteriuria. Patients should irrigate daily to evacuate intestinal mucus. This has been shown to decrease the incidence of bladder stones. It is less clear whether irrigation decreases the incidence of bacteriuria and/or symptomatic urinary tract infection (UTI). NaCl has been traditionally used as an irrigant presumably because of concerns of electrolyte disturbances when hypotonic solutions are exposed to the intestine. However, the dwell time during irrigation is very short and unlikely to cause electrolyte abnormalities. There is not a placebo (ie, no irrigation) arm in this study. Results are shown in Fig 2 and Table 2 in the original article. The significance of difference in nitrite positivity is unclear because not all bacteria metabolize nitrate. The difference did not translate into a decreased number of positive urine cultures, although there were fewer symptomatic UTIs (fever or abdominal discomfort) in the water irrigation group. There is not a proven benefit of water over saline, but given the safety and simplicity water should be the preferred irrigation solution.

D. E. Coplen, MD

Pelvic endometriosis and hydroureteronephrosis
Carmignani L, Vercellini P, Spinelli M, et al (Univ of Milan, Italy)
Fertil Steril 93:1741-1744, 2010

Objective.—To assess whether routine renal ultrasonography may be recommended in all patients with pelvic endometriosis, in order to avoid silent ureteral involvement of the disease.

Design.—Retrospective descriptive study.

Settings.—Tertiary center for the treatment of endometriosis at the Department of Obstetrics and Gynecology of the State University of Milan, Milan, Italy.

Patient(s).—Seven-hundred-fifty patients with a primary diagnosis of endometriosis, between January 2005 and July 2007.

Intervention(s).—Routine urinary ultrasound; recording of patient history, signs, and symptoms; gynecologic examination; blood and urinary analyses; magnetic resonance imaging; spiral multislice computerized tomography.

Main Outcome Measure(s).—Symptoms and signs of ureterohydronephrosis; diagnosis of ureterohydronephrosis.

Result(s).—Twenty-three patients (3%) of all 750 patients with endometriosis had associated ureterohydronephrosis diagnosed at renal ultrasound. Symptoms secondary to ureteral and renal involvement were present in 10 patients (43.5%); 6 reported lumbar pain (26.1%) and 4 patients (17.4%) had renal colic.

Conclusion(s).—In our study, the high number (56.5%) of asymptomatic ureteral involvement in patients with known pelvic endometriosis seems to warrant the need for further investigations regarding the possibility to avoid the high percentage of silent renal losses. Unfortunately there appears to be no specific risk factor to allow for early suspicion nor a validated preventive diagnostic and therapeutic program. It remains to be evaluated whether urinary ultrasound ensures a beneficial cost-benefit ratio if employed on a routine basis.

▶ In consideration of the prevalence of endometriosis, this study presents some interesting data. The authors correctly surmise that their relatively high prevalence rate of hydronephrosis is because of bias from a tertiary referral center. Nevertheless, the findings of silent hydronephrosis in more than half of the patients (and absence of hematuria in *all* affected patients) underscore the importance of screening the upper urinary tract in these at-risk relatively young patients. It is reassuring that most patients responded to urinary reconstruction.

E. S. Rovner, MD

12 Neurogenic Bladder/ Urinary Diversion

Children and youth with myelomeningocele's independence in managing clean intermittent catheterization in familiar settings
Donlau M, Imms C, Mattsson GG, et al (Vuxenhabiliteringen Landstinget i Östergötland, Linkoping, Sweden; La Trobe Univ and Murdoch Children's Res Inst, Melbourne, Victoria, Australia; Linköping Univ, Sweden)
Acta Paediatr 100:429-438, 2011

Aim.—To examine the ability of children and youth with myelomeningocele to independently manage clean intermittent catheterization.

Methods.—There were 50 participants with myelomeningocele (5–18 years); 13 of them had also participated in a previous hospital-based study. Their abilities and interest in completing the toilet activity were examined at home or in school using an interview and the Canadian Occupational Performance Measure (COPM). Actual performance was observed and rated. Background variables were collected from medical records and KatAD+E tests.

Results.—In total, 48% were observed to perform the toilet activity independently, in comparison with 74% who self-reported independence. Univariate analyses found KatAD+E could predict who was independent. COPM failed to do so. Ability to remain focused and ambulation were predictors of independence, but age, sex and IQ were not. Multivariable analysis found time to completion to be the strongest predictor of independence. Four children were independent in their familiar environment, but not in the hospital setting, and six of 13 children maintained focus only in their familiar environment.

Conclusions.—Interviews were not sufficiently accurate to assess independence in the toilet activity. Instead, observations including time to completion are recommended. The execution of the toilet activity is influenced by the environmental context.

▶ Even though most children with myelomeningocele (MMC) reported the ability to independently manage clean intermittent catheterization, direct observation confirmed that only a minority were successful on an independent basis. These results question whether children and youth with MMC should be evaluated with self-reporting instruments. Because most children cannot function independently, it is imperative that family and social situations are appropriately evaluated to assure compliance with the recommended management plan. This assessment also becomes very important during transition from teenage to adult care.

D. E. Coplen, MD

Irrigation of Continent Catheterizable Ileal Pouches: Tap Water Can Replace Sterile Solutions Because It Is Safe, Easy, and Economical
Birkhäuser FD, Zehnder P, Roth B, et al (Univ of Bern, Switzerland)
Eur Urol 59:518-523, 2011

Background.—Continent catheterizable ileal pouches require regular irrigations to reduce the risk of bacteriuria and urinary tract infections (UTIs).

Objective.—Our aim was to compare the UTI rate, patient friendliness, and costs of standard sterile irrigation versus irrigation with tap water.

Design, Setting, and Participants.—Twenty-three patients participated in a prospective randomized two-arm crossover single-center trial. Aseptic intermittent self-catheterization (ISC) combined with sterile sodium chloride (NaCl) 0.9% irrigation was compared with clean ISC and irrigation with tap water (H_2O) during two study periods of 90 d each.

Intervention.—Patients underwent daily pouch irrigations with NaCl 0.9% solution or tap water.

Measurements.—Urine nitrite dipstick tests were evaluated daily; urine culture (UC) and patient friendliness were evaluated monthly. Costs were documented.

Results and Limitations.—A total of 3916 study days with nitrite testing and irrigation were analyzed, 1876 (48%) in the NaCl arm and 2040 (52%) in the H_2O arm. In the NaCl arm, 418 study days (22%) with nitrite-positive dipsticks were recorded, 219 d (11%) in the H_2O arm, significantly fewer ($p = 0.01$). Of the 149 UCs, 96 (64%) were positive, 48 in each arm, revealing a total of 16 different germs. All patients preferred the H_2O method. Monthly costs were up to 20 times lower in the H_2O arm.

Conclusions.—Pouch irrigation with sterile NaCl 0.9% solution and tap water had comparable rates of positive UC. Irrigation with tap water significantly lowered the incidence of nitrite-positive study days and was substantially less costly and more patient friendly than NaCl irrigation. We therefore recommend the use of tap water (or bottled water) instead of sterile NaCl 0.9% solution for daily irrigation of continent catheterizable ileal pouches.

Trial Registration.—Australian New Zealand Clinical Trials Registry, ACTRN12610000618055, http://www.ANZCTR.org.au/ACTRN126100 00618055.aspx.

▶ Intestinal segments are commonly used for lower urinary tract reconstruction. Because of ongoing intestinal mucus production, it is often necessary for patients to irrigate their bladders or pouches postoperatively to prevent complications such as poor urine drainage or stone formation. In addition, some patients with indwelling catheters will develop a large amount of sediment, and irrigation can help these catheters to drain adequately. The sterile irrigant fluid (saline or water) is typically used for irrigations, but this use has never made much sense to me because the urine will be chronically colonized with bacteria as a result of the regular catheterizations. I have frequently recommended the use of tap water for irrigation in these patients. This study confirms my impression that this practice is safe and cost effective.

J. Q. Clemens, MD

Imaging-Guided Suprapubic Bladder Tube Insertion: Experience in the Care of 549 Patients
Cronin CG, Prakash P, Gervais DA, et al (Massachusetts General Hosp, Boston)
AJR Am J Roentgenol 196:182-188, 2011

Objective.—Symptomatic bladder outlet obstruction and neurogenic bladder are common conditions that frequently necessitate suprapubic insertion of a bladder tube. The purpose of this study was to describe an experience with minimally invasive imaging-guided percutaneous suprapubic bladder tube placement and the clinical and technical success and complications encountered.

Materials and Methods.—A total of 585 primary suprapubic bladder tube insertions and 439 exchanges of suprapubic bladder tubes were performed on 549 patients (469 men, 80 women; mean age, 66 years; range, 15–106 years). The details of percutaneous tube placement (indication, tube type, size at insertion and change, and method of insertion) were retrospectively recorded.

Results.—The technical success rate for primary suprapubic bladder tube insertion was 99.6% (547/549) and for exchanges was 92.3% (405/439). The clinical success rate for primary insertion was 98.1% (572/583), and symptoms were unresolved in 1.9% (11/583). Minor complications occurred in 7.2% (42/583) of cases at tube insertion and in 4.8% (21/439) at exchange. There was one major complication (a patient needed surgery because the small bowel was traversed by a catheter), and there was no procedure-related mortality.

Conclusion.—Radiologic imaging-guided percutaneous suprapubic bladder tube placement is a safe and effective procedure.

▶ I typically do not ask interventional radiology to place elective suprapubic tubes for me, but apparently, it is commonplace at some institutions. This large series documents the safety of this approach. In those with previous abdominal surgery or obese patients, it may be a safer option because of the use of imaging guidance to assist with accurate tube placement. Another advantage is the avoidance of heavier sedation that may be required for tube placement in the operating room. Disadvantages include the increased radiation exposure consequent to the imaging guidance and the requirement for the patient to coordinate the procedure with a separate specialty group. The authors tended to place small diameter catheters initially (mean size 12F), which subsequently required upsizing in the radiology suite. Future catheter changes were then performed via the mature tract in the urology office or at home.

J. Q. Clemens, MD

Intravesical Electromotive Botulinum Toxin Type A Administration—Part II: Clinical Application
Kajbafzadeh A-M, Ahmadi H, Montaser-Kouhsari L, et al (Tehran Univ of Med Sciences, Iran; Charles R. Drew Univ of Medicine and Sciences, Los Angeles, CA)
Urology 77:439-445, 2011

Objectives.—To assess the effect of electromotive botulinum toxin type A administration on urodynamic variables, urinary/fecal incontinence, and vesicoureteral reflux (VUR) due to refractory neurogenic detrusor overactivity in children with myelomeningocele.

Methods.—A total of 15 children (mean age 7.8 years) were included. Using a specially designed catheter, 10 IU/kg of electromotive botulinum toxin type A was inserted into the distended bladder. While connected to the indwelling catheter and 2 dispersive pads, a pulsed current generator delivered 10 mA for 15 minutes. The urodynamic parameters, including reflex volume, maximal bladder capacity, maximal detrusor pressure, and end-fill pressure, and the urinary/fecal incontinence status and VUR grade were evaluated before and at 1, 4, and 9 months after treatment.

Results.—The mean reflex volume and maximal bladder capacity had increased considerably (99 ± 35 mL versus 216 ± 35 mL and 121 ± 39 mL versus 262 ± 41 mL, respectively; $P < .001$). In contrast, the mean maximal detrusor pressure and end-fill pressure had significantly decreased (75 ± 16 cm H_2O versus 39 ± 10 cm H_2O and 22 ± 7 cm H_2O versus 13 ± 2 cm H_2O) after treatment. The difference was statistically significant ($P < .001$). Urinary incontinence improved in 12 patients (80%). The VUR grade substantially decreased in 7 of the 12 children (mean VUR grade 2.25 ± 1.3 versus 1.37 ± 0.7; $P = .001$), and none of the children required surgical intervention. Fecal incontinence was alleviated in 10 (83.3%) of the 12 children. Skin erythema and burning sensation were observed in 6 children.

Conclusions.—The results of our study have shown that electromotive botulinum toxin type A administration is a feasible and safe method with no need for anesthesia. This novel delivery system resulted in considerable improvement in the urodynamic parameters, urinary/fecal incontinence, and VUR in patients with refractory neurogenic detrusor overactivity.

▶ In this nonrandomized noncontrolled clinical trial, electromotive administration of botulinum toxin A (Dysport) was shown to be efficacious both symptomatically and urodynamically in 15 children with neurogenic voiding dysfunction secondary to myelomeningocele. The method of administration is clearly different from that reported previously in studies using botulinum toxin in a therapeutic manner for treatment of lower urinary tract dysfunction. Prior studies used botulinum toxin injected directly into the detrusor muscle using multiple needle injection sites.

If additional studies confirm these findings, this could substantially improve the patient acceptance of botulinum toxin, which is not only limited by financial and regulatory considerations but also by the discomfort and inconvenience of intravesical needle injection. Currently, in the United States, botulinum toxin A is under clinical development for utilization in both neurogenic and idiopathic detrusor overactivities. It is unclear whether the findings in this study of pediatric neurogenic voiding dysfunction could and would translate into other types of adult neurogenic voiding dysfunction or could withstand the rigors of a randomized placebo controlled trial. Nevertheless, these results are promising.

E. S. Rovner, MD

Urodynamic Profile of Diabetic Patients With Lower Urinary Tract Symptoms: Association of Diabetic Cystopathy With Autonomic and Peripheral Neuropathy
Bansal R, Agarwal MM, Modi M, et al (Postgraduate Inst of Med Education and Res, Chandigarh, India)
Urology 77:699-705, 2011

Objectives.—To evaluate the association between diabetic cystopathy (DC) and neuropathy (autonomic and peripheral) in patients with diabetes mellitus (DM) presenting with lower urinary tract symptoms (LUTS).

Methods.—Men with DM who presented with bothersome LUTS were enrolled from January 2008 to June 2009. Their demographic and clinical profiles were noted. Multichannel urodynamic studies were performed using the Solar Silver digital urodynamic apparatus. Hand and foot sympathetic skin responses, and motor and sensory nerve-conduction velocity studies were performed using the Meditronic electromyographic/evoked potentials system.

Results.—A total of 52 men (mean age 61.3 ± 12.1 years, DM duration 11.0 ± 7.5 years) completed the study protocol. Of these 52 men, abnormal sympathetic skin responses, motor and sensory nerve-conduction velocity studies, and combined neuropathy (all 3 tests abnormal) were noted in 80.7% 57.7%, 57.7%, and 51.9%, respectively. Urodynamic studies showed impaired first sensation (>250 mL), increased capacity (>600 mL), detrusor underactivity, detrusor overactivity, high postvoid residual urine volume (more than one third of capacity), and bladder outlet obstruction (Abrams-Griffiths number >40) in 23.1%, 25.0%, 78.8%, 38.5%, 65.4%, and 28.8% of the men, respectively. Both sensory and motor DC correlated with abnormal motor and sensory nerve-conduction velocity studies ($P = .015$ and $P = .005$, respectively). Only motor DC correlated with abnormal sympathetic skin responses ($P = .015$). The correlations were stronger in the presence of combined neuropathy (sensory DC, $P = .005$; motor DC, $P = .0001$).

Conclusions.—Men with DM and LUTS can present with varied urodynamic findings, apart from the classic sensory or motor cystopathy. A large proportion of these patients will have electrophysiologic evidence of neuropathy, and electrophysiologic evidence of neuropathy can moderately predict the presence of cystopathy.

▶ The typical urodynamic and clinical pattern of the presentation of diabetic cystopathy has been challenged over the last few years. The classical description of a sensory deficit leading to bladder overdistention clearly is not always the end result from long-term diabetes. These authors demonstrate a wide variety of urodynamic abnormalities in the study. More than 80% of these individuals demonstrated objective evidence of diabetic neuropathy on neurological testing, suggesting that these were, in fact, somewhat severely affected individuals. It is important to note that their symptomatology could not be correlated with urodynamic findings, which supports work of prior authors. Although most of the patients demonstrated detrusor underactivity and increased postvoid residual on urodynamics, there were a significant number of patients (almost 40%) with detrusor overactivity as well. It is clear that the patients with diabetes and lower urinary tract symptoms warrant further urodynamic investigation as to optimally evaluate the cause of their symptoms and direct appropriate therapy.

E. S. Rovner, MD

A 20-year follow-up of the mesh wallstent in the treatment of detrusor external sphincter dyssynergia in patients with spinal cord injury
Abdul-Rahman A, Ismail S, Hamid R, et al (Royal Natl Orthopaedic Hosp, Stanmore, London, UK)
BJU Int 106:1510-1513, 2010

Objective.—To assess the long-term (20 years) effectiveness of the UroLume wallstent™ (Pfizer Inc., UK) in the treatment of detrusor external sphincter dyssynergia (DESD) in patients with spinal cord injury (SCI).

Patients and Methods.—Twelve patients with quadriplegia secondary to SCI underwent external striated sphincter stenting with the UroLume wallstent in place of sphincterotomy for DESD ≈ 20 years ago. The mean (range) age was 41.8 (26–65) years. Eleven patients had cervical level injury whilst one had a thoracic injury. All the patients were shown to have high-pressure neurogenic detrusor overactivity and DESD with incomplete emptying on preoperative video-cystometrograms (VCMG).

Results.—Six of the 12 patients have now been followed-up for a mean (range) of 20 (19–21) years. Of the remaining six, two were lost to follow-up at 1 and 3 years, but both remained free of complications during that time. Two patients developed encrustation causing obstruction, requiring stent removal within 1 year of insertion. Another patient with an adequately functioning stent died 7 years after stent insertion from a chest infection. The twelfth patient developed bladder cancer 14 years after stent insertion and underwent cystectomy with urinary diversion. VCMG follow-up of the six patients showed a significantly sustained reduction of maximum detrusor pressure and duration of detrusor contraction at the 20-year follow-up. Five of these six patients developed bladder neck dyssynergia of varying degrees as shown on VCMG within the first 9 years of follow-up. All were successfully treated with bladder neck incision (BNI) where the last BNI needed was at 12 years. We did not encounter any problem with stent migration, urethral erosion, erectile dysfunction or autonomic dysreflexia.

Conclusion.—Urethral stenting using the UroLume wallstent is effective in the management of DESD in patients with SCI and provides an acceptable long-term (20-year follow-up) alternative to sphincterotomy. The failures manifest within the first few years and can be managed easily with stent removal without any significant problems. Bladder neck dyssynergia was the long-term complication which was treated successfully with BNI. It has no significant interference with erectile function, being reversible, minimally invasive and has a shorter hospital stay.

▶ It is indeed rare that a 20-year follow-up for any surgical intervention for voiding dysfunction is published. This is a small case series of patients with 2 of the 12 patients having been lost to the follow-up. Nevertheless, this article provides some insight into management. Neurogenic voiding dysfunction secondary to high spinal cord injury is a difficult and challenging clinical scenario. There are few options for these individuals with limited upper extremity function. The goal of management in this patient population is to minimize complications, reduce intravesical storage pressures, maintain satisfactory bladder emptying, protect the upper urinary tract, and minimize iatrogenic complications. It is remarkable that none of the individuals who were followed for the duration of the study demonstrated upper urinary tract deterioration, autonomic dysreflexia, or new onset erectile dysfunction. It is also remarkable that only 2 patients in this study developed encrustation of the stent, which is much lower than that reported in studies using stents for treatment of urethral strictures. This implies a considerable difference in the pathophysiology related to the complications of encrustation in these 2 patient populations.

E. S. Rovner, MD

13 Neurogenic Reconstruction

Comparison of Bladder Outlet Procedures Without Augmentation in Children With Neurogenic Incontinence

Snodgrass W, Darbei T (Univ of Texas Southwestern Med Ctr and Children's Med Ctr, Dallas)
J Urol 184:1775-1780, 2010

Purpose.—We compared continence results of the bladder neck sling vs the Leadbetter-Mitchell bladder neck procedure plus fascial sling in children with neurogenic urinary incontinence.

Materials and Methods.—We compared consecutive patients who received a 360-degree tight bladder neck sling to subsequent, similar patients who underwent a Leadbetter-Mitchell bladder neck procedure plus fascial sling involving a 50% reduction in bladder neck and proximal urethral diameter before a 360-degree tight sling. All patients underwent simultaneous appendicovesicostomy and none had undergone prior or simultaneous augmentation. All patients followed similar preoperative and postoperative protocols for urodynamic evaluation and anticholinergic therapy with data maintained prospectively.

Results.—After surgery 46% of 35 sling cases did not require pads vs 82% of 17 Leadbetter-Mitchell cases with a sling (p = 0.02). Mean followup was 28 months in sling and 13 months in Leadbetter-Mitchell cases. Initial urodynamics done approximately 6 months postoperatively were similar in the 2 cohorts and no patient had hydronephrosis. Transient low grade reflux occurred in 2 Leadbetter- Mitchell cases, of which 1 with increased intravesical pressures early after surgery that caused trabeculation received increased medical management. Augmentation was not done in any patient except 1 previously reported on after a sling.

Conclusions.—Patients undergoing Leadbetter-Mitchell procedure plus fascial sling were significantly less likely to require pads postoperatively than those with a sling alone. Adverse bladder changes have not required augmentation to date.

▶ Achieving continence in children with a neurogenic bladder and decreased outlet resistance is often a challenge. The bladder neck is often widely open and external compression (bladder neck sling [BNS] or artificial sphincter) achieves appropriate mucosal coaptation some of the time. The authors compare consecutive series of BNS with bladder neck narrowing performed presumably after the authors assessed their initial experience and wanted to improve results. The results are better in the latter group, although the 2 groups are not entirely comparable. Many of the children in the isolated sling group have functional bladder capacities of less than 100 to 150 mL as defined by volume less than 40 cm H_2O. That being said, in my experience, continence is better after this adjunct to BNS. There is no correlation between the detrusor leak point pressure and postoperative continence. Very importantly, the authors again show that continence can be achieved without concomitant bladder augmentation in a large proportion of children with neurogenic incontinence. In this series, a concomitant catheterizable channel was constructed in all children because of the possibility of catheterization difficulties secondary to bladder neck angulation by the sling. Another recent series shows excellent continence after a modified bladder neck reconstruction and no difficulty with transurethral catheterization.[1]

D. E. Coplen, MD

Reference

1. Churchill BM, Bergman J, Kristo B, Gore JL. Improved continence in patients with neurogenic sphincteric incompetence with combination tubularized posterior urethroplasty and fascial wrap: the lengthening, narrowing and tightening procedure. *J Urol.* 2010;184:1763-1767.

14 Vesicoureteral Reflux

The Swedish Reflux Trial in Children: I. Study Design and Study Population Characteristics

Brandström P, Esbjörner E, Herthelius M, et al (Univ of Gothenburg, Göteborg, Sweden; Örebro Univ Hosp, Sweden; Karolinska Univ Hosp, Huddinge, Sweden; et al)

J Urol 184:274-279, 2010

Purpose.—We compared the rates of febrile urinary tract infection, kidney damage and reflux resolution in children with vesicoureteral reflux treated in 3 ways, including antibiotic prophylaxis, endoscopic therapy and surveillance with antibiotics only for symptomatic urinary tract infection.

Materials and Methods.—Children 1 to younger than 2 years with grade III–IV reflux were recruited into this prospective, open, randomized, controlled, multicenter study and followed for 2 years after randomization. The main study end points were recurrent febrile urinary tract infection, renal status on dimercapto-succinic acid scintigraphy and reflux status. Outcomes were analyzed by the intent to treat principle.

Results.—During a 6-year period 128 girls and 75 boys entered the study. In 96% of cases reflux was detected after urinary tract infection. The randomization procedure was successful and resulted in 3 groups matched for relevant factors. Recruitment was slower than anticipated but after patients were entered adherence to the protocol was good. Of the children 93% were followed for the intended 2 years without a treatment arm change. All except 2 patients completed 2-year followup scintigraphy.

Conclusions.—Recruitment was difficult but a substantial number of children were entered and randomly assigned to 3 groups with similar basic characteristics. Good adherence to the protocol made it possible to address the central study questions (Figs 1 and 2).

▶ The appropriate use of antibiotic prophylaxis in children with recurrent urinary tract infections (UTIs) and/or of vesicoureteral reflux is currently the subject of much debate. There are very few well-designed clinical trials that compare antibiotic prophylaxis and placebo. Most recently published studies show no benefit in children with low-grade reflux (I-III/V)[1-3] with the exception of some gender differences. Only one trial randomized a small number of patients with grade IV reflux (33 patients) and showed no difference in the rate of recurrent febrile UTIs and scarring.[4] The Prevention of Recurrent Urinary Tract Infection in Children with Vesicoureteric Reflux and Normal Renal Tracts

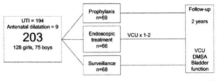

FIGURE 1.—Overall protocol design. (Reprinted from Brandström P, Esbjörner E, Herthelius M, et al. The Swedish Reflux Trial in Children: I. Study Design and Study Population Characteristics. *J Urol.* 2010;184:274-279, Copyright 2010, with permission from American Urological Association.)

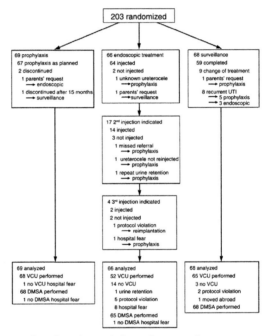

FIGURE 2.—Patient flow chart. Arrows indicate change to other treatment arm. (Reprinted from Brandström P, Esbjörner E, Herthelius M, et al. The Swedish Reflux Trial in Children: I. Study Design and Study Population Characteristics. *J Urol.* 2010;184:274-279, Copyright 2010, with permission from American Urological Association.)

trial randomized 576 children with UTIs, and 40% of them had reflux.[5] There was a modest reduction in the incidence of UTI on prophylaxis, with treatment of 14 children with antibiotic prophylaxis required to prevent one UTI.

The Swedish Reflux Trial is reported in a series of 5 articles. The study evaluates the 3 most important end points in a patient with reflux (recurrent infections, renal scarring, and reflux resolution). Recruitment was difficult and stopped after 6 years. The enrollment goal at study initiation was 330 infants aged between 1 and 2 years with grade III and IV reflux. There were 203 evaluable patients with complete follow-up. The study design is discussed in part I and detailed in Fig 1. The patient flow is shown in Fig 2. The trial was not placebo controlled, and there was no verification that parents were actually giving the prophylaxis to children, although children with breakthrough UTIs in general had bacteria resistant to the antibiotic. The strengths of the study include (1) a nationalized health care system that allows capture of system interactions, (2) renal scintigraphy at study entry and conclusion, (3) follow-up voiding cystourethrograms obtained in more than 90% of children, and (4) excellent protocol adherence.

Because reflux is a spectrum of disease, the Swedish Trial does not answer all reflux management questions. However, it is clear that antibiotic prophylaxis is not for all patients but has a benefit in others. Males older than 1 year with dilating reflux do not appear to have a benefit. However, there is likely a benefit in some if not the majority of females with dilating reflux because they have a higher incidence of infections and new scarring.

D. F. Coplen, MD

References

1. Garin EH, Olavarria F, Garcia Nieto V, Valenciano B, Campos A, Young L. Clinical significance of primary vesicoureteral reflux and urinary antibiotic prophylaxis after acute pyelonephritis: a multicenter, randomized, controlled study. *Pediatrics.* 2006;117:626-632.
2. Roussey-Kesler G, Gadjos V, Idres N, et al. Antibiotic prophylaxis for the prevention of recurrent urinary tract infection in children with low grade vesicoureteral reflux: results from a prospective randomized study. *J Urol.* 2008;179:674-679.
3. Montini G, Rigon L, Zucchetta P, et al. Prophylaxis after first febrile urinary tract infection in children? A multicenter, randomized, controlled, noninferiority trial. *Pediatrics.* 2008;122:1064-1071.
4. Pennesi M, Travan L, Peratoner L, et al. Is antibiotic prophylaxis in children with vesicoureteral reflux effective in preventing pyelonephritis and renal scars? A randomized, controlled trial. *Pediatrics.* 2008;121:e1489-e1494.
5. Craig JC, Simpson JM, Williams GJ, et al. Antibiotic prophylaxis and recurrent urinary tract infection in children. *N Engl J Med.* 2009;361:1748-1759.

The Swedish Reflux Trial in Children: II. Vesicoureteral Reflux Outcome
Holmdahl G, Brandström P, Läckgren G, et al (Univ of Gothenburg, Göteborg, Sweden; Uppsala Univ Children's Hosp, Sweden)
J Urol 184:280-285, 2010

Purpose.—We compared reflux status in children with dilating vesicoureteral reflux treated in 3 groups, including low dose antibiotic prophylaxis, endoscopic therapy and a surveillance group on antibiotic treatment only for febrile urinary tract infection.

Materials and Methods.—A total of 203 children 1 to younger than 2 years with grade III–IV reflux were recruited into this open, randomized, controlled trial. Endoscopic treatment was done with dextranomer/ hyaluronic acid copolymer. The main end point was reflux status after 2 years. Data were analyzed by the intent to treat principle.

Results.—Reflux status improved in all 3 treatment arms. Of patients in the prophylaxis, endoscopic and surveillance groups 39%, 71% and 47%,

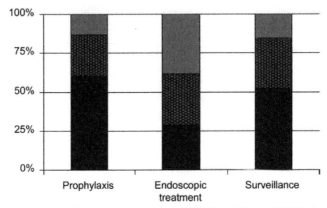

FIGURE 1.—VUR status after 2 years in treatment groups. Red bars indicate no VUR. Red and black bars indicate grade I–II VUR. Black bars indicate grade II–IV VUR. For interpretation of the references to color in this figure legend, the reader is referred to web version of this article. (Reprinted from Holmdahl G, Brandström P, Läckgren G, et al. The Swedish reflux trial in children: II. vesicoureteral reflux outcome. *J Urol.* 2010;184:280-285, Copyright 2010, with permission from American Urological Association.)

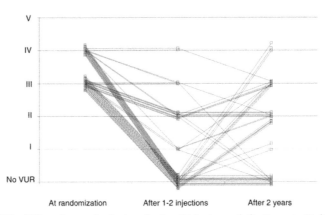

FIGURE 3.—VUR grade at randomization, after 1 or 2 injections and after 2 years in 66 children with endoscopic treatment. (Reprinted from Holmdahl G, Brandström P, Läckgren G, et al. The Swedish reflux trial in children: II. vesicoureteral reflux outcome. *J Urol.* 2010;184:280-285, Copyright 2010, with permission from American Urological Association.)

respectively, had reflux resolution or downgrading to grade I–II after 2 years. This was significantly more common in the endoscopic than in the prophylaxis and surveillance groups (p = 0.0002 and 0.0030, respectively). After 1 or 2 injections 86% of patients in the endoscopic group had no or grade I–II reflux but recurrent dilating reflux was seen in 20% after 2 years.

Conclusions.—Endoscopic treatment resulted in dilating reflux resolution or downgrading in most treated children. After 2 years endoscopic treatment results were significantly better than the spontaneous resolution rate or downgrading in the prophylaxis and surveillance groups. However, of concern is the common reappearance of dilating reflux after 2 years (Figs 1 and 3).

▶ This is the second of the 5 articles on the Swedish Reflux Trial addressing reflux resolution. As could be predicted, the children undergoing endoscopic correction of reflux had a lower incidence of reflux at the end of the study (Fig 1). There was resolution of reflux or downgrading in close to 50% of children in the other 2 groups. The initial success rate of endoscopic correction is much lower than has been reported in some centers. This may be because of higher reflux grade and coexisting voiding dysfunction. The authors state that there was no correlation of endoscopic success with injected volume. It is concerning that 13 patients with improved reflux after 1 injection had recurrence of a higher grade of reflux for cause (or end) of study voiding cystourethrography (Fig 3). As such, less than 50% of children in this group had no reflux, and 25% still had dilating reflux (Fig 1). Because follow-up in this series is only 2 years, continued deterioration in efficacy over time would make up-front endoscopic treatment less appealing. I think it is unlikely that the recurrence rate will continue to increase unless the population includes a large percentage of dysfunctional voiders.

D. E. Coplen, MD

The Swedish Reflux Trial in Children: III. Urinary Tract Infection Pattern

Brandström P, Esbjörner E, Herthelius M, et al (Univ of Gothenburg, Göteborg, Sweden; Örebro Univ Hosp, Sweden; Karolinska Univ Hosp, Huddinge, Sweden)
J Urol 184:286-291, 2010

Purpose.—We evaluated the difference in the febrile urinary tract infection rate in small children with dilating vesicoureteral reflux randomly allocated to 3 management alternatives, including antibiotic prophylaxis, endoscopic treatment or surveillance only as the control.

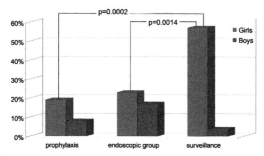

FIGURE 1.—Febrile UTI recurrence rate by gender and treatment group. (Reprinted from Brandström P, Esbjörner E, Herthelius M, et al. The Swedish reflux trial in children: III. urinary tract infection pattern. *J Urol.* 2010;184:286-291, Copyright 2010, with permission from American Urological Association.)

TABLE 1.—Recurrent Febrile UTIs by Gender and Treatment

| | No. Pts With UTI/Total No. (No. UTIs) | |
	Girls	Boys
Prophylaxis	8/43 (11)	2/26 (2)
Endoscopic	10*/43 (14)	4*/23 (4)†
Surveillance	24/42 (42)	1/26 (2)
Totals	42/128 (67)	7/75 (8)

*No worse VUR outcome after 1 injection than in those without recurrence (31% and 25% with still dilating VUR, respectively).
†Two UTIs developed within 3 days of urethral instrumentation.

TABLE 3.—Recurrent Febrile UTIs in Girls by VUR Status at 2 years

| | | No. Recurrence | |
2-Yr VUR Grade	No	Yes	Totals
No VUR	22	5	27
I	4	2	6
II	22	5	27
III	24	19	43
IV	8	8	16
Total No.	80	39	119*

*Two-year VCU not done in 9 girls (Mantel Haenszel chi-square test p = 0.0095).

Materials and Methods.—At 23 centers a total of 203 children were included in the study, including 128 girls and 75 boys 1 to younger than 2 years. Vesicoureteral reflux grade III in 126 cases and IV in 77 was detected after a febrile urinary tract infection (194) after prenatal screening (9). Voiding cystourethrography and dimercapto-succinic acid scintigraphy were done before randomization and after 2 years. The febrile urinary tract infection rate was analyzed by the intent to treat principle.

Results.—We noted a total of 67 febrile recurrences in 42 girls and a total of 8 in 7 boys (p = 0.0001). There was a difference in the recurrence rate among treatment groups in girls with febrile infection in 8 of 43 (19%) on prophylaxis, 10 of 43 (23%) with endoscopic therapy and 24 of 42 (57%) on surveillance (p = 0.0002). In girls the recurrence rate was associated with persistent reflux after 2 years (p = 0.0095). However, reflux severity (grade III or IV) at study entry did not predict recurrence.

Conclusions.—In this randomized, controlled trial there was a high rate of recurrent febrile urinary tract infection in girls older than 1 year with dilating vesicoureteral reflux at study entry but not in boys. Antibiotic prophylaxis and endoscopic treatment decreased the infection rate (Fig 1, Tables 1 and 3).

▶ This article addresses recurrence of urinary tract infections (UTIs) in the Swedish reflux trial. Boys had a lower rate of infection than girls in all treatment groups (Table 1). This may seem surprising given that most males in the study were not circumcised. However, studies show a higher risk of UTI only before 6 months of age, and the study population was older than 1 year. In girls, recurrence was more frequent in the surveillance group when compared with the prophylaxis and endoscopy groups (Fig 1). The recurrent UTIs were more likely to occur in children with high-grade reflux (Table 3). It may be true that endoscopy decreases the overall number of infections by correcting dilating reflux, but in this study that subset of patients was maintained on prophylaxis until imaging showed resolution/improvement in the reflux. Thus, with regard to prevention of infection, those 2 arms of the study are actually very similarly managed. If a decision is made for prophylaxis, then endoscopic correction is a reasonable alternative to get the child off antibiotics if the parents are medication averse.

D. E. Coplen, MD

The Swedish Reflux Trial in Children: V. Bladder Dysfunction

Sillén U, Brandström P, Jodal U, et al (Univ of Gothenburg, Göteborg, Sweden; et al)
J Urol 184:298-304, 2010

Purpose.—We investigated the prevalence and types of lower urinary tract dysfunction in children with vesicoureteral reflux grades III and IV, and related improved dilating reflux, renal damage and recurrent urinary tract infection to dysfunction.

Materials and Methods.—A total of 203 children between ages 1 to less than 2 years with reflux grades III and IV were recruited into this open, randomized, controlled, multicenter study. Voiding cystourethrography and dimercapto-succinic acid scintigraphy were done at study entry and 2-year followup. Lower urinary tract function was investigated by noninvasive methods, at study entry with 4-hour voiding observation in 148 patients and at 2 years by structured questionnaire and post-void residual flow measurement in 161.

Results.—At study entry 20% of patients had lower urinary tract dysfunction, characterized by high bladder capacity and increased post-void residual urine. At 2 years there was dysfunction in 34% of patients. Subdivision into groups characteristic of children after toilet training revealed that 9% had isolated overactive bladder and 24% had voiding phase dysfunction. There was a negative correlation between dysfunction at 2 years and improved dilating reflux (p = 0.002). Renal damage at study entry and followup was associated with lower urinary tract dysfunction at 2 years (p = 0.001). Recurrent urinary tract infections were seen in 33% of children with and in 20% without dysfunction (p = 0.084).

Conclusions.—After toilet training a third of these children with dilating reflux had lower urinary tract dysfunction, mainly voiding phase problems. Dysfunction was associated with persistent reflux and renal damage

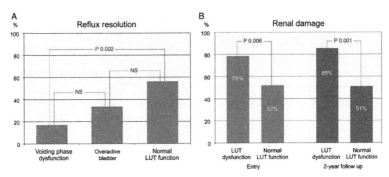

FIGURE 3.—*A*, VUR improvement by LUT function at 2-year followup. *B*, renal damage at study entry and 2-year followup by LUT function at 2 years. (Reprinted from Sillén U, Brandström P, Jodal U, et al. The Swedish Reflux Trial in Children: V. Bladder Dysfunction. *J Urol.* 2010;184:298-304, Copyright 2010, with permission from American Urological Association.)

while dysfunction at study entry did not predict the 2-year outcome (Fig 3).

▶ Any study dealing with urinary tract infections must address the possible influence of voiding dysfunction on clinical outcomes. In the Swedish Reflux Trial, infant males with reflux are more likely to have large bladder capacities, high voiding pressures, and high postvoid residuals. As external sphincter coordination improves, voiding normalizes and reflux resolves. While voiding dysfunction is hard to address prior to toilet training, it is important that it is detected and treated in older children with urinary tract infections and reflux. Failure to treat is associated with persistent reflux and a higher incidence of renal damage (Fig 3).

D. E. Coplen, MD

The Swedish Reflux Trial in Children: IV. Renal Damage

Brandström P, Nevéus T, Sixt R, et al (Univ of Gothenburg, Göteborg, Sweden; Uppsala Univ Children's Hosp, Sweden)
J Urol 184:292-297, 2010

Purpose.—We compared the development of new renal damage in small children with dilating vesicoureteral reflux randomly allocated to antibiotic prophylaxis, endoscopic treatment or surveillance as the control group.

Materials and Methods.—Included in the study were 128 girls and 75 boys 1 to younger than 2 years with grade III−IV reflux. Voiding cystourethrography and dimercapto-succinic acid scintigraphy were done before randomization and after 2 years. Febrile urinary tract infections were recorded during followup. Data analysis was done by the intent to treat principle.

Results.—New renal damage in a previously unscarred area was seen in 13 girls and 2 boys. Eight of the 13 girls were on surveillance, 5 received

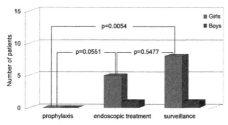

FIGURE 1.—New renal damage in children with dilating VUR by treatment arm. (Reprinted from Brandström P, Nevéus T, Sixt R, et al. The Swedish Reflux Trial in Children: IV. Renal Damage. *J Urol.* 2010;184:292-297, Copyright 2010, with permission from American Urological Association.)

endoscopic therapy and none were on prophylaxis (p = 0.0155). New damage was more common in children with than without febrile recurrence (11 of 49 or 22% vs 4 of 152 or 3%, p <0.0001).

Conclusions.—In boys the rate of new renal damage was low. It was significantly higher in girls and most common in the control surveillance group. There was also a strong association between recurrent febrile UTIs and new renal damage in girls (Fig 1).

▶ Prevention of reflux is a primary goal in reflux management. In the Swedish Reflux Trial, most children had an abnormal [99m]technetium dimercaptosuccinic acid (DMSA) scan at trial entry. The incidence was much larger in males (60% vs 23%), so it is likely that much of this was congenital scarring/dysplasia that is frequently seen in male infants with reflux. The end-of-study DMSA scan did show more new renal damage in girls in the endoscopic and surveillance groups (Fig 1). The overall rate of new damage was very low. Only girls on surveillance had a statistically higher rate of new renal scarring when compared with the prophylaxis group. Given that the incidence of infections (part III) and new scarring (part IV) in males is low, prophylaxis may be of benefit to decrease morbidity in males with reflux and recurrent urinary tract infections (UTIs). Because girls are more likely to have recurrent infections and a higher incidence of new scars (though small), prophylaxis is advisable, although one must remember that most children with recurrent UTIs did not develop a new scar during the 2-year follow-up.

D. E. Coplen, MD

High Grade Primary Vesicoureteral Reflux in Boys: Long-Term Results of a Prospective Cohort Study

Alsaywid BS, Saleh H, Deshpande A, et al (Univ of Sydney, New South Wales, Australia)
J Urol 184:1598-1603, 2010

Purpose.—We evaluated the incidence of new permanent defects in boys with grade 4 or 5 vesicoureteral reflux, identified the risk factors for new permanent defects and reviewed the outcome of different management approaches by assessing the rates of urinary tract infection and new permanent defects.

Materials and Methods.—This prospective cohort study recruited patients from July 1995 to December 2006. Study inclusion criteria were male gender and grade 4 or 5 primary vesicoureteral reflux. Patients were divided into 2 groups by presentation mode, including group 1—prenatal reflux diagnosis and group 2—reflux diagnosed after investigation for urinary tract infection. All patients underwent initial renal ^{99m}Tc-dimercapto-succinic acid scan evaluation. Continuous antibiotic prophylaxis was given in all patients until at least age 2 years. Surgical correction for reflux was done in 28 patients and 76 were circumcised. Followup included renal ^{99m}Tc-dimercapto-succinic acid scan with renal ultrasound at age 12 months with repeat ^{99m}Tc-dimercapto-succinic acid scan at ages 2 and 4 years.

Results.—Included in our study were 151 patients (206 high grade refluxing renal units) with a median age at diagnosis of 1.9 months (range 1 day to 8.8 years). Median age at first followup was 14 months (range 3 months to 3 years) and at next followup it was 39 months (range 10 months to 11.3 years). There were 52 boys (34%) in group 1 and 99 (66%) in group 2. Baseline perfusion defects on initial renal ^{99m}Tc-dimercapto-succinic acid scan were identified in 41 of 52 boys (78.8%) in group 1 and in 74 of 99 (74.7%) in group 2. During followup new permanent defects developed in 8 of 52 boys (15%) in group 1 and in 10 of 99 (10%) in group 2. In 18 patients a total of 20 renal units showed new permanent defects, including 13 in kidneys with baseline perfusion defects and 7 in previously normal kidneys (p >0.9). In groups 1 and 2 combined infection developed before and after circumcision in 62 of 137 (45.2%) and 5 of 74 cases (6.7%), respectively (p <0.001). New permanent defects were seen in 4 of 76 circumcised (5.2%) and in 14 of 137 uncircumcised boys (10.2%) (p >0.3).

Conclusions.—Baseline perfusion defects were seen on ^{99m}Tc-dimercapto-succinic acid scan at presentation in 115 of our 151 patients (76%) independent of presentation mode. New permanent defects developed in abnormal and previously normal kidneys, and were associated with urinary tract infection. Being circumcised was associated with fewer urinary tract infections and a lower incidence of observed new permanent defects (5.2% vs 10.2%).

▶ Nearly three-fourths of the males with high-grade reflux in this study had renal cortical defects, regardless of presentation after urinary tract infection (UTI) or prenatal diagnosis. Most of these defects are congenital dysplasia and not acquired renal scars. This would imply, although not definitively show, that screening boys with prenatal hydronephrosis for reflux may not decrease the incidence of scars. The authors show that new renal scarring in males with high-grade reflux is related to breakthrough UTIs. All boys were maintained on prophylaxis until 2 years of age. Infections were most related to circumcision status. The authors do not separate out the incidence of infections after stopping prophylaxis and/or toilet training. There was actually a higher incidence of UTIs after surgery, but presumably 100% of these boys had infections before surgery. Clearly, the goal is preventing infections that might lead to scarring. Surgical correction has a role, but prophylaxis and circumcision seem to be very protective in this population.

D. E. Coplen, MD

Pediatric Vesicoureteral Reflux Guidelines Panel Summary Report: Clinical Practice Guidelines for Screening Siblings of Children With Vesicoureteral Reflux and Neonates/Infants With Prenatal Hydronephrosis
Skoog SJ, Peters CA, Arant BS Jr, et al (American Urological Association Education and Res, Inc, Linthicum, MD)
J Urol 184:1145-1151, 2010

Purpose.—The American Urological Association established the Vesicoureteral Reflux Guideline Update Committee in July 2005 to update the management of primary vesicoureteral reflux in children guideline. The Panel defined the task into 5 topics pertaining to specific vesicoureteral reflux management issues, which correspond to the management of 3 distinct index patients and the screening of 2 distinct index patients. This report summarizes the existing evidence pertaining to screening of siblings and offspring of index patients with vesicoureteral reflux and infants with prenatal hydronephrosis. From this evidence clinical practice guidelines are developed to manage the clinical scenarios insofar as the data permit.

Materials and Methods.—The Panel searched the MEDLINE® database from 1994 to 2008 for all relevant articles dealing with the 5 chosen guideline topics. The database was reviewed and each abstract segregated into a specific topic area. Exclusions were case reports, basic science, secondary reflux, review articles and not relevant. The extracted article to be accepted should have assessed a cohort of children, clearly stating the number of children undergoing screening for vesicoureteral reflux. Vesicoureteral reflux should have been diagnosed with a cystogram and renal outcomes assessed by nuclear scintigraphy. The screening articles were extracted into data tables developed to evaluate epidemiological factors, patient and renal outcomes, and results of treatment. The reporting of meta-analysis of observational studies elaborated by the MOOSE group was followed. The extracted data were analyzed and formulated into evidence-based recommendations regarding the screening of siblings and offspring in index cases with vesicoureteral reflux and infants with prenatal hydronephrosis.

Results.—In screened populations the prevalence of vesicoureteral reflux is 27.4% in siblings and 35.7% in offspring. Prevalence decreases at a rate of 1 screened person every 3 months of age. The prevalence is the same in males and females. Bilateral reflux prevalence is similar to unilateral reflux. Grade I–II reflux is estimated to be present in 16.7% and grade III–V reflux in 9.8% of screened patients. The estimate for renal cortical abnormalities overall is 19.3%, with 27.8% having renal damage in cohorts of symptomatic and asymptomatic children combined. In asymptomatic siblings only the rate of renal damage is 14.4%. There are presently no randomized, controlled trials of treated vs untreated screened siblings with vesicoureteral reflux to evaluate health outcomes as spontaneous resolution, decreased rates of urinary infection, pyelonephritis or renal scarring.

In screened populations with prenatal hydronephrosis the prevalence of vesicoureteral reflux is 16.2%. Reflux in the contralateral nondilated kidney accounted for a mean of 25.2% of detected cases for a mean prevalence of 4.1%. In patients with a normal postnatal renal ultrasound the prevalence of reflux is 17%. The prenatal anteroposterior renal pelvic diameter was not predictive of reflux prevalence. A diameter of 4 mm is associated with a 10% to 20% prevalence of vesicoureteral reflux. The prevalence of reflux is statistically significantly greater in females (23%) than males (16%) (p=0.022). Reflux grade distribution is approximately a third each for grades I–II, III and IV–V. The estimate of renal damage in screened infants without infection is 21.8%. When stratified by reflux grade renal damage was estimated to be present in 6.2% grade I–III and 47.9% grade IV–V (p <0.0001). The risk of urinary tract infection in patients with and without prenatal hydronephrosis and vesicoureteral reflux could not be determined. The incidence of reported urinary tract infection in patients with reflux was 4.2%.

Conclusions.—The meta-analysis provided meaningful information regarding screening for vesicoureteral reflux. However, the lack of randomized clinical trials for screened patients to assess clinical health outcomes has made evidence-based guideline recommendations difficult. Consequently, screening guidelines are based on present practice, risk assessment, meta-analysis results and Panel consensus.

▶ The original reflux guidelines published by the American Urological Association in 1997 did not address screening of asymptomatic populations that have been shown to have a higher incidence of vesicoureteral reflux (VUR). In theory, screening allows treatment to prevent urinary tract infections (UTIs), pyelonephritis, and renal scarring. The incidence of reflux in asymptomatic siblings averages 28%, although the range is quite large (Fig 1 in the original article). It is well known that the reflux spontaneously resolves, so it is not surprising that the detection rate decreases as patient age increases. The incidence of VUR in infants with prenatally detected renal dilation (prenatal hydronephrosis [PNH]) is lower—16% with a broad range (Fig 3 in the original article). In the sibling screening group, there is little available evidence correlating reflux and renal scarring. There is evidence that infants with PNH and renal cortical abnormalities are much more likely to have high-grade reflux (Fig 4 in the original article). There is no evidence showing that infants with VUR detected after febrile UTI have a different outcome (infections, scarring, etc) than those detected by screening. Because of the lack of consistent data, screening is predominantly an option based on family history, presence of renal scarring, and the magnitude of hydronephrosis. If an observational approach is chosen, families must be aware that a urine sample should be obtained when their child has an unexplained fever, and preemptive treatment pending culture results is advisable to decrease morbidity.

D. E. Coplen, MD

Summary of the AUA Guideline on Management of Primary Vesicoureteral Reflux in Children
Peters CA, Skoog SJ, Arant BS Jr, et al (American Urological Association Education and Res, Inc, Linthicum, MD)
J Urol 184:1134-1144, 2010

Purpose.—The American Urological Association established the Vesicoureteral Reflux Guideline Update Committee in July 2005 to update the management of primary vesicoureteral reflux in children guideline. The Panel defined the task into 5 topics pertaining to specific vesicoureteral reflux management issues, which correspond to the management of 3 distinct index patients and the screening of 2 distinct index patients. This report summarizes the existing evidence pertaining to children with diagnosed reflux including those young or older than 1 year without evidence of bladder and bowel dysfunction and those older than 1 year with evidence of bladder and bowel dysfunction. From this evidence clinical practice guidelines were developed to manage the clinical scenarios insofar as the data permit.

Materials and Methods.—The Panel searched the MEDLINE® database from 1994 to 2008 for all relevant articles dealing with the 5 chosen guideline topics. The database was reviewed and each abstract segregated into a specific topic area. Exclusions were case reports, basic science, secondary reflux, review articles and not relevant. The extracted article to be accepted should have assessed a cohort of children with vesicoureteral reflux and a defined care program that permitted identification of cohort specific clinical outcomes. The reporting of meta-analysis of observational studies elaborated by the MOOSE (Metaanalysis Of Observational Studies in Epidemiology) group was followed. The extracted data were analyzed and formulated into evidence-based recommendations.

Results.—A total of 2,028 articles were reviewed and data were extracted from 131 articles. Data from 17,972 patients were included in this analysis. This systematic meta-analysis identified increasing frequency of urinary tract infection, increasing grade of vesicoureteral reflux and presence of bladder and bowel dysfunction as unique risk factors for renal cortical scarring. The efficacy of continuous antibiotic prophylaxis could not be established with current data. However, its purported lack of efficacy, as reported in selected prospective clinical trials, also is unproven owing to significant limitations in these studies. Reflux resolution and endoscopic surgical success rates are dependent upon bladder and bowel dysfunction. The Panel then structured guidelines for clinical vesicoureteral reflux management based on the goals of minimizing the risk of acute infection and renal injury, while minimizing the morbidity of testing and management. These guidelines are specific to children based on age as well as the presence of bladder and bowel dysfunction. Recommendations for long-term followup based on risk level are also included.

Conclusions.—Using a structured, formal meta-analytic technique with rigorous data selection, conditioning and quality assessment, we attempted to structure clinically relevant guidelines for managing vesicoureteral reflux in children. The lack of robust prospective randomized controlled trials limits the strength of these guidelines but they can serve to provide a framework for practice and set boundaries for safe and effective practice. As new data emerge, these guidelines will necessarily evolve.

▶ In 1997, the first American Urological Association (AUA) guideline addressing the management of vesicoureteral reflux (VUR) was published. Since that time, there have been several published studies that call into question the routine use of antibiotic prophylaxis in all children with reflux. In the last decade, endoscopic treatment of reflux has also been adopted as a treatment modality. The current guidelines address evaluation and management of (1) infants with VUR, (2) children older than 1 year with VUR, and (3) children with VUR and coexisting bowel and bladder dysfunction (BBD). They also address the appropriate follow-up of children with VUR and appropriate interventions for children who fail medical management (breakthrough urinary tract infection [UTI]).

Unfortunately, there is a lack of robust randomized trials addressing reflux management. Specifically, the efficacy (or lack thereof) of continuous antibiotic prophylaxis cannot be established based on the limitations of studies. For example, the consensus panel recommends prophylaxis in children younger than 1 year with VUR and a history of UTI. This is based on the higher potential morbidity (renal scarring, need for hospitalization, etc) in the younger age group and not necessarily on a proven better outcome. It is clear that the presence of BBD plays a large role in recurrent infections (Fig 4 in the original article) and decreases the likelihood of reflux resolution (Fig 5 in the original article). Children with VUR, infections, and BBD should be placed on prophylaxis while the elimination pattern is modified. In older children with reflux and no BBD, the panel states that prophylaxis and observational management are both reasonable options in the absence of significant renal scarring.

The guidelines are summarized in this excellent review. The complete guidelines are in the public domain on the AUA Web site (http://www.auanet.org/content/guidelines-and-quality-care/clinical-guidelines.cfm?sub=vur2010) and should be read by any urologist managing VUR in infants and children. Those looking for a fixed set of rules will be disappointed. Reflux is a complex problem, and chosen management must take into account reflux grade, status of the renal parenchyma, patient age, infection history, elimination history, and family compliance with recommendations. No 2 patients are alike, and as the conclusion in the abstract states, they "provide a framework for practice and set boundaries for safe and effective practice."

D. E. Coplen, MD

15 Male Incontinence/ Voiding Dysfunction

Treatment for Postprostatectomy Incontinence: Is This as Good as It Gets?
Penson DF (Vanderbilt Univ, Nashville, TN)
JAMA 305:197-198, 2011

Background.—A relatively common complication after the treatment of localized prostate cancer is urinary dysfunction, with stress urinary incontinence a common occurrence after radical prostatectomy. Even 5 years after surgery, 14% to 28% of patients still report incontinence. New technologies developed to improve this outcome have yet to show benefit. An analysis of behavioral therapy as a method to improve the rate of incontinence after radical prostatectomy raised questions about the effectiveness of all current approaches.

Study Details.—A randomized clinical trial conducted by Goode et al compared 8 weeks of behavioral therapy with or without biofeedback and pelvic floor electrical stimulation with delayed treatment (control). Weekly episodes of urinary incontinence in men whose incontinence had been present for 1 to 17 years were measured. The relative reduction was 55% in the behavioral therapy group and 24% in the control group. In addition, 90% of the men in the behavioral therapy group but only 10% of the men in the control group reported better or much better urinary leakage status than before treatment. Mean urinary leakage episodes declined from 28 to 13 per week with behavioral therapy. In addition, the American Urological Association (AUA-7) symptom index score was improved by 2.5 points with the behavioral intervention. After 6 and 12 months, the AUA-7 symptom score had improved by 4 points in the intervention group.

Analysis.—The improvements reported in this study represent minimal changes. It is questionable whether men would feel satisfied because they had only 2 episodes of urinary incontinence each week. In addition, the 2.5-point improvement in AUA-7 symptom index score represents a slight improvement only, with the 4-point improvement representing the threshold for moderate improvement. Although behavioral therapy appears to improve urinary incontinence after prostatectomy, the degree of improvement is only slightly better than no treatment.

Conclusions.—It may be wise to rethink how best to treat men with post-prostatectomy urinary incontinence. Primary prevention, consisting of increased use of active surveillance in patients with lower-risk disease and selective application of aggressive interventions in patients with worse prognostic variables, may be a better strategy. The use of prostate-specific antigen (PSA) screening identifies many clinically indolent prostate cancers, with rates between 23% and 42%. Aggressive interventions are often undertaken in response to patients', family members', and clinicians' preconceived ideas about cancer in general and prostate cancer in particular; because of financial concerns; and as a result of other obstacles to pursuing active surveillance. If the goal is to reduce the incidence of complications such as urinary incontinence associated with the treatment of localized prostate cancer, it may be best to follow a course of PSA testing and serial prostate biopsies with aggressive treatment delayed until the patient reaches specific pathologic or biochemical milestones.

▶ Randomized controlled trials have suggested that the use of behavioral therapy (pelvic floor muscle exercises and bladder control strategies) may hasten the recovery of urinary control after radical prostatectomy. This study is unique in that it examined the efficacy of behavioral therapy (8 weeks) for postprostatectomy incontinence that had persisted for more than 12 months after surgery (range, 1-17 years). The mean number of weekly incontinence episodes was approximately 26, and many of the men indicated that they had previously tried pelvic floor muscle exercises for the symptoms. Despite this, the active treatment was more effective than the control, and the effects persisted to at least 1 year. Only 16% of men became completely dry, but there were clinically meaningful improvements in quality of life and incontinence severity measures. It would be interesting to know if these effects were dependent on the type of baseline symptoms (stress incontinence vs mixed incontinence), but the author did not analyze this. Furthermore, the study was conducted by an experienced group of investigators who have a long-standing interest in the study of behavioral therapy, and therefore the results may not be generalizable to the types of behavioral therapy that are offered in a community setting. In men with long-standing postprostatectomy incontinence, it is common to proceed directly to surgical therapy, but this study suggests that behavioral therapy should also be considered in these patients.

J. Q. Clemens, MD

Patient-reported reasons for discontinuing overactive bladder medication
Benner JS, Nichol MB, Rovner ES, et al (IMS Health, Falls Church, VA; Univ of Southern California, Los Angeles, CA; Med Univ of South Carolina, Charleston; et al)
BJU Int 105:1276-1282, 2010

Objective.—To evaluate patient-reported reasons for discontinuing antimuscarinic prescription medications for overactive bladder (OAB).

Patients and Methods.—A phase 1 screening survey was sent to a representative sample of 260 000 households in the USA to identify patients using antimuscarinic agents for OAB. A detailed phase-2 follow-up survey was sent to 6577 respondents with one or more antimuscarinic prescriptions for OAB in the 12 months before the phase 1 survey. The follow-up survey included questions about demographics, clinical characteristics, antimuscarinic use, beliefs about OAB, treatment expectations, OAB symptom bother, and pre-coded reasons for discontinuation. Patients who reported discontinuing one or more OAB medication during the 12 months before phase 2 were grouped by reason, using latent class analysis (LCA); the Lo-Mendell-Rubin likelihood statistical test was used to determine the number of classes. Conditional probabilities of reasons for discontinuation were calculated for each class. Multivariable logistic regression was used to assess the influence of demographic and clinical characteristics on class assignment.

Results.—In all, 162 906 (63%) and 5392 (82%) useable responses were returned in phases 1 and 2, respectively; the demographics were similar in respondents and nonrespondents in both phases. In all, 1322 phase 2 respondents (24.5%) reported discontinuing one or more antimuscarinic drugs during the 12 months before phase 2. LCA identified two classes (Lo-Mendell-Rubin statistic, $P = 0.01$) based on reasons for discontinuation. Most respondents (89%) reported discontinuing OAB medication primarily due to unmet treatment expectations and/or tolerability; many respondents in this class switched to a new antimuscarinic agent. A smaller group (11%) indicated a general aversion to taking medication. Age, sex, race, income, and history of incontinence were not predictive of class assignment.

Conclusions.—Expectations about treatment efficacy and side-effects are the most important considerations in discontinuing OAB medications for most patients. Interventions to promote realistic expectations about treatment efficacy and side-effects might enhance adherence.

▶ Why do patients discontinue medications for overactive bladder at such a high rate? Prior published data suggest that less than 20% of the patients started on an overactive bladder medication are still taking the medication at the end of 1 year. However, long term studies sponsored by pharmaceutical companies suggest that persistence rates at 1 and 2 years may be as high as 70% to 90%. How we can reconcile these 2 differences? This article provides some insight into possible explanations. It is interesting that cost or amount of co-pay was only the sixth most common reason for discontinuing medication, whereas unrealized expectations was by far the most common reason. Would an alteration or adjustment of expectations in our patients at the time that the medication is prescribed improve long-term use of these medications? Or would such an alteration of expectations simply diminish their level of disappointment and not have any impact on long-term utilization?

E. S. Rovner, MD

Complications of the AdVance Transobturator Male Sling in the Treatment of Male Stress Urinary Incontinence

Bauer RM, Mayer ME, May F, et al (Ludwig-Maximilian Univ, Munich, Germany)
Urology 75:1494-1498, 2010

Objective.—To evaluate prospectively the complication rate of the retrourethral transobturator sling (AdVance sling) for the functional treatment of male stress urinary incontinence (SUI).

Methods.—In 230 patients with SUI due to nonintrinsic sphincter deficiency (without direct sphincter lesion) after radical prostatectomy (n = 213), radical cystoprostatectomy with ileal neobladder (n = 2) and transurethral resection of the prostate (n = 15) a retrourethral transobturator sling was implanted. Patients were followed up for a median of 17 months (range, 4-42 months) with regard to intraoperative, early postoperative, and midterm postoperative complications.

Results.—Overall complication rate of the AdVance sling was 23.9%. Despite one accidental sling misplacement, no intraoperative complication occurred. Forty-nine patients (21.3%) experienced urinary retention postsurgery. Two slings were explanted (0.9%), 1 due to initial wrong placement and the other due to a symphysitis, attributed to a Guillain-Barré syndrome and not to a sling infection. One sling was transected (0.4%) due to slippage of the sling with obstruction of the urethra. Further complications were local wound infection (0.4%), urinary infection with fever (0.4%), and persistent moderate perineal pain (0.4%). There was no correlation between postoperative acute urinary retention and age at sling implantation, time of incontinence before sling implantation, preoperative daily pad use, or prior invasive incontinence treatment, respectively.

Conclusions.—The retrourethral transobturator AdVance sling is a safe treatment option for male nonintrinsic sphincter deficiency SUI, with the main postoperative complication being transient acute urinary retention. Severe intra- and postoperative complications are rare and sling explantation rate is very low.

▶ Male slings represent an emerging and viable alternative to the artificial urinary sphincter and other treatments for some individuals with postprostatectomy stress urinary incontinence. Overall, the complications that were seen in this study were, for the most part, minor. Urinary retention was the most common complication that resolved in almost all patients following a course of intermittent catheterization with a mean duration of catheterization of 27 days. Persistent perineal pain was quite low in this study as compared with other male sling procedures, with only 1 patient reporting persistent chronic perineal pain. Only 2 patients required sling explantation; one was done for urethral erosion of the sling material, and the other was explanted because of long-term urinary retention. Efficacy data were not reported in this article.

E. S. Rovner, MD

Response to fesoterodine in patients with an overactive bladder and urgency urinary incontinence is independent of the urodynamic finding of detrusor overactivity

Nitti VW, Rovner ES, Bavendam T (New York Univ Med Ctr; Med Univ of South Carolina, Charleston; Pfizer Inc, NY)
BJU Int 105:1268-1275, 2009

Objective.—To determine whether the presence of detrusor overactivity (DO) in patients with overactive bladder (OAB) and urgency urinary incontinence (UUI) is a predictor of the response to treatment with fesoterodine.

Patients and Methods.—This phase 2 randomized, multicentre, placebo-controlled trial consisted of a 1-week placebo run-in phase followed by an 8-week double-blind period. Eligible for the study were men and women aged 18—78 years with symptoms or signs of OAB with UUI; they were stratified into two balanced strata depending on the outcome of a baseline urodynamic assessment. By using this particular study design it was possible to investigate whether there were differences between the strata. The primary endpoint was the change from baseline to week 8 in mean voids/24 h. Secondary endpoints were the changes in UUI episodes/week, and for those patients with DO at baseline, the mean changes in volume at first involuntary contraction associated with a feeling of urgency, first desire to void, and strong desire to void, and change in maximum cystometric capacity. Because there were few patients the secondary analyses were considered exploratory.

Results.—Overall, there were linear dose-response relationships for placebo and the fesoterodine groups for the reduction in the number of voids/24 h and UUI episodes/week. Compared with the placebo group, the least squares mean changes from baseline to week 8 in both variables were significantly improved in patients receiving fesoterodine 4 mg ($P = 0.045$ and 0.040, respectively), 8 mg ($P < 0.001$ for both), and 12 mg ($P < 0.001$ for both). There were no significant differences in treatment responses, as measured by both variables between patients with and without DO. For patients with DO, the mean volume at the first desire to void improved in all fesoterodine treatment groups and worsened in the placebo group.

Conclusions.—Regardless of the presence of DO, the response to fesoterodine treatment was dose-proportional and associated with significant improvements in OAB symptoms, indicating that the response to OAB pharmacotherapy in patients with UUI was independent of the urodynamic diagnosis of DO.

▶ There is accumulating evidence that the response to various interventions for overactive bladder is independent of the finding of detrusor overactivity on pre-intervention urodynamics. The findings in this study, specifically that response to antimuscarinic therapy is not contingent on the finding of bladder overactivity, are similar to previous findings and studies looking at tolterodine and oxybutynin.

Additional studies have demonstrated that injection of OnabotulinumtoxinA and sacral neuromodulation are likewise not dependent on the finding of detrusor overactivity prior to intervention. The reasons for this remain unclear, but it may be that at least a component of the overactive bladder syndrome, that of urinary urgency, is unrelated to detrusor overactivity but instead related to aberrant afferent signal mechanisms arising from the bladder urothelium or suburothelial layers. If such abnormal afferent signaling truly exists in patients with overactive bladder and interventions such as antimuscarinic therapy and other well-described interventions demonstrate efficacy, future interventions directed at these currently poorly defined mechanisms may offer additional therapeutic options in the future.

E. S. Rovner, MD

16 Benign Prostatic Hyperplasia

Epidemiology and Biomarkers

Low Dose Oral Desmopressin for Nocturnal Polyuria in Patients With Benign Prostatic Hyperplasia: A Double-Blind, Placebo Controlled, Randomized Study
Wang C-J, Lin Y-N, Huang S-W, et al (Saint Martin De Porres Hosp, Chiayi, Taiwan, R.O.C.)
J Urol 185:219-223, 2011

Purpose.—We evaluated the long-term efficacy and safety of low dose oral desmopressin in elderly patients with benign prostatic hyperplasia with more than nocturnal voids and nocturnal polyuria more than 30% of total daily urine volume.

Materials and Methods.—Eligible patients with benign prostatic hyperplasia older than 65 years with nocturia, nocturnal polyuria and International Prostate Symptom Score 14 or greater were included in the study. All patients received placebo or 0.1 mg desmopressin orally at bedtime. Patients were required to visit the outpatient clinic from the first visit, and after 1, 3, 6 and 12 months of treatment. Patients maintained flow volume charts and used diaries to record voiding data throughout the study. During followup urinalysis, urine sodium, urine osmolality, serum electrolytes, prostate specific antigen, International Prostate Symptom Score, quality of life, transrectal ultrasonography of prostate, uroflowmetry and post-void residual urine volume were performed at each visit.

Results.—A total of 115 patients were enrolled in the study and randomized as 58 in the placebo group and 57 in the desmopressin group. Desmopressin significantly decreased nocturnal urine output and the number of nocturia episodes, and prolonged the first sleep period (p <0.01). Compared to before treatment desmopressin gradually decreased serum sodium and induced statistically but not clinically significant hyponatremia after 12 months of treatment. No serious systemic complications were found during medication.

Conclusions.—Low dose oral desmopressin is an effective and well tolerated treatment for nocturnal polyuria in the lower urinary tract symptoms of patients with benign prostatic hyperplasia. Long-term desmopressin therapy gradually decreases serum sodium and it might induce hyponatremia even in patients without initial hyponatremia. For long-term desmopressin administration serum sodium should be assessed carefully, at least at 1 week after treatment.

▶ Nocturia can be very bothersome in a subset of elderly men with benign prostatic hyperplasia and associated lower urinary tract symptoms. Desmopressin is a synthetic analog of arginine vasopressin that is indicated for the treatment of primary nocturnal enuresis (PNE) and central diabetes insipidus. In this study, desmopressin led to a decrease of 2 or more voids in most men (Fig in the original article). This was related to a decrease in nocturnal urine output. This indicates that nocturnal polyuria was the main cause of nocturia in the study population. The authors state that this improvement translated to significant change in quality of life in the treatment arm compared with the placebo group, although this conclusion must be challenged because the exact questionnaire used to assess quality of life is not detailed. There was no difference between the 2 groups in the International Prostate Symptom Score. Perhaps the men were better rested but still had significant daytime symptoms. The safety of desmopressin has been shown in children. While the 0.1-mg dose used in this study is very low compared with that used in children treated for PNE, hyponatremia developed in both treatment arms. This stresses the importance of close follow-up and the need for long-term safety data in elderly patients.

D. E. Coplen, MD

17 Bladder Cancer

International Phase III Trial Assessing Neoadjuvant Cisplatin, Methotrexate, and Vinblastine Chemotherapy for Muscle-Invasive Bladder Cancer: Long-Term Results of the BA06 30894 Trial

International Collaboration of Trialists on behalf of the Medical Research Council Advanced Bladder Cancer Working Party (now the National Cancer Research Institute Bladder Cancer Clinical Studies Group), the European Organisation for Research and Treatment of Cancer Genito-Urinary Tract Cancer Group, the Australian Bladder Cancer Study Group, the National Cancer Institute of Canada Clinical Trials Group, Finnbladder, Norwegian Bladder Cancer Study Group, and Club Urologico Espanol de Tratamiento Oncologico Group (Cardiff Univ, UK; European Organisation for Res and Treatment of Cancer, Brussels, Belgium; Cleveland Clinic Taussing Cancer Inst, OH; et al)

J Clin Oncol 29:2171-2177, 2011

Purpose.—This article presents the long-term results of the international multicenter randomized trial that investigated the use of neoadjuvant cisplatin, methotrexate, and vinblastine (CMV) chemotherapy in patients with muscle-invasive urothelial cancer of the bladder treated by cystectomy and/or radiotherapy. Nine hundred seventy-six patients were recruited between 1989 and 1995, and median follow-up is now 8.0 years.

Patients and Methods.—This was a randomized phase III trial of either no neoadjuvant chemotherapy or three cycles of CMV.

Results.—The previously reported possible survival advantage of CMV is now statistically significant at the 5% level. Results show a statistically significant 16% reduction in the risk of death (hazard ratio, 0.84; 95% CI, 0.72 to 0.99; P = .037, corresponding to an increase in 10-year survival from 30% to 36%) after CMV.

Conclusion.—We conclude that CMV chemotherapy improves outcome as first-line adjunctive treatment for invasive bladder cancer. Two large randomized trials (by the Medical Research Council/European Organisation for Research and Treatment of Cancer and Southwest Oncology Group) have confirmed a statistically significant and clinically relevant survival benefit, and neoadjuvant chemotherapy followed by definitive local therapy should be viewed as state of the art, as compared with cystectomy or radiotherapy alone, for deeply invasive bladder cancer.

▶ Neoadjuvant cisplatin, methotrexate, and vinblastine (CMV) saves lives. Patients enrolled had clinical T2, T3, or T4 disease and received 3 cycles on

CMV followed by local treatment. They demonstrated a 16% reduction in risk of death with a hazard ratio of 0.84 (95% confidence interval, 0.72-0.99; $P = .037$). The Kaplan-Meier curve for overall survival for both radiation therapy (Fig 3A in the original article) and radical cystoprostatectomy (Fig 3B in the original article) favors the chemotherapy arm. The magnitude of improvement in survival is actually larger than in prior studies.

This study demonstrates that there is a clear survival advantage for patients receiving CMV. This is yet another randomized trial demonstrating that neoadjuvant chemotherapy for bladder cancer saves lives. The preponderance of the evidence favors this approach. Critics will (correctly) point out that lumping radiation therapy or radical cystectomy as their local control modality is a shortcoming to this article. Still, both surgery and radiation therapy cohorts benefited in keeping with the concept that occult metastatic disease kills patients. While, this study does not address which is better, adjuvant or neoadjuvant, it clearly provides strong evidence that we should strive to give chemotherapy to all of our patients with invasive bladder cancer because it is now well recognized that it will improve their outcomes.

A. S. Kibel, MD

Treatment of Muscle Invasive Bladder Cancer: Evidence From the National Cancer Database, 2003 to 2007
Fedeli U, Fedewa SA, Ward EM (Veneto Region, Castelfranco Veneto, Italy; American Cancer Society, Atlanta, GA)
J Urol 185:72-78, 2011

Purpose.—We describe nationwide treatment patterns of muscle invasive bladder cancer, investigated determinants of cystectomy and provide contemporary trends in process of care measures in patients undergoing cystectomy.

Materials and Methods.—We selected 40,388 patients 18 to 99 years old diagnosed with muscle invasive (stages II to IV) bladder cancer in 2003 to 2007 from the National Cancer Database. Treatment included cystectomy, neoadjuvant and adjuvant chemotherapy, chemotherapy without surgery and radiation therapy. In patients undergoing cystectomy we retrieved the procedure type (partial vs radical), lymphadenectomy extent and 30-day followup. Cystectomy determinants were assessed by Poisson regression with robust error variance. Perioperative mortality was analyzed by multilevel logistic regression.

Results.—The proportion of patients treated with cystectomy (42.9%) and radiation therapy (16.6%) remained stable with time while the incidence of those who received chemotherapy increased from 27.0% in 2003 to 34.5% in 2007 due to an increase in neoadjuvant chemotherapy and chemotherapy without surgery. The cystectomy rate decreased with age and was lower in racial/ethnic minorities (especially black patients), uninsured or Medicaid patients, patients residing in the South and Northeast, and those treated at nonteaching/research hospitals. The partial cystectomy rate decreased and lymphadenectomy extent increased with time. The perioperative mortality rate was 2.6% and it was higher at low vs very high volume hospitals (OR 1.71, 95% CI 1.26–2.32).

Conclusions.—Recent nationwide data confirm ongoing improvements in process of care measures in patients who undergo cystectomy but also show marked differences in treatment patterns for muscle invasive bladder cancer by patient age, race, insurance status, geographic area and facility type

▶ I firmly believe that we are in a period of transition in the management of muscle invasive bladder cancer. This is clearly a deadly disease of an order of magnitude significantly higher than renal cell and prostate cancers, at least how the vast majority of patients present in 2011. Fedeli et al present an excellent overview of where we are today in 2011. They used the National Cancer Database to identify more than 40 000 patients who were diagnosed with muscle-invasive bladder cancer. The take-home message from the article is that we need to do a better job. A minority of the patients were actually treated with cystectomy at approximately 42%, which to my mind is the standard of care. Factors associated with decreased utilization of cystectomy were age (older patients), ethnicity (minority populations, particularly African Americans), the uninsured and Medicaid patients, specific geographic areas, and, lastly, those treated at nonteaching hospitals. The good news is that the number of patients receiving chemotherapy appeared to increase substantially from approximately 27% to 34%, and the rate of lymphadenectomy in the patients undergoing cystectomy actually appears to be increasing. Lastly, it is always striking, but the perioperative mortality rate was quite high at approximately 2.6%. Mortality is substantially lower in high-volume hospitals.

How do these data help the average urologic surgeon? Well, the first thing is that this is a disease that appears to be best treated in high-volume centers that do at least 14 cystectomies or more per year. High-volume centers are most likely to treat the patient aggressively with both neoadjuvant and adjuvant chemotherapies as well as radical cystectomy. The more-intense treatment does not appear to be associated with higher perioperative mortality rate. In fact, the 30-day mortality was almost double in low-volume compared with very-high-volume hospitals.

The rest of the data are harder to interpret. Yes, older patients should be considered for cystectomy. With good monitoring, radical cystectomy can be done in patients in their 80s and 90s. Still, it is obvious that many elderly patients cannot tolerate such an invasive procedure. The fact that uninsured or Medicaid patients and ethnic minorities are less likely to undergo surgical intervention is clearly multifactorial. These are individuals who are possibly being discriminated against because of the inability to pay. However, alternatively, this may be a population more resistant to socioeconomic reasons for undergoing an aggressive intervention. In addition, they would be much less likely to seek care promptly again for socioeconomic reasons, and this may ultimately lead to decreased ability to perform optimal care. Because of these barriers, these are populations of patients we must strive to educate so that they receive optimal care.

A. S. Kibel, MD

A Population-Based Competing-Risks Analysis of the Survival of Patients Treated With Radical Cystectomy for Bladder Cancer
Lughezzani G, Sun M, Shariat SF, et al (Univ of Montreal Health Ctr, Quebec, Canada; Weill Med College of Cornell Univ, Ithaca, NY; et al)
Cancer 117:103-109, 2011

Background.—Patients treated with radical cystectomy represent a very heterogeneous group with respect to cancer-specific and other-cause mortality. Comorbidities and comorbidity-associated events represent very important causes of mortality in those individuals. The authors examined the rates of cancer-specific and other-cause mortality in a population-based radical cystectomy cohort.

Methods.—The authors identified 11,260 patients treated with radical cystectomy for urothelial carcinoma of the urinary bladder between 1988 and 2006 within 17 Surveillance, Epidemiology, and End Results registries. Patients were stratified into 20 strata according to patient age and tumor stage at radical cystectomy. Smoothed Poisson regression models were fitted to obtain estimates of cancer-specific and other-cause mortality rates at specific time points after radical cystectomy.

Results.—After stratification according to disease stage and patient age, cancer-specific mortality emerged as the main cause of mortality in all patient strata. Nonetheless, at 5 years after radical cystectomy, between 8.5% and 27.1% of deaths were attributable to other-cause mortality. The 3 most common causes of other-cause mortality were other malignancies, heart disease, and chronic obstructive pulmonary disease. The most prominent effect on cancer-specific mortality was exerted by locally advanced bladder cancer stages. Conversely, age was the main determinant of other-cause mortality. Interestingly, even after adjusting for bladder cancer pathologic stage, cancer-specific mortality was higher in older individuals than their younger counterparts.

Conclusions.—The current study provides a valuable graphical aid for prediction of cancer-specific and other-cause mortality according to disease stage and patient age. It can help clinicians to better stratify the risk-benefit ratio of radical cystectomy. Hopefully, these findings will be considered in treatment decision making and during informed consent before radical cystectomy.

▶ If you are only willing to operate on healthy patients, then you should not be taking care of patients with bladder cancer. The most striking thing about this article is that almost 50% of the patients are dead at 5 years, and these are the healthier patients, those who are suitable for major surgery. While bladder cancer was the main cause of mortality, it is not surprising that the next 3 were other malignancies, heart disease, and chronic obstructive pulmonary disease, the other side effects of smoking. How will this alter management? I think that particular attention should be paid to other comorbid conditions that don't necessarily preclude surgery but may influence other aspects of medical care. This is a patient population that in general is resistant to seeking care. Any opportunity to improve their general health will pay dividends. Clearly, a thorough and meticulous operation that cures the patient of disease but the patient dies of a preventable medical event shortly thereafter is not a success.

A. S. Kibel, MD

18 Cryptorchidism

Intra-Abdominal Testis: Histological Alterations and Significance of Biopsy
AbouZeid AA, Mousa MH, Soliman HA, et al (Ain Shams Univ, Cairo, Egypt)
J Urol 185:269-274, 2011

Purpose.—Intra-abdominal testes represent only 5% of undescended testes. Review of the literature reveals that few data exist on the histological analysis of intra-abdominal testes. We studied histological alterations in intra-abdominal testes in relation to patient age at orchiopexy.

Materials and Methods.—A total of 57 boys underwent laparoscopy for impalpable undescended testes between October 2002 and June 2005. Testicular biopsies were taken from intra-abdominal testes, fixed in 3% glutaraldehyde, embedded in Epon, sectioned at 1 micron thickness and stained with toluidine blue. Histomorphometric analysis was performed by light microscopy. Effect of age at operation on histological evaluation of abdominal testes was also studied.

Results.—Testicular biopsies from 29 patients with intra-abdominal testes showed the histological alterations of decreased mean diameter of seminiferous tubules, germinal cell depletion (55%) and presence of microliths (6.9%).

Conclusions.—As age at orchiopexy increases, deviation from the norm is more evident and absence of germ cells on biopsy becomes more pronounced, reaching a rate of 93% after age 3 years. Further studies on orchiopexy with or without biopsy in the first few months of life would likely improve our understanding and treatment of cryptorchidism.

▶ The authors show (Table in the original article) age-related perturbation of germ cells in abdominal undescended testes. Germ cells were identified in no boy older than 5 years (Figure 3 in the original article). This raises the question of whether or not intra-abdominal orchiopexy is of benefit in an older boy with a normally descended contralateral testicle. In boys with bilateral undescended testes and intra-abdominal testes, orchiopexy should be performed as early as possible. It is unknown if this will decrease the risk of infertility in these patients.

D. E. Coplen, MD

Modified Scrotal (Bianchi) Mid Raphe Single Incision Orchiopexy for Low Palpable Undescended Testis: Early Outcomes

Cloutier J, Moore K, Nadeau G, et al (Université Laval, Quebec, Canada)
J Urol 185:1088-1092, 2011

Purpose.—We compared the results of low transscrotal mid raphe orchiopexy, high scrotal incision (Bianchi) and conventional inguinal approach in patients with palpable undescended testes.

Materials and Methods.—Orchiopexies performed between January 2003 and September 2009 with a minimum 3-month followup were included. Low scrotal incision (group 1) and high scrotal incision (group 2) were compared to the traditional inguinal 2-incision technique (group 3). We retrospectively reviewed operative time, success as defined by mid or lower scrotal position of the testis, and complications at 12 weeks and 1 year postoperatively.

Results.—A total of 286 orchiopexies were performed in 214 patients with palpable undescended testes. Group 1 included 81 patients with 125 undescended testes. Group 2 consisted of 44 patients with 60 undescended testes. Group 3 included 89 patients with 101 undescended testes. Postoperatively the testes were located in a good position within the scrotum in 99% of patients in group 1, 98% in group 2 and 100% in group 3. Mean ± SD operative time for unilateral undescended testes was significantly shorter for low transscrotal compared to inguinal orchiopexy (28 ± 10 vs 37 ± 12 minutes, p <0.0001) but equivalent to a high scrotal incision (27 ± 10 minutes, p = 0.59). For all 160 children followed for 1 year no long-term atrophy or secondary reascent was observed.

Conclusions.—Low transscrotal mid raphe orchiopexy appears to be an excellent alternative to high scrotal incision or standard inguinal orchiopexy for low palpable undescended testes, especially bilateral cases.

▶ This is a nonrandomized and noncontrolled comparison of 3 surgical approaches to palpable undescended testes that were in the upper third of the scrotum at the time of surgery. The authors do not identify what percentage of undescended testes are amenable to a scrotal approach at their institution. The children in the inguinal orchiopexy group had a much higher incidence of patent processus (68% vs 19% and 22% in groups 1 and 2, respectively). Because the operating surgeon chose the approach, the testes were almost certainly higher prior to surgery in group 3. Success was equivalent in all the groups. The only other end point evaluated was surgical time. The scrotal approach was quicker, but most patients in the group 3 required the additional time to isolate and divide the patent processus. There was no assessment comparing postoperative pain and recovery in the 3 groups. Presumably, cosmesis is better with the midline scrotal incision. The modified scrotal approach is clearly applicable in a subset of patients with undescended testes. High ligation of a patent processus may be difficult through a scrotal incision, but an inguinal approach can be added if the scrotal exposure is inadequate. A scrotal approach is appropriate for the very low (scrotal) undescended testicle.

D. E. Coplen, MD

Diagnostic Performance of Ultrasound in Nonpalpable Cryptorchidism: A Systematic Review and Meta-analysis
Tasian GE, Copp HL (Univ of California, San Francisco)
Pediatrics 127:119-128, 2011

Context.— Ultrasound is frequently obtained during the presurgical evaluation of boys with nonpalpable undescended testes, but its clinical utility is uncertain.

Objective.— To determine the diagnostic performance of ultrasound in localizing nonpalpable testes in pediatric patients.

Methods.— English-language articles were identified by searching Medline, Embase, and the Cochrane Library. We included studies of subjects younger than 18 years who had preoperative ultrasound evaluation for nonpalpable testes and whose testis position was determined by surgery. Data on testis location determined by ultrasound and surgery were extracted by 2 independent reviewers, from which ultrasound performance characteristics (true-positives, falsepositives, false-negatives, and true-negatives) were derived. Metaanalysis of 12 studies (591 testes) was performed by using a randomeffects regression model; composite estimates of sensitivity, specificity, and likelihood ratios were calculated.

Results.— Ultrasound has a sensitivity of 45% (95% confidence interval [CI]: 29—61) and a specificity of 78% (95% CI: 43—94). The positive and negative likelihood ratios are 1.48 (95% CI: 0.54—4.03) and 0.79 (95% CI: 0.46—1.35), respectively. A positive ultrasound result increases and negative ultrasound result decreases the probability that a nonpalpable testis is located within the abdomen from 55% to 64% and 49%, respectively. Significant heterogeneity limited the precision of these estimates, which was attributable to variability in the reporting of selection criteria, ultrasound methodology, and differences in the proportion of intraabdominal testes.

Conclusions.— Ultrasound does not reliably localize nonpalpable testes and does not rule out an intraabdominal testis. Eliminating the use of ultrasound will not change management of nonpalpable cryptorchidism but will decrease health care expenditures.

▶ Primary care physicians often obtain imaging to evaluate boys with nonpalpable testes. Ultrasonography, CT, or MRI cannot reliably identify the absence of a testicle. Exploration is still required in the presence of a negative test. Exploration is also required if the testis is identified in an abnormal location. Localization of the testicle rarely, if ever, changes the surgical approach. Imaging in the evaluation of undescended testes is rarely, if ever, indicated.

D. E. Coplen, MD

The testicular regression syndrome—do remnants require routine excision?

Bader MI, Peeraully R, Ba'ath M, et al (Alder Hey Children's NHS Foundation Trust, Liverpool, UK)
J Pediatr Surg 46:384-386, 2011

Aim.—Excision of testicular remnants is debatable in the scenario where hypoplastic vas and vessels can be seen entering a closed internal ring during laparoscopy for impalpable testes. We aimed to establish how frequently excised remnants have identifiable testicular tissue and, hence, malignant potential.

Methods.—This study is a retrospective review of all excised testicular remnants in children with impalpable testis. Specimens that were excised for indications other than testicular regression syndrome were excluded. Pathology reports of excised specimens were reviewed, and the presence of multiple histologic features was noted. Histologic confirmation of testicular/paratesticular tissue required the presence of 1 or more of the following: seminiferous tubules, germ cells, Sertoli cells, Leydig cells, vas deferens, or epididymal structures. *Malignancy potential* was defined by the presence of germ cells or seminiferous tubules. All patients with seminiferous tubules were further examined by a single histopathologist.

Results.—A total of 208 testicular remnants from 206 children were excised over the 11-year period (1999-2009). Histologic evidence confirmed excision of testicular/paratesticular tissue in 180 cases (87%). Seminiferous tubules were noted in 27 (15%), and germ cells were present in 19 (11%) cases.

Conclusion.—Viable germ cells were found in 11% of examined remnants, which, in our opinion, justifies their removal.

▶ The authors report histologic findings in atrophic gonads identified during laparoscopic and/or inguinal exploration for nonpalpable undescended testes. They do not report on the position of the gonads, although typically the gonads are located in the scrotum. They conclude that the presence of germ cells warrants excision of all gonads. However, an atrophic scrotal gonad is likely at no higher risk for testicular cancer than a man with a palpably normal descended testicle. If hypoplastic cord structures are identified at the internal ring during laparoscopy, there are only relative reasons to proceed with inguinal exploration and excision of an atrophic gonad.

D. E. Coplen, MD

19 Genital Ambiguity

Sexual Function and Surgical Outcome in Women with Congenital Adrenal Hyperplasia Due to *CYP21A2* Deficiency: Clinical Perspective and the Patients' Perception

Nordenström A, Frisén L, Falhammar H, et al (Karolinska Univ Hosp, Stockholm, Sweden; Karolinska Institutet, Stockholm, Sweden; et al)

J Clin Endocrinol Metab 95:3633-3640, 2010

Context.—Females with congenital adrenal hyperplasia (CAH) due to a CYP21A2 deficiency are exposed to androgens during fetal development, resulting in virilization of the external genitalia. Little is known about how these women feel that the disease has affected their lives regarding surgery and psychosexual adaptation.

Objective.—Our objective was to investigate the correlation between the surgical results, the self-perceived severity of the disease, and satisfaction with sexual life and relate the results to the CYP21A2 genotype.

Design and Participants.—Sixty-two Swedish women with CAH and age-matched controls completed a 120-item questionnaire, and a composite score for sexual function was constructed. The surgical outcome, including genital appearance and clitoral sensitivity, was evaluated by clinical examination. The patients were divided into four CYP21A2 genotype groups.

Results.—The sexual function score, but not for genital appearance, was higher in the patients satisfied with their sexual life. This was also true of the patients who were satisfied with the surgical result. There were discrepancies between the patients' perception of the impact of the condition on their sexual life and what health professionals would assume from clinical examination. The patients in the null genotype group scored lower on sexual function and satisfaction with their sexual life and had more surgical complications, also compared with the slightly less severe I2-splice genotype group.

Conclusion.—Our data show that the null genotype group was considerably more affected by the condition than the other groups and should be regarded as a subgroup, both psychologically and from a surgical perspective. Genotyping adds clinically valuable information.

▶ Females with congenital adrenal hyperplasia (CAH) are known to have some degree of behavioral masculinization secondary to prenatal androgen exposure. Any evaluation of outcomes is potentially influenced by the genotype and the timing and type of surgical reconstruction. For example, in this patient population, there were 5 different clitoral managements (no operation, partial resection, subcutaneous recession with or without partial resection, and amputation) and 4 different approaches to the vagina. As one can imagine, the type of initial surgery is directly related to sensitivity. For these patients, function seems to be more important than genital appearance. With regard to sexual function, it is difficult to ascertain if differences in sexual function are related to the degree of virilization at presentation or adverse outcomes from neonatal surgery, because most adult females with a poor outcome were severely virilized and had surgery in the first year of life. Evaluation and management of CAH requires a multidisciplinary team that provides both medical and psychological support of the patients and parents throughout life.

D. E. Coplen, MD

Should Male Gender Assignment be Considered in the Markedly Virilized Patient With 46,XX and Congenital Adrenal Hyperplasia?
Lee PA, Houk CP, Husmann DA (Indiana Univ School of Medicine, Indianapolis; Med College of Georgia, Augusta; Mayo Clinic, Rochester, MN)
J Urol 184:1786-1792, 2010

Purpose.—We assess the outcome in 46,XX men with congenital adrenal hyperplasia who were born with Prader 4 or 5 genitalia and assigned male gender at birth.

Materials and Methods.—After receiving institutional review board approval and subject consent we reviewed the medical records of 12 men 35 to 69 years old with 46,XX congenital adrenal hyperplasia, of whom 6 completed social and gender issue questionnaires.

Results.—All subjects were assigned male gender at birth, were diagnosed with virilizing congenital adrenal hyperplasia at age greater than 3 years and indicated a male gender identity with sexual orientation to females. Ten of the 12 subjects had always lived as male and 2 who were reassigned to female gender in childhood subsequently self-reassigned as male. Nine of the 12 men had long-term female partners, including 7 married 12 years or more. The 3 subjects without a long-term female partner included 1 priest, 1 who was reassigned female gender, married, divorced and self-reassigned as male, and 1 with a girlfriend and sexual activity. All except the priest and the subject who was previously married when female indicated a strong libido and frequent orgasmic sexual activity. Responses to self-esteem, masculinity, body image, social adjustment and symptom questionnaires suggested adjustments related to the extent of familial and social support.

Conclusions.—Outcome data on severely masculinized 46,XX patients with congenital adrenal hyperplasia who were assigned male gender at birth indicate male gender identity in adulthood with satisfactory male sexual function in those retaining male genitalia. In men who completed questionnaires results were poorer in those lacking familial/social support. Male gender of rearing may be a viable option for parents whose children are born with congenital adrenal hyperplasia, a 46,XX karyotype and male genitalia, although positive parental and other support, and counseling are needed for adjustment.

▶ The current general understanding is that virilized 46XX newborns should be raised as female because there is good potential for fertility and female gender identity. There are, however, potential issues in severely virilized 46XX patients with congenital adrenal hyperplasia. This subset is more likely to exhibit male behaviors and less likely to have sexual interaction with men. The authors provide adult outcome data in patients raised as male. Many of these were diagnosed at an older age (3-10 years of age) and the male gender assignment was not questioned at the time of diagnosis. The results are compelling, but the denominator is not known. Are excluded patients dissatisfied with their male gender assignment? Are there similar patients who are satisfied with a female gender? Quite honestly the outcome in neither group has been adequately studied in a longitudinal fashion. This article drives home the point that a multi-disciplinary evaluation and assessment is required at diagnosis and that caregivers need to be honest with families regarding the available outcome data. Additionally, families need to be supported during and after the decision-making process.

D. E. Coplen, MD

20 Hypospadias

Management of hypospadias cripples with two-staged Bracka's technique
Gill NA, Hameed A (Shaikh Zayed Hosp, Lahore, Pakistan)
J Plast Reconstr Aesthet Surg 64:91-96, 2011

Patients labelled as 'hypospadias cripples' pose a challenge to reconstructive surgeons because of the complexity of the problem and limited options for reconstruction. The two-staged Bracka method is a versatile technique that is relatively easy to learn and applicable in difficult cases of salvage hypospadias. Over a period of 8 years, we applied this technique to 100 patients with hypospadias cripples who had previously undergone multiple (3–16) procedures. In the first stage, a full-thickness graft of skin or buccal mucosa was used for urethral plate reconstruction after release of chordee. Stage II was carried out at least 6 months after the first procedure. Meatal opening at the tip of the glans was achieved in 94 patients, straightening of the penis in 96 and proper urinary stream in 92 patients. Fistula formation occurred in nine patients. In our opinion, the two-staged Bracka technique is a useful strategy to deal with the myriad abnormalities encountered in crippled hypospadias. This technique not only creates a neourethra successfully, but also gives the penis a near-normal shape and appearance.

▶ The authors report a large series of staged correction of complicated reoperative hypospadias. The average number of prior surgeries was 5. It is a little bit surprising that adequate preputial skin (39 patients) was available for grafting after that many prior surgeries. Buccal mucosa was used in 34 patients. The authors do not state why they chose postauricular or inner arm in 27 patients as opposed to buccal mucosa. The results are good and are not influenced by the grafted tissue. The incidence of fistula and stricture was lower in the preputial group, although this was not statistically significant. Follow-up was at least 1 year in all patients but 5 years in only one-third. Because half of the patients were prepubertal, longer follow-up is required to assure that complications do not develop with pubertal penile growth. By default, staged reconstruction means that 2 additional surgeries are required in a patient who has already had multiple procedures. These outcomes demonstrate the utility of a staged approach.

D. E. Coplen, MD

Critical Outcome Analysis of Staged Buccal Mucosa Graft Urethroplasty for Prior Failed Hypospadias Repair in Children

Leslie B, Lorenzo AJ, Figueroa V, et al (Hosp for Sick Children and Univ of Toronto, Ontario, Canada)

J Urol 185:1077-1082, 2011

Purpose.—Although staged buccal mucosa graft urethroplasty is a well accepted technique for salvage urethroplasty, there are few reports on this procedure for redo hypospadias repair in children.

Materials and Methods.—We reviewed patients who underwent staged buccal mucosa graft urethroplasty for redo hypospadias repair. Age, quality of graft before tubularization, meatal position, presence of balanitis xerotica obliterans and complications were recorded.

Results.—A total of 30 patients underwent 32 repairs during a 5-year period. Mean age at first stage was 7 years (range 1 to 17) and mean interval between stages was 9.3 months (5 to 13). Mean followup after second stage was 25 months (range 10 to 46). Meatal position before first stage was proximal in 44% of patients, mid shaft in 39% and distal in 16%. Nine patients had biopsy proved balanitis xerotica obliterans. There were no donor site complications. Four patients underwent a redo grafting procedure. Complications after second stage occurred in 11 of 32 repairs (34%), consisting of urethral stenosis in 5, glanular dehiscence in 3 and urethrocutaneous fistula in 3. A third of the patients had some degree of graft fibrosis/induration after the first stage. These patients were prone to more complications at second stage (9 of 11, 82%), compared to patients without these unfavorable findings (4 of 21, 19%; p <0.001). Presence of balanitis xerotica obliterans and meatal position were not significant factors associated with adverse outcomes.

Conclusions.—Staged buccal mucosa graft urethroplasty is a suitable technique for salvage urethroplasty. Complications after second stage were seen in approximately a third of patients, mainly those with fibrotic/indurated grafts.

▶ One-third of patients had a complication requiring additional surgery after a planned staged reconstruction of failed hypospadias. This complication rate is much higher than in several other series. This may be related to the small number of patients (30) and large number of operating surgeons (5). Most complications occurred in hindsight in a subset of patients with small areas of fibrosis or induration at the graft site (Fig 4 in the original article). This is clearly a subjective assessment but reinforces the importance of the grafting technique and the postprocedure assessment. There should be a low threshold to repeat the graft before construction of the urethra if there is any question regarding the adequacy of the template. Poor take is related to thickness of the graft, trauma to the graft during harvest, scarring and impaired vascularity of the recipient bed, and inadequate immobilization of the graft during initial healing. Buccal mucosa is a good but imperfect graft material. Careful reading of this article highlights the potential pitfalls and will hopefully translate to improved outcomes.

D. E. Coplen, MD

Water Consumption and Use, Trihalomethane Exposure, and the Risk of Hypospadias
Iszatt N, Nieuwenhuijsen MJ, Nelson P, et al (Imperial College London, UK; Phrisk Ltd, London, UK)
Pediatrics 127:e389-e397, 2011

Objectives.—Hypospadias is a congenital anomaly that affects up to 70 in 10 000 males. Ingestion of drinking-water—disinfection byproducts such as trihalomethanes (THMs) has been associated with hypospadias in a small sample. We examined risk of hypospadias and exposure to THMs through water consumption and use.

Methods.—Between September 2000 and March 2003, we interviewed mothers of 471 boys with hypospadias and 490 controls in southeast England about maternal water consumption, dishwashing, showering, bathing and swimming. We obtained residential THM concentrations from the water companies and linked them by using Geographical Information Systems, which provided data on 468 case-subjects and 485 controls.

Results.—THM exposures, except for ingestion of $\geq$6 μg/day of bromodichloromethane (odds ratio [OR]: 1.65 [95% confidence interval (CI): 1.02—2.69]), were not associated with risk of hypospadias. Elevated risk of hypospadias was associated with estimates of consumption of cold tap water at home (OR: 1.71 [95% CI: 1.07—2.76]), total water (OR: 1.70 [95% CI: 1.09—2.67]), bottled water (OR: 1.64 [95% CI: 1.09—2.48]), and total fluid (OR: 1.55 [95% CI: 1.01—2.39]) for the highest versus the lowest categories; the first 2 showed dose-response trends.

Conclusions.—Evidence for an association between maternal water consumption and risk of hypospadias did not seem to be explained by THM exposure. Factors that influence maternal water consumption or other contaminants in tap or bottled water might explain this finding. It is important that women maintain an adequate fluid intake during pregnancy.

▶ The incidence of hypospadias may be increasing. The purported increase is likely secondary to a combination of environmental and maternal issues. It has been shown that advanced maternal age and the use of assisted reproductive techniques are associated with a higher incidence of hypospadias. Endocrine disrupting chemicals that leach from plastic bottles (phthalates) have been implicated in hypospadias. The authors evaluate whether or not trihalomethanes (THMs) (a reaction between chlorine disinfectants and natural organic matter in the water supply) are associated with hypospadias. Exposure can be both via ingestion and absorption. The questionnaires assessing water consumption were also filled out 2 to 6 years after delivery. Because this is a case-control study, it is difficult to control water intake and exposure, although, presumably, the 2 arms were equally good or bad at reporting. The authors show a small increased risk of hypospadias related to increased water intake (odds ratio, 1.55). Whether this is from THM, phthalates, or an undetermined component is unclear. Certainly, water intake is important and should not be restricted based on the findings of this study.

D. E. Coplen, MD

21 Infertility

Finasteride-associated male infertility

Chiba K, Yamaguchi K, Li F, et al (Kobe Univ Graduate School of Medicine, Japan)

Fertil Steril 95:1786.e9-1786.e11, 2011

Objective.—To describe a male patient with finasteride-associated infertility.

Design.—Case report.

Setting.—Tertiary-care clinic for male infertility.

Patient(s).—A patient with azoospermia who had been taking finasteride (1-mg dose) for 1 year for androgenic alopecia. He had been diagnosed with oligospermia 5 years before.

Intervention(s).—Discontinuation of finasteride.

Main Outcome Measure(s).—Improvement of semen parameters.

Result(s).—After cessation of finasteride, the patient's semen volume increased immediately, and sperm concentration was up to more than 10×10^6/mL 16 weeks after stopping finasteride. He is now trying to achieve pregnancy by intrauterine insemination.

Conclusion(s).—Cessation of finasteride improved spermatogenesis and allowed the couple to attempt less-invasive fertility therapy. In this case, the patient had impaired spermatogenesis before he started the drug. In such patients, the drug may further decrease spermatogenesis. We suggest that drug cessation could be taken into consideration for infertile male patients with impaired semen parameters who are taking finasteride at a 1 mg dose.

▶ Androgens are crucial in spermatogenesis, although the exact role of testosterone and/or dihydrotestosterone in spermatogenesis is unknown. Men with 5α-reductase deficiency have decreased ejaculate volumes secondary to prostatic and seminal vesicle hypoplasia. A prior double-blind placebo controlled trial showed no appreciable effect of finasteride on seminal parameters in men with normal spermatogenesis.[1] The authors show (Fig 1 in the original article) improved seminal parameters after stopping finasteride that was being used for alopecia. Whether this improvement will lead to pregnancy is unclear. This suggests that finasteride may affect the semen in men with a preexisting abnormality. Cessation of low dose finasteride should be considered in infertile men.

D. E. Coplen, MD

Reference

1. Overstreet JW, Fuh VL, Gould J, et al. Chronic treatment with finasteride daily does not affect spermatogenesis or semen production in young men. *J Urol.* 1999;162:1295-1300.

22 Urinary Tract Infection

Predicting the Need for Radiologic Imaging in Adults with Febrile Urinary Tract Infection

van Nieuwkoop C, Hoppe BPC, Bonten TN, et al (Loidon Univ Mcd Ctr, the Netherlands; et al)

Clin Infect Dis 51:1266-1272, 2010

Background.—Radiologic evaluation of adults with febrile urinary tract infection (UTI) is frequently performed to exclude urological disorders. This study aims to develop a clinical rule predicting need for radiologic imaging.

Methods.—We conducted a prospective, observational study including consecutive adults with febrile UTI at 8 emergency departments (EDs) in the Netherlands. Outcomes of ultrasounds and computed tomographs of the urinary tract were classified as "urgent urological disorder" (pyonephrosis or abscess), "nonurgent urologic disorder," "normal," and "incidental nonurological findings." Urgent and nonurgent urologic disorders were classified as "clinically relevant radiologic findings." The data of 5 EDs were used as the derivation cohort, and 3 EDs served as the validation cohort.

Results.—Three hundred forty-six patients were included in the derivation cohort. Radiologic imaging was performed for 245 patients (71%). A prediction rule was derived, being the presence of a history of urolithiasis, a urine pH ≥ 7.0, and/or renal insufficiency (estimated glomerular filtration rate, ≤ 40 mL/min/1.73 m^3). This rule predicts clinically relevant radiologic findings with a negative predictive value (NPV) of 93% and positive predictive value (PPV) of 24% and urgent urological disorders with an NPV of 99% and a PPV of 10%. In the validation cohort ($n = 131$), the NPV and PPV for clinically relevant radiologic findings were 89% and 20%, respectively; for urgent urological disorders, the values were 100% and 11%, respectively. Potential reduction of radiologic imaging by implementing the prediction rule was 40%.

Conclusions.—Radiologic imaging can selectively be applied in adults with febrile UTI without loss of clinically relevant information by using a simple clinical prediction rule.

► Fewer than 50% of children with a febrile urinary tract infection (UTI) have renal obstruction or an abscess at presentation. Consequently, it is not surprising that

237

only 6% of patients had a radiological abnormality related to the UTI. An additional 13% had nonurgent urological disorders. Whether or not the incidence of abnormality is higher in adults being evaluated in an estrogen receptor when compared with a febrile UTI managed in a primary care office cannot be determined from this study. The suggested algorithm is applied during the acute evaluation. As applied, a large number of patients have unnecessary imaging. With an appropriate follow-up plan, imaging can safely be delayed in patients who fail to improve on standard therapy. The authors argue that their approach identifies those who will fail treatment and require intervention. This study gives no evidence showing that early imaging results in an improvement in clinical outcomes. A more extensive analysis is required to determine the cost-effectiveness of each approach.

D. E. Coplen, MD

Cranberry Juice Fails to Prevent Recurrent Urinary Tract Infection: Results From a Randomized Placebo-Controlled Trial

Barbosa-Cesnik C, Brown MB, Buxton M, et al (Univ of Michigan School of Public Health, Ann Arbor; et al)
Clin Infect Dis 52:23-30, 2011

Background.—A number of observational studies and a few small or open randomized clinical trials suggest that the American cranberry may decrease incidence of recurring urinary tract infection (UTI).

Methods.—We conducted a double-blind, placebo-controlled trial of the effects of cranberry on risk of recurring UTI among 319 college women presenting with an acute UTI. Participants were followed up until a second UTI or for 6 months, whichever came first. A UTI was defined on the basis of the combination of symptoms and a urine culture positive for a known uropathogen. The study was designed to detect a 2-fold difference between treated and placebo groups, as was detected in unblinded trials. We assumed 30% of participants would experience a UTI during the follow-up period.

Results.—Overall, the recurrence rate was 16.9% (95% confidence interval, 12.8%−21.0%), and the distribution of the recurrences was similar between study groups, with the active cranberry group presenting a slightly higher recurrence rate (20.0% vs 14.0%). The presence of urinary symptoms at 3 days, 1−2 weeks, and at ≥1 month was similar between study groups, with overall no marked differences.

Conclusions.—Among otherwise healthy college women with an acute UTI, those drinking 8 oz of 27% cranberry juice twice daily did not experience a decrease in the 6-month incidence of a second UTI, compared with those drinking a placebo.

▶ Recurrent urinary tract infections (UTIs) are potentially associated with significant morbidity. Behavioral modification, probiotics, postcoital antibiotics, and daily prophylaxis are all potential modalities to decrease infections. Cranberry juice is a natural product that might decrease the number of UTIs.

Unfortunately, while proanthocyanidin is felt to be the active ingredient, it is really unknown if another component might be important. Prior nonblinded studies have shown a decrease in the number of UTIs when compared with placebo and nearly the same efficacy as daily prophylaxis. Some of these studies were performed in patients with a documented history of recurrent UTI, while this study did not necessarily stratify based on the number of prior infections. In this study, the dose (volume) of cranberry juice did not decrease the number of symptomatic UTIs. Because the active ingredient is not known, it is difficult to know if this absence of effect is present for increased volumes of cranberry juice. Even though this is a negative study, additional study of this and other natural compounds in the prevention is important.

D. E. Coplen, MD

Cranberry Juice Fails to Prevent Recurrent Urinary Tract Infection: Results From a Randomized Placebo-Controlled Trial
Barbosa-Cesnik C, Brown MB, Buxton M, et al (Univ of Michigan School of Public Health, Ann Arbor; et al)
Clin Infect Dis 52:23-30, 2011

Background.—A number of observational studies and a few small or open randomized clinical trials suggest that the American cranberry may decrease incidence of recurring urinary tract infection (UTI).

Methods.—We conducted a double-blind, placebo-controlled trial of the effects of cranberry on risk of recurring UTI among 319 college women presenting with an acute UTI. Participants were followed up until a second UTI or for 6 months, whichever came first. A UTI was defined on the basis of the combination of symptoms and a urine culture positive for a known uropathogen. The study was designed to detect a 2-fold difference between treated and placebo groups, as was detected in unblinded trials. We assumed 30% of participants would experience a UTI during the follow-up period.

Results.—Overall, the recurrence rate was 16.9% (95% confidence interval, 12.8%−21.0%), and the distribution of the recurrences was similar between study groups, with the active cranberry group presenting a slightly higher recurrence rate (20.0% vs 14.0%). The presence of urinary symptoms at 3 days, 1−2 weeks, and at ≥1 month was similar between study groups, with overall no marked differences.

Conclusions.—Among otherwise healthy college women with an acute UTI, those drinking 8 oz of 27% cranberry juice twice daily did not experience a decrease in the 6-month incidence of a second UTI, compared with those drinking a placebo.

▶ Cranberry ingredients are thought to reduce the binding of *Escherichia Coli* to uroepithelial cells, and thereby, may reduce the incidence of urinary tract infections (UTIs). This study suggests that cranberry juice is no more effective than placebo juice in preventing UTI recurrence. However, the authors point out that the active ingredient in cranberry juice is uncertain and that it is possible that the placebo juice may have contained an active ingredient such as ascorbic acid. Other studies have suggested that cranberry treatment is beneficial, so at this time, the role of this treatment in UTI prevention is not clear. Of note, a low-calorie cranberry juice was used in this study. I do not routinely recommend cranberry for UTI prevention, but if a patient brings up the topic, I tend to suggest the use of cranberry capsules, which contain fewer calories than standard cranberry juice.

J. Q. Clemens, MD

Executive Summary: International Clinical Practice Guidelines for the Treatment of Acute Uncomplicated Cystitis and Pyelonephritis in Women: A 2010 Update by the Infectious Diseases Society of America and the European Society for Microbiology and Infectious Diseases
Gupta K, Hooton TM, Naber KG, et al (Veterans Affairs Boston Health Care System and Boston Univ School of Medicine, MA; Univ of Miami, FL; Technical Univ of Munich, Germany; et al)
Clin Infect Dis 52:561-564, 2011

A Panel of International Experts was convened by the Infectious Diseases Society of America (IDSA) in collaboration with the European Society for Microbiology and Infectious Diseases (ESCMID) to update the 1999 Uncomplicated Urinary Tract Infection Guidelines by the IDSA. Co-sponsoring organizations include the American Congress of Obstetricians and Gynecologists, American Urological Association, Association of Medical Microbiology and Infectious Diseases—Canada, and the Society for Academic Emergency Medicine. The focus of this work is treatment of women with acute uncomplicated cystitis and pyelonephritis, diagnoses limited in these guidelines to premenopausal, non-pregnant women with no known urological abnormalities or co-morbidities. The issues of in vitro resistance prevalence and the ecological adverse effects of antimicrobial therapy (collateral damage) were considered as important factors in making optimal treatment choices and thus are reflected in the rankings of recommendations.

▶ These evidence-based guidelines focus on the treatment of urinary tract infection (UTI) in females. The treatment of recurrent cystitis, UTI in pregnancy, prevention of UTI, and the appropriate diagnosis of UTI are not addressed. Some knowledge of the local resistance rates of uropathogens causing UTIs is important when determining empiric therapy. Based on expert opinion derived from clinical and in vitro data, an antibiotic may be used if there is less than 20% resistance. There is level A-I evidence supporting the use of nitrofurantoin monohydrate (100 mg bid for 5 days) and trimethoprim-sulfamethoxazole (160/800) twice daily for 3 days in the treatment of acute cystitis. The quinolones and β-lactamases are highly efficacious (level A-I evidence) but should be considered alternative antimicrobials for acute cystitis. Both agents should be reserved for severe infections and are associated with potentially more side effects. Ampicillin and Amoxil have poor efficacy based on current sensitivity patterns unless *Enterococcus* is the pathogen. Because nitrofurantoin also treats *Enterococcus*, Ampicillin should not be used.

Given the increased potential morbidity associated with febrile UTIs, empiric treatment with ciprofloxacin is recommended when resistance prevalence is less than 10% in the community. For patients treated as an outpatient, a single parenteral dose of Ceftriaxone or and aminoglycoside should be considered pending culture results if resistance prevalence is high. Oral trimethoprim-sulfamethoxazole for 14 days is an effective treatment for pyelonephritis when cultures document sensitivity. Patients who are admitted for treatment should be treated with parenterals. An understanding of these recommendations will hopefully decrease the use of broad-spectrum antibiotics, decrease the development of resistant bacteria, and limit the adverse effects of antibiotic use.

D. E. Coplen, MD

A program to limit urinary catheter use at an acute care hospital
Rothfeld AF, Stickley A (Hollywood Presbyterian Med Ctr, Los Angeles, CA)
Am J Infect Control 38:568-571, 2010

Background.—Urinary catheters are the major cause of catheter-associated urinary tract infections (CAUTIs) and often may be unnecessary. We attempted to reduce the number of CAUTIs by limiting the use of urinary catheters.

Methods.—The number of catheters and CAUTIs were recorded during a control period of 7 months. A program was implemented limiting these catheters to patients who had urinary tract obstruction, orders for hourly output measurements, breakdown of skin in areas exposed to urine in patients with documented urinary tract infections, or urine- associated skin irritation that was unresponsive to barrier measures. In patients who did not meet these criteria, the physician was asked for a catheter removal order, and superabsorbent pads or diapers were used. Urinary catheter use and CAUTIs were then recorded during a subsequent 5-month intervention period. Nursing personnel were queried regarding their experience after 4 months of the intervention period.

Results.—Urinary catheter use decreased by 42% (*P* < .01), and the incidence of CAUTIs decreased by 57% (*P* < .05). There was some improvement in nursing satisfaction.

Conclusion.—Limiting urinary catheter use can reduce the incidence of CAUTI with no deterioration in nursing satisfaction.

▶ Center for Medicare and Medicaid has recently instituted new policies in which additional inpatient expenses incurred as a result of certain preventable medical complications will not be reimbursed by Medicare. One of these so-called never events is the development of nosocomial catheter-associated urinary tract infections (UTIs). The authors of this study implemented a program to reduce urinary catheter use in a 60-bed ICU step-down unit. Patients without clear indications for indwelling catheters were managed with absorbable pads or diapers, which were weighed to assess urine output. The new program resulted in a significant reduction in the rate of catheter-associated UTIs, defined as the presence of > 100 000 organisms/mL after the third day of hospitalization.

This study emphasizes some of the difficulties in the detection and management of catheter-associated UTIs. It is well documented that bacteriuria is almost universal in patients with indwelling catheters and that treatment is not indicated in the absence of symptoms. In this study, the authors actually demonstrated a reduction in bacteriuria, not UTIs. Further information about clinical symptoms would be required to determine which of the patients with bacteriuria had clinical evidence of symptomatic bacteriuria requiring treatment. Unfortunately, the distinction between asymptomatic bacteriuria and a true catheter-associated UTI is lost on most clinicians (and policy makers).

J. Q. Clemens, MD

No increased risk of adverse pregnancy outcomes in women with urinary tract infections: a nationwide population-based study
Chen Y-K, Chen S-F, Li H-C, et al (Taipei County Hosp, Taiwan; Taipei Med Univ, Taiwan)
Acta Obstet Gynecol Scand 89:882-888, 2010

Objective.—To examine the risk of adverse pregnancy outcomes (low birthweight (LBW), preterm birth, and small-for-gestational age (SGA)) in pregnant women with urinary tract infections (UTIs) using a 3-year nationwide population-based database, simultaneously taking characteristics of infant and mother into consideration.

Design.—Retrospective cross-sectional study.

Setting.—Taiwan.

Sample.—In total, 42,742 mothers with UTIs and 42,742 randomly selected mothers were included.

Methods.—Conditional logistic regression analyses to investigate the risk of LBW, preterm birth, and SGA, comparing these two cohorts.

Main Outcome Measures.—LBW, preterm birth, and SGA.

Results.—Pearson χ^2 tests show that there were significant differences in the prevalence of preterm births (<37 weeks) (7.2%, 7.7 vs. 8.3%, $p = 0.006$) and SGA infants (<10th percentile) (16.1%, 16.5 vs. 18.9%, $p = 0.003$) among pregnant women who were not exposed to UTIs, those exposed to antepartum non-pyelonephritic UTIs and those exposed to pyelonephritis. However, after adjusting for potential confounding factors, the odd ratios (ORs) for LBW were not statistically significant for mothers exposed to antepartum non-pyelonephritic UTIs, compared to women who were not diagnosed with UTIs; neither for <34 or <37 weeks nor SGA <10th percentile and <2 SDs. Similarly, compared to women who were not exposed to UTIs, the adjusted ORs for LBW, <34 weeks, <37 weeks, SGA

<10th centile, and <2 SD did not reach a significant level for mothers exposed to pyelonephritis.

Conclusions.—Women exposed to antepartum pyelonephritis or non-pyelonephritic UTIs were not at increased risk of having LBW, preterm, and SGA babies, compared to mothers who did not experience UTIs.

▶ The rate of asymptomatic bacteriuria is the same in pregnant women as it is in nonpregnant women. However, because of anatomic and functional changes that occur during pregnancy, asymptomatic bacteriuria in pregnancy is much more likely to cause pyelonephritis. The traditional teaching is that pyelonephritis during pregnancy conveys a greater risk of low birthweight and preterm delivery. This is the rationale for the routine screening for asymptomatic bacteriuria that occurs during pregnancy.

In this article, the authors conducted a retrospective cohort study for the period 2001-2003 using 2 nationwide population-based data sets in Taiwan. They identified women who were diagnosed with urinary tract infections (UTIs) during pregnancy (n = 42 742), and matched them at a 1:1 ratio with women who had no UTI diagnoses during pregnancy. Comprehensive national birth registry data were used to identify infants born with adverse outcomes (low birthweight, preterm deliveries, or small-for-gestational age), and the risk of these adverse outcomes was compared between the 2 groups. Initial univariate statistical analysis indicated a slight risk of adverse pregnancy outcomes in pregnant women with UTIs or pyelonephritis. However, after controlling for potential confounding factors (maternal age, education level, marital status, monthly income, parity, infant gender, presence of gestational hypertension, diabetes, or anemia) the associations were no longer observed. The authors point out that the association between maternal UTIs and adverse pregnancy outcomes were largely derived from older studies that did not control for important confounding factors and which did not use contemporary antibiotic treatments for the UTIs. Their conclusion seems appropriate: "Early prenatal screening for UTIs and treatment for women found to be bacteriuric are still needed, but patients need not panic about adverse pregnancy outcomes brought on by UTIs."

J. Q. Clemens, MD

23 Pediatric Urinary Tract Infection

Imaging Strategy for Infants With Urinary Tract Infection: A New Algorithm

Preda I, Jodal U, Sixt R, et al (Univ of Gothenburg, Göteborg, Sweden)

J Urol 185:1046-1052, 2011

Purpose.—We analyzed clinical data for prediction of permanent renal damage in infants with first time urinary tract infection.

Materials and Methods.—This population based, prospective, 3-year study included 161 male and 129 female consecutive infants with first time urinary tract infection. Ultrasonography and dimercapto-succinic acid scintigraphy were performed as acute investigations and voiding cystourethrography within 2 months. Late scintigraphy was performed after 1 year in infants with abnormality on the first dimercapto-succinic acid scan or recurrent febrile urinary tract infections. End point was renal damage on the late scan.

Results.—A total of 270 patients had end point data available, of whom 70 had renal damage and 200 did not. Final kidney status was associated with C-reactive protein, serum creatinine, temperature, leukocyturia, non-Escherichia coli bacteria, anteroposterior diameter on ultrasound and recurrent febrile urinary tract infections. In stepwise multiple regression analysis C-reactive protein, creatinine, leukocyturia, anteroposterior diameter and non E.coli bacteria were independent predictors of permanent renal damage. C-reactive protein 70 mg/l or greater combined with anteroposterior diameter 10 mm or greater had sensitivity of 87% and specificity of 59% for renal damage. An algorithm for imaging of infants with first time urinary tract infection based on these results would have eliminated 126 acute dimercapto-succinic acid scans compared to our study protocol, while missing 9 patients with permanent renal damage.

Conclusions.—C-reactive protein can be used as a predictor of permanent renal damage in infants with urinary tract infection and together with anteroposterior diameter serves as a basis for an imaging algorithm.

▶ The prevention of significant renal scarring should be the primary goal in the management of urinary tract infections (UTIs) in children. Historically, imaging was focused on reflux detection. Reflux management was based on grade and,

245

perhaps, infections, while there was less attention placed on the renal paren-chyma. In an alternative approach, a dimercapto-succinic acid scan (DMSA) is obtained in all children with a febrile UTI. A voiding cystourethrography is obtained if inflammation is identified on the DMSA. In this study the authors evaluate C-reactive protein (CRP) as a surrogate for renal inflammation. This in conjunction with dilation of the renal pelvis (a reasonable surrogate for dilating vesicoureteral reflux [VUR] in their population but, in most studies, not a very good discriminator standing alone) correctly identified 87% of patients with renal scarring (Fig 2 in the original article). Based on their data they suggest a management algorithm (Fig 3 in the original article). With long-term follow-up in their patient population, only 5 of 20 patients with a recurrent febrile UTI would not have had further acute phase imaging in the algorithm. All of these children had a normal late-phase DMSA, and only one had VUR. CRP is easier to obtain than DMSA in the acute phase. Further evaluation of this and other biomarkers may simplify the evaluation of children with febrile UTIs.

D. E. Coplen, MD

Febrile Infants With Urinary Tract Infections at Very Low Risk for Adverse Events and Bacteremia

Schnadower D, for the American Academy of Pediatrics Pediatric Emergency Medicine Collaborative Research Committee (Columbia Univ College of Physicians and Surgeons, NY; et al)

Pediatrics 126:1074-1083, 2010

Background.—There is limited evidence from which to derive guidelines for the management of febrile infants aged 29 to 60 days with urinary tract infections (UTIs). Most such infants are hospitalized for ≥48 hours. Our objective was to derive clinical prediction models to identify febrile infants with UTIs at very low risk of adverse events and bacteremia in a large sample of patients.

Methods.—This study was a 20-center retrospective review of infants aged 29 to 60 days with temperatures of ≥38°C and culture-proven UTIs. We defined UTI by growth of ≥50 000 colony-forming units (CFU)/mL of a single pathogen or ≥10 000 CFU/mL in association with positive urinalyses. We defined adverse events as death, shock, bacterial meningitis, ICU admission need for ventilator support, or other substantial complications. We performed binary recursive partitioning analyses to derive prediction models.

Results.—We analyzed 1895 patients. Adverse events occurred in 51 of 1842 (2.8% [95% confidence interval (CI): 2.1%−3.6%)] and bacteremia in 123 of 1877 (6.5% [95% CI: 5.5%−7.7%]). Patients were at very low risk for adverse events if not clinically ill on emergency department (ED) examination and did not have a high-risk past medical history (prediction model sensitivity: 98.0% [95% CI: 88.2%−99.9%]). Patients were at lower risk for bacteremia if they were not clinically ill on ED examination, did not have a high-risk past medical history, had a peripheral band count of <1250 cells per μL, and had a peripheral absolute neutrophil count of ≥1500 cells per μL (sensitivity 77.2% [95% CI: 68.6%– 84.1%]).

Conclusion.—Brief hospitalization or outpatient management with close follow-up may be considered for infants with UTIs at very low risk of adverse events.

▶ The American Academy of Pediatrics guidelines recommend hospitalization of infants younger than 2 months who have a urinary tract infection (UTI). The predominant reason for this recommendation is concerns regarding acute adverse events and the potential for bacteremia. Prior studies have shown that older children with bacteremia at the time of a UTI can be safely treated on an outpatient basis with low risk of short-term (return to the hospital) or long-term sequela (renal scarring). The data show that infants younger than 60 days who do not appear clinically ill at the time of emergent evaluation and have no prior medical history can perhaps be managed in a similar fashion. Most infants in this study met these criteria. A compromise may be observation in the hospital for 23 hours after evaluation. If there is a reliable home environment, children can be discharged from the emergency room with close follow-up. Certainly a prolonged hospitalization is not required in most infants with a febrile UTI.

D. E. Coplen, MD

5-Year Prospective Results of Dimercapto-Succinic Acid Imaging in Children With Febrile Urinary Tract Infection: Proof That the Top-Down Approach Works
Herz D, Merguerian P, McQuiston L, et al (Dartmouth-Hitchcock Med Ctr, Lebanon, NH)
J Urol 184:1703-1709, 2010

Purpose.—Evaluation in children after febrile urinary tract infection involves voiding cystourethrogram, which emphasizes urinary reflux rather than renal risk. We believe that early dimercapto-succinic acid renal scan after febrile urinary tract infection predicts clinically significant reflux and which children should undergo voiding cystourethrogram. The criticism of this approach is that some reflux and preventable renal damage would be missed. This study validates the use of initial dimercapto-succinic scan and presents 5-year renal outcomes.

Materials and Methods.—We prospectively studied children with febrile urinary tract infection using initial dimercapto-succinic acid renal scan, voiding cystourethrogram and renal/bladder ultrasound. Children with anatomical or neurological genitourinary abnormality and protocol failures were excluded from analysis. Dimercapto-succinic acid scan was repeated at 6 months if initially abnormal. Followup was done every 6 months in all children for at least 5 years.

Results.—A total of 121 children fit study inclusion criteria and completed the 5-year study. Overall 88 initial dimercapto-succinic acid scans (73%) were abnormal and 78 children (64%) had urinary reflux. The OR of having clinically significant reflux predicted by abnormal initial scan was 35.4. Abnormal followup scan did not predict clinically significant reflux. Overall subsequent urinary tract infection developed in 32 patients (26.5%) and 27 (85%) had an abnormal initial scan. No child with a normal initial scan had clinically significant reflux.

Conclusions.—Dimercapto-succinic acid scan can predict clinically significant reflux and children at greatest renal risk. Initial dimercapto-succinic acid scan should be done in all children after febrile urinary tract infection while voiding cystourethrogram should be reserved for those with an abnormal initial dimercapto-succinic acid scan.

▶ The evaluation and management of infants and children with febrile urinary tract infections is changing. Over the last 20 years, a voiding cystourethrogram has been part of the standard evaluation as recommended by the American Academy of Pediatrics and American Urological Association. Up to 40% of studied children will have reflux. Using this approach, it is clear that we overdiagnose and overtreat reflux. Some are low grade and not likely associated with recurrent infection. Other children with higher grades may not be at risk for renal scarring but may experience the morbidity of repeated febrile illnesses. The top-down approach hypothesizes that (99m) technetium-dimercapto-succinic acid (DMSA) scan will detect children at risk for renal injury (scarring). In theory, this group should be treated more aggressively. The authors show that most patients with reflux were identified with a positive DMSA scan. The average age for first febrile urinary tract infection (mean 3.6/median 2.4 years) is much older than is typically seen in clinical practice. Most of these children are toilet trained, and this makes it very likely that the children have some degree of voiding dysfunction as an etiologic factor in their infections. Based on that alone, one could argue that behavioral modification (not identification and treatment of reflux) is the most important therapy to prevent recurrent infections and renal scarring. I think the real imaging debate is in infants who are more likely to have an anatomic cause of infection (obstruction/reflux).

D. E. Coplen, MD

24 Pediatric Imaging

Assessment of Parental Satisfaction in Children Undergoing Voiding Cystourethrography Without Sedation

Sandy NS, Nguyen HT, Ziniel SI, et al (Children's Hosp Boston and Harvard Med School, MA)
J Urol 185:658-662, 2011

Purpose.—Approximately 50,000 children undergo voiding cystourethrography annually. There is a recent trend toward using sedation or delaying voiding cystourethrography due to the anticipated distress to the patient. We hypothesized that with adequate preparation and proper techniques to minimize anxiety, voiding cystourethrography can be performed without sedation. We assessed parental satisfaction associated with patient and parent experience of voiding cystourethrography without sedation.

Materials and Methods.—We used a 33-question survey to evaluate parental satisfaction with patient and parent experience of voiding cystourethrography without sedation. Children were divided into 3 groups according to toilet training status. Statistical analysis was performed using Stata®.

Results.—A total of 200 surveys were completed. Of the children 54% were not toilet trained. Of the parents 90% reported adequate preparation. More than half of parents classified the experience of voiding cystourethrography as equivalent to or better than a physical examination, immunization, ultrasound and prior catheterization. Most parents were satisfied with the ability of the child to tolerate the procedure and considered the experience better than expected. Children in the process of toilet training had the most difficulty with the procedure, correlating with lower levels of parental satisfaction.

Conclusions.—Voiding cystourethrography performed with adequate preparation and support can be tolerated without sedation. Children in the process of toilet training and females tolerate the procedure least.

▶ The voiding cystourethrogram is the gold standard for detection of vesicoureteral reflux. Unfortunately, the urethral catheterization is invasive, uncomfortable, and a source of great anxiety for children and their parents. Randomized placebo controlled trials evaluating conscious sedation during cystography show benefit in selected children, with only a small minority benefitting from treatment. Because of the lack of efficacy, parent/child education and distraction techniques have been used. A certified child life specialist is an invaluable adjunct during a cystogram or other invasive testing/procedures.

Parental talking and touching, using comfort items from home, playing with toys during the procedure, and watching digital video disks effectively decrease anxiety. The parents should be present and should participate in comforting their child. The authors evaluate parental satisfaction. It would be more interesting if they had evaluated satisfaction in the children who were undergoing the testing.

D. E. Coplen, MD

25 Pediatric Urology

Are Antibiotics Necessary for Pediatric Epididymitis?
Santillanes G, Gausche-Hill M, Lewis RJ (LAC + USC Med Ctr, Los Angels;
Harbor — UCLA Med Ctr, Torrance)
Pediatr Emerg Care 27:174-178, 2011

Objectives. To determine the percentage of cases of epididymitis in
pediatric patients that is of bacterial cause and to identify factors that
predict a positive urine culture.

Methods.—We conducted a retrospective chart review of patients diagnosed with acute epididymitis or epididymo-orchitis in 1 pediatric emergency department for 11 years. Charts were reviewed for historical,
physical, laboratory, and radiologic data. A positive urine culture was
used to identify patients with a bacterial cause of epididymitis.

Results.—A total of 160 patient records were initially identified as
having a diagnosis of epididymitis; of these, 20 met exclusion criteria or
did not have records available for review and 140 cases of epididymitis
were reviewed. Patients' age ranged from 2 months to 17 years, with
a median age of 11 years. Of these patients, 91% received empiric antibiotic therapy. Also, of these patients, 97 (69%) had a urine culture sent, of
whom 4 (4.1%; 95% confidence interval, 1.1%−10.2%) were positive. Of
the 4 positive urine cultures, 3 had organisms not sensitive to usual empiric
therapy for urinary tract infections. The boys with positive urine cultures
were not significantly different from the other patients in age, maximum
temperature, or number of white blood cells on urinalysis.

Conclusions.—Given the low incidence of urinary tract infections in
boys with epididymitis, in prepubertal patients, antibiotic therapy can
be reserved for young infants and those with pyuria or positive urine
cultures. Because it is difficult to predict which patients will have a positive
urine culture, urine cultures should be sent on all pediatric patients with
epididymitis.

▶ The authors correlate the clinical diagnosis of epididymitis and urine cultures in
children. The majority of these boys were prepubertal. In the absence of coexisting
abnormalities (neurogenic bladder, bladder exstrophy, ectopic ureter, etc) that
predispose to urinary tract infections, bacterial epididymitis is very rare. As
expected, only 4 patients in this study had a positive culture. In this population,
the clinical diagnosis of epididymal inflammation is correct, but the most common
etiology is mechanical. The inflammation is secondary to torsion of a testicular/
epididymal appendage that is adjacent to the epididymis. The inflammation and

251

pain typically persist for 5 to 7 days and resolve without antibiotics. The authors' conclusion that prepubertal patients with epididymitis should be placed on antibiotics is not based on data presented in the article. Antibiotics should be selectively used in prepubertal children with voiding symptoms, pyuria, or predisposing syndromic/anatomic issues. Postpubertal males should be checked for sexually transmitted diseases and treated based on laboratory findings.

D. E. Coplen, MD

26 Quality Improvement

Overprescription of Postoperative Narcotics: A Look at Postoperative Pain Medication Delivery, Consumption and Disposal in Urological Practice
Bates C, Laciak R, Southwick A, et al (Univ of Utah Health Sciences Ctr, Salt Lake City; et al)
J Urol 185:551-555, 2011

Purpose.—Prescription narcotic abuse is a significant social problem. Surplus medication following surgery is 1 source of prescription diversion. We assessed prescribing practices, consumption and disposal of prescribed narcotics after urological surgery.

Materials and Methods.—Surveys were administered to a 3-month consecutive sample of adult patients who underwent surgery performed by full and adjunct University of Utah Urology faculty. Surveys were performed 2 to 4 weeks postoperatively. With the exception of the investigators, prescribing physicians had no prior knowledge of the study. Data collected included perception of pain control, type and quantity of medication prescribed, quantity of leftover medication, refills needed, disposal instructions and surplus medication disposition.

Results.—Overall 47% of 586 patients participated in the study. Hydrocodone was prescribed most commonly (63%), followed by oxycodone (35%), and 86% of the patients were satisfied with pain control. Of the dispensed narcotics 58% was consumed and 12% of patients requested refills. A total of 67% of patients had surplus medication from the initial prescription and 92% received no disposal instructions for surplus medication. Of those patients with leftover medication 91% kept the medication at home while 6% threw it in the trash, 2% flushed it down the toilet and less than 1% returned it to a pharmacy.

Conclusions.—Overprescription of narcotics is common and retained surplus medication presents a readily available source of opioid diversion. It appears that no entity on the prescribing or dispensing ends of prescription opioid delivery is fulfilling the responsibility to accurately educate patients on proper surplus medication disposal. Surgeons should analyze prescribing practices and consider decreasing the quantity of postoperative narcotics prescribed.

▶ The authors address narcotic use after a variety of urologic procedures (refer to Fig in the original article). As might be expected, most patients did not use all the prescribed medication. A nonvalidated pain questionnaire was used to assess patient satisfaction with analgesia. Because only a small minority of patients (12%) actually refilled their prescription, the majority was satisfied but some were perhaps overmedicated. From a societal standpoint, the larger concern is the management of the leftover narcotics. The potential for abuse by patients, relatives, or others with access to the medicine cabinet cannot be underestimated. Overprescribing is likely a result of convenience. A larger quantity results in less time spent answering the phone and calling in refills. In the pediatric population, it is well known that acetaminophen and ibuprofen effectively manage pain in the vast majority of children. Research is warranted to give procedure-specific recommendations regarding reasonable medication quantities given to adults postoperatively.

D. E. Coplen, MD

Evaluating an Evidence-Based Bundle for Preventing Surgical Site Infection: A Randomized Trial

Anthony T, Murray BW, Sum-Ping JT, et al (Veterans Affairs North Texas Health Care System, Dallas)
Arch Surg 146:263-269, 2011

Objective.—To determine if an evidence-based practice bundle would result in a significantly lower rate of surgical site infections (SSIs) when compared with standard practice.

Design.—Single-institution, randomized controlled trial with blinded assessment of main outcome. The trial opened in April 2007 and was closed in January 2010.

Setting.—Veterans Administration teaching hospital.

Patients.—Patients who required elective transabdominal colorectal surgery were eligible. A total of 241 subjects were approached, 211 subjects were randomly allocated to 1 of 2 interventions, and 197 were included in an intention-to-treat analysis.

Interventions.—Subjects received either a combination of 5 evidenced-based practices (extended arm) or were treated according to our current practice (standard arm). The interventions in the extended arm included (1) omission of mechanical bowel preparation; (2) preoperative and intraoperative warming; (3) supplemental oxygen during and immediately after surgery; (4) intraoperative intravenous fluid restriction; and (5) use of a surgical wound protector.

Main Outcome Measure.—Overall SSI rate at 30 days assessed by blinded infection control coordinators using standardized definitions.

Results.—The overall rate of SSI was 45% in the extended arm of the study and 24% in the standard arm ($P=.003$). Most of the increased number of infections in the extended arm were superficial incisional SSIs (36% extended arm vs 19% standard arm; $P=.004$). Multivariate analysis suggested that allocation to the extended arm of the trial conferred a 2.49-fold risk (95% confidence interval, 1.36-4.56; $P=.003$) independent of other factors traditionally associated with SSI.

Conclusions.—An evidence-based intervention bundle did not reduce SSIs. The bundling of interventions, even when the constituent interventions have been individually tested, does not have a predictable effect on outcome. Formal testing of bundled approaches should occur prior to implementation.

▶ The general surgery literature is replete with research related to the prevention of surgical site infections (SSIs), while the urologic literature is sparse in this regard. Consequently, it is common for findings in the general surgery literature to be translated and adopted as best practices for urology as well. Surprisingly, this article found that the use of a panel of accepted infection control measures (omission of mechanical bowel prep, preoperative and intraoperative warming, supplemental oxygen during surgery, intraoperative fluid restriction, and use of a surgical wound protector) was associated with an increased risk for the development of SSI after colorectal surgery. The accompanying editorial comment suggests that adherence to a panel of quality measures, or checklist, may divert attention away from other important but unmeasured aspects of infection prevention.

J. Q. Clemens, MD

27 Training

A Survey of Ethically Challenging Issues in Urological Practice
Klausner AP, King AB, Velasquez M, et al (Virginia Commonwealth Univ Health System, Richmond)
J Urol 185:1407-1411, 2011

Purpose.—We surveyed ethical attitudes among urological and nonurological practitioners, allowing for thought and discussion regarding ethical issues in a larger audience.

Materials and Methods.—With input from an academic urologist, a senior medical student and a hospital ethics committee member, a survey was created which asked for multiple choice responses to 3 demographic questions (practice type, age, location) and 10 ethically challenging clinical questions. Surveys were distributed online or via mail to 5 groups including academic urologists, urologists in private practice, medical students, hospital risk managers/attorneys and members of a bioethical society. Surveys were analyzed according to demographic variables.

Results.—Surveys were sent out to 1,447 individuals and 340 responses were received (24%). There were statistically significant differences in the responses to several questions based on practice type, age and practice location. There was a lack of consistency in answer choices with greater than 50% agreeing on a single answer choice for only 4 of 10 questions (40%).

Conclusions.—This is the first study to our knowledge which attempts to objectively categorize ethical attitudes in a broad based survey of urologists and nonurologists, and challenges members of our profession to study their own responses to these ethical issues.

▶ The Accreditation Council for Graduate Medical Education has identified core competencies that residents are supposed to acquire during training. These include patient care, medical knowledge, practice-based learning and improvement, system-based practice, professionalism, and interpersonal skills and communication. The tools for teaching some of these competencies are poorly developed. The principles of ethics, patient privacy (Health Insurance Portability and Accountability Act), and state laws affect patient care and treatment. The authors presented 10 different patient management/ethical scenarios to physicians, medical students, legal staff, and bioethicists and evaluated the responses. The questions can be found online (http://www.vcu.edu/urology/pdf/ethics_survey.pdf). The questions deal with patient privacy, power of attorney, disclosure, and medico-legal issues. There was management consensus on very few of the questions (Fig 2 in the original article). There are multiple reasons for the disparity, including differences in training and/or inadequate fund of knowledge in the groups. For example, question 13 deals with disclosure of a sexually transmitted disease to the father of a 16 year old. Medical students, risk management staff, and bioethicists correctly answered that a father is not entitled to this information, while only 55% of practicing physicians knew this was the correct approach. However, the paucity of information in a 3 to 4 sentence clinical scenario may lead to ambiguity and difficulty ascertaining the most appropriate management. For example, question 12 deals with complex consent issues where almost everyone would consult a hospital legal counsel or ethics committee prior to disclosure to family. Unfortunately, these options were not potential answers. These large differences suggest that the teaching of ethics needs to be improved. Additionally, tools for evaluation of a physician's understanding of these same issues need to be enhanced.

D. E. Coplen, MD

28 Trauma

A Conservative Approach to Testicular Rupture in Adolescent Boys
Cubillos J, Reda EF, Gitlin J, et al (Cohen Children's Med Ctr of New York-Long Island Jewish Health System; Westchester Med Ctr, Valhalla, New York)
J Urol 184:1733-1738, 2010

Purpose.—Management for blunt trauma with breach of the renal capsule or bladder (extraperitoneal) has largely become nonsurgical since a conservative approach proved to be effective and safe. Currently the recommendation for managing testicular rupture is surgical exploration and débridement or orchiectomy. We report outcomes in boys diagnosed with testicular rupture and treated without surgical intervention.

Materials and Methods.—In the last year we conservatively treated 7 consecutive boys with delayed presentation of testicular rupture after blunt scrotal trauma. Patients were treated with scrotal support, antibiotics to prevent abscess, rest, analgesics and serial ultrasound. We report clinical information and outcomes.

Results.—The 7 boys were 11 to 14 years old and presented 1 to 5 days after injury. Trauma was to the left testis in 3 cases and to the right testis in 4. Patients presented with mild to moderate pain and similar scrotal swelling. Ultrasound findings consistently revealed hematocele and increased echogenicity. Blood flow was present in the injured portion of the testes in 3 cases and to the remainder of the affected testicle in 6 of the 7 boys. In the remaining boy an adequate waveform was not seen in either testicle, which the radiologist thought was secondary to prepubertal status. Other findings included scrotal edema, irregular contour and seminiferous tubule extrusion. Followup was greater than 6 months in all cases. Five boys were seen at the office and the 2 remaining had telephone followup. In all cases hematocele resolved, testicular size stabilized without atrophy and echogenicity normalized in the 5 patients with followup ultrasound. One patient required surgical repair of hydrocele 4 months after trauma but no other patient needed surgical exploration. No abscess or infection developed.

Conclusions.—A conservative approach in a select group of adolescent boys with testicular rupture can result in resolution of the fracture and maintenance of testicular architectural integrity.

▶ Testicular rupture after blunt trauma has typically been deemed a relative surgical emergency to decrease morbidity, expedite healing, and prevent testicular loss. Surgical repair may also result in earlier recovery and a return to normal activity. There is a small risk of orchiectomy and perhaps testicular injury (atrophy) from the debridement and repair. The primary advantage of a nonoperative approach is avoiding unnecessary surgery. In the acute setting, the diagnosis of testicular rupture may not be clearly evident on ultrasound (US). There is only a small hematocele and no definite disruption of the tunica or extrusion of tubules. If the testicle is viable on US, then with appropriate parental counseling expectant management is reasonable. Intractable discomfort, expanding hematoma, and suspicion for infection/abscess formation are indications for delayed exploration. If there is a delayed presentation and the patient is clinically well, conservative treatment may be reasonable even when imaging is conclusive.

D. E. Coplen, MD

Instituting a Conservative Management Protocol for Pediatric Blunt Renal Trauma: Evaluation of a Prospectively Maintained Patient Registry
Fitzgerald CL, Tran P, Burnell J, et al (Detroit Med Ctr, MI)
J Urol 185:1058-1064, 2011

Purpose.—Retrospective studies show that even high grade pediatric renal trauma can be safely managed conservatively. We evaluated a prospective patient registry at our level 1 pediatric trauma center, where patients with renal trauma were treated with an institutional review board approved conservative blunt renal trauma protocol. Standardized treatment included a trial of expectant management for all stable cases.

Materials and Methods.—We identified 39 children with blunt renal trauma treated between 2003 and 2008. A strict conservative approach was used, ie nonoperative management in cases that were hemodynamically stable or had a favorable response with up to 2 units of blood transfused and no operative renal lesion on imaging. Adult imaging protocols were followed and exploratory laparotomy for nonrenal causes did not alter course of expectant renal management. Outcomes evaluated were injury grade, hematuria, operative management, length of stay and associated injuries.

Results.—Based on the American Association for the Surgery of Trauma organ injury severity scale, 13 patients were considered to have grade I disease, 8 grade II, 11 grade III, 6 grade IV and 1 grade V. Conservative management resulted in a 97% nonoperative rate and a single renorrhaphy.

Conclusions.—Using a prospective patient registry, this study demonstrates that conservative treatment of blunt pediatric renal trauma is safe and effective. Also, serious renal injuries are not missed by applying adult diagnostic imaging protocols in children.

▶ The authors prospectively evaluate a blunt renal trauma management algorithm (Figure in the original article). They use an adult imaging protocol (gross hematuria, microscopic hematuria with shock, deceleration injury, or associated injury requiring imaging). Because all patients did well with conservative management, it is conceivable that a significant injury was missed by not imaging all the patients. Because all did well, perhaps detection was not needed. Nonoperative management was successful in all but one child. This conclusion must be tempered by the fact that only one child had a grade V renal injury. The authors also report data (Table 2 in the original article) from a retrospective evaluation of renal trauma previously reported at the same institution. In combination, 15 of 19 patients with grades IV and V trauma were managed expectantly. Long-term functional outcomes are not available in any of these children. Hemodynamically stable children with blunt renal injuries can be treated using conservative protocols.

D. E. Coplen, MD

Intermediate-Term Follow-Up of Patients Treated With Percutaneous Embolization for Grade 5 Blunt Renal Trauma
Stewart AF, Brewer ME Jr, Daley BJ, et al (Univ of Tennessee Graduate School of Medicine, Knoxville)
J Trauma 69:468-470, 2010

Background.—The short-term efficacy and safety of percutaneous embolization for the treatment of hemodynamically unstable patients with grade 5 renal injuries secondary to blunt trauma has been previously established; however, there has been no published intermediate-term follow-up. The purpose of this study is to report intermediate-term follow-up and complications for this treatment modality.

Methods.—A retrospective study was performed to determine intermediate-term outcomes in an observational cohort of patients who underwent percutaneous embolization for the management of grade 5 blunt renal trauma. Demographic and perioperative data were obtained. Follow-up was performed via mail and/or phone questionnaires.

Results.—Between October 2004 and July 2008, 10 hemodynamically unstable patients with grade 5 blunt renal trauma were treated with percutaneous embolization. Mean age of the cohort was 29 years (range, 5-50). Mean follow-up via phone and/or mail questionnaires was 2.7 years (1.5–5.1 years). One patient reported a new diagnosis of hypertension, which is well controlled by a single antihypertensive medication. There were no reported complications of refractory hypertension, altered renal function, new urolithiasis, chronic pain, urine leak, arteriovenous fistula, or pseudoaneurysm. No other procedures were required after the initial embolization for their renal trauma.

Conclusions.—Management of grade 5 renal injuries with percutaneous embolization is safe and is not associated with intermediate-term adverse events.

▶ The authors describe interventional management of both severe renal crush (shattered kidney) and renal pedicle injuries. In the past, these were lumped together as grade V renal injuries. Currently, grade V includes only renal pedicle injury. Segmental vascular injuries with or without collecting system injury are classified as grade IV. Regardless of the staging system, a hemodynamically unstable patient who does not require exploration for other organ injuries embolization can effectively control bleeding. The end point with main renal artery embolization is essentially the same as that with exploration and nephrectomy. The major limitation of this study is that the authors' follow-up is solely based on a patient questionnaire. None of the patients had a physical examination or laboratory test to assess renal function. There is no radiographic follow-up after initial hospital discharge. Based on this, we can conclude that embolization is safe in the short term and does not seem to be associated with any clinically apparent long-term sequelae.

D. E. Coplen, MD

Revision of Current American Association for the Surgery of Trauma Renal Injury Grading System
Buckley JC, McAninch JW (Lahey Clinic Med Ctr, Burlington, MA; San Francisco General Hosp, CA)
J Trauma 70:35-37, 2011

Background.—We propose a revision of the original 1989 renal organ injury system established by the American Association for the Surgery of Trauma based on our institution's >25-year longitudinal experience. Our goal is to expand the current grading system to include segmental vascular injuries and ureteral pelvic injuries and to establish a more rigorous definition of severe grade IV and V renal injuries.

Methods.—We retrospectively reviewed our prospectively gathered contiguous renal database of 3,580 renal injuries to describe a revised renal grading injury scale based on clinical renal salvage outcomes. We focused on the mechanism of injury, the stability of the patient, radiographic imaging, associated nonrenal injuries, and clinical salvage outcome data.

Results.—No changes were made in the definition of grade I to III injuries. The revised grade IV classification includes all collecting system, renal pelvis injuries and segmental arterial and/or venous injuries. The revised grade V classification is limited to main renal artery and/or vein injuries, including laceration, avulsion, and thrombosis. We compared the nephrectomy rate and clinical renal salvage rate between the original 1989 renal organ injury system with our revised renal injury staging classification.

Conclusion.—The revised renal injury staging classification provides complete and clear definitions of renal trauma while still performing its fundamental objective to reflect increasingly complex renal injuries. Uniform language and classification of renal injuries will enhance discussion, clinical investigation, and research of renal trauma.

▶ The authors revise the renal injury staging classification. Improved imaging technology allows more accurate identification of the location and severity of renal injury. There is no collecting system injury in grades I, II, and III injuries.

In grade III injury, the renal laceration is greater than 1 cm and into the renal medulla. Grade IV is now any collecting system injury or segmental venous or arterial injury. Previously, grade V was the somewhat nebulous shattered kidney. It now includes only vascular injuries to the renal pedicle. A kidney with grade V injury is almost never salvageable because of time delays between injury and evaluation. Because most renal injuries are grade I, this new classification will likely impact only the management of the most serious renal injuries.

D. E. Coplen, MD

29 Varicocele

Does Varicocele Repair Improve Male Infertility? An Evidence-Based Perspective From a Randomized, Controlled Trial

Abdel-Meguid TA, Al-Sayyad A, Tayib A, et al (King Abdulaziz Univ Med City, Jeddah, Saudi Arabia)
Eur Urol 59:455-461, 2011

Background.—Randomized controlled trials (RCTs) addressing varicocele treatment are scarce and have conflicting outcomes.

Objective.—To determine whether varicocele treatment is superior or inferior to no treatment in male infertility from an evidence-based perspective.

Design, Setting, and Participants.—A prospective, nonmasked, parallel-group RCT with a one-to-one concealed-to-random allocation was conducted at the authors' institution from February 2006 to October 2009. Married men 20-39 yr of age who had experience infertility ≥1 yr, had palpable varicoceles, and with at least one impaired semen parameter (sperm concentration <20 million/ml, progressive motility <50%, or normal morphology <30%) were eligible. Exclusions included subclinical or recurrent varicoceles, normal semen parameters, and azoospermia. Sample size analysis suggested 68 participants per arm.

Intervention.—Participants were randomly allocated to observation (the control arm [CA]) or subinguinal microsurgical varicocelectomy (the treatment arm [TA]). Semen analyses were obtained at baseline (three analyses) and at follow-up months 3, 6, 9, and 12. The mean of each sperm parameter at baseline and follow-ups was determined.

Measurements.—We measured the spontaneous pregnancy rate (the primary outcome), changes from baseline in mean semen parameters, and the occurrence of adverse events (AE—the secondary outcomes) during 12-mo follow-up; $p < 0.05$ was considered significant.

Results and Limitations.—Analysis included 145 participants (CA: $n = 72$; TA: $n = 73$), with a mean age plus or minus standard deviation of 29.3 ± 5.7 in the CA and 28.4 ± 5.7 in the TA ($p = 0.34$). Baseline characteristics in both arms were comparable. Spontaneous pregnancy was achieved in 13.9% (CA) versus 32.9% (TA), with an odds ratio (OR) of 3.04 (95% confidence interval [CI], 1.33−6.95) and a number needed to treat (NNT) of 5.27 patients (95% CI, 1.55−8.99). In CA within-arm analysis, none of semen parameters revealed significant changes from baseline (sperm concentration [$p = 0.18$], progressive motility [$p = 0.29$], and normal morphology [$p = 0.05$]). Conversely, in

TA within-arm analysis, the mean of all semen parameters improved significantly in follow-up versus baseline ($p < 0.0001$). In between-arm analysis, all semen parameters improved significantly in the TA versus CA ($p < 0.0001$). No AEs were reported.

Conclusions.—Our RCT provided level 1b evidence of the superiority of varicocelectomy over observation in infertile men with palpable varicoceles and impaired semen quality, with increased odds of spontaneous pregnancy and improvements in semen characteristics within 1-yr of follow-up.

▶ Although varix repair has been widely performed in the management of male infertility, questions regarding efficacy have not been answered. There are trials showing improved semen characteristics and pregnancy rates, while others show no benefit. In this trial, 3 abnormal semen analyses were required in addition to infertility after a year of unprotected intercourse and a palpable varicocele. Compliance with the protocol was excellent in both arms. Patients who explicitly elected or rejected surgery were excluded from randomization. Baseline and treatment outcomes are shown in Table 2 in the original article. Spontaneous pregnancy was the primary outcome in the study and is shown in Table 3 in the original article. Improved seminal parameters and an increased chance of spontaneous pregnancy are present within 1 year after varicocelectomy. As can be seen, varicocele repair was beneficial in 1 in 5 men (number needed to treat, 5.27). While the pregnancy outcome is not perfect, these data do support treatment of a varicocele in men with infertility, a palpable varicocele and impaired semen quality.

D. E. Coplen, MD

Percutaneous retrograde endovascular occlusion for pediatric varicocele
Fayad F, Sellier N, Chabaud M, et al (Hôpital Saint-Camille, Bry sur Marne Cedex, France; AP-HP-Hôpital Jean Verdier, Bondy, France; AP-HP — Groupe Hospitalier Armand Trousseau — La Roche-Guyon, Cedex, Paris, France; et al)
J Pediatr Surg 46:525-529, 2011

Background/Purpose.—The aim of this study was to assess whether percutaneous retrograde endovascular occlusion (PREVO) is effective and safe for the treatment of varicocele in pediatric patients.

Methods.—We retrospectively studied 71 children who underwent PREVO for left-sided varicocele. The primary outcome was the proportion of varicocele-free patients 6 months after PREVO as assessed by ultrasonography.

Results.—Seventy-one boys with left-sided grade III varicocele underwent PREVO at a mean age of 13.2 years. PREVO was performed under local anesthesia in all boys but 2, who required general anesthesia. The procedure was technically feasible in 68 (96%) patients. In the remaining 3 patients, the internal spermatic vein could not be catheterized. Minor short-term complications occurred in 6 patients and resolved fully. No major complications or deaths were recorded. The proportion of varicocele-free patients 6 months after PREVO was 93% (66/71) overall and 97% (66/68) in the patients whose PREVO procedure was feasible. No clinical recurrence was observed during the mean follow-up of 17.5 months.

Conclusions.—Percutaneous retrograde endovascular occlusion is an effective minimally invasive approach for varicocele treatment in pediatric patients. It can be safely performed on an outpatient basis under local anesthesia.

▶ The authors evaluate the feasibility and efficacy of radiographic embolization in the treatment of pediatric varicocele. The primary indication for intervention was scrotal pain. In my experience, adolescents rarely have pain related to a varix. Regardless, the authors safely and successfully perform embolization in adolescents using local anesthesia. It is unclear if a different population of boys with a varix was referred to urologists, resulting in a selection bias that facilitated these excellent results. An advantage of embolization when compared with either inguinal or retroperitoneal varicocelectomy is the very low risk of postoperative hydrocele. The incidence should be close to zero because the embolization does not risk injury to lymphatics. When indicated there are multiple approaches to varicocele management. Embolization is an excellent option and may be the preferred approach in males with a prior history of inguinal surgery that may have compromised some of the redundant testicular blood supply.

D. E. Coplen, MD

Article Index

Chapter 1: Clinical Outcomes

Chapter 2: Endourology and Stone Disease

Chapter 3: Transplantation

Chapter 4: Female Urology

Chapter 5: Renal Tumors

Chapter 6: Urothelial Cancer

Chapter 7: Prostate Cancer

Chapter 8: Testicular Cancer

Chapter 9: Sexual Function

Chapter 10: Urethral Reconstruction

Chapter 11: Urinary Reconstruction

Chapter 12: Neurogenic Bladder/Urinary Diversion

Chapter 13: Neurogenic Reconstruction

Chapter 14: Vesicoureteral Reflux

Chapter 15: Male Incontinence/Voiding Dysfunction

Chapter 16: Benign Prostatic Hyperplasia

Chapter 17: Bladder Cancer

Chapter 18: Cryptorchidism

Author Index

Printed and bound by CPI Group (UK) Ltd, Croydon, CR0 4YY

08/05/2025

01864678-0005